364 Days
of Healthy Eating

(because nobody is perfect)

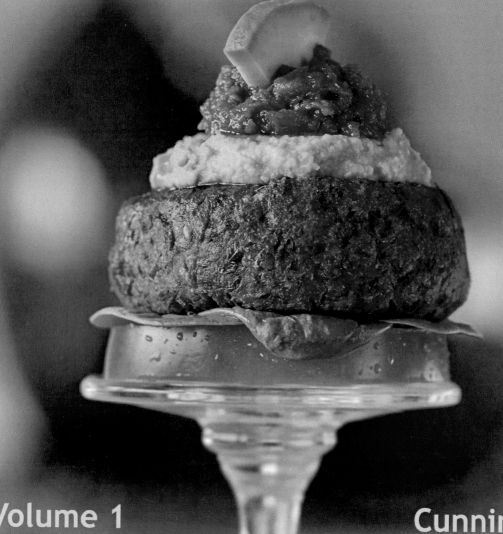

Volume 1

Karen
Cunningham

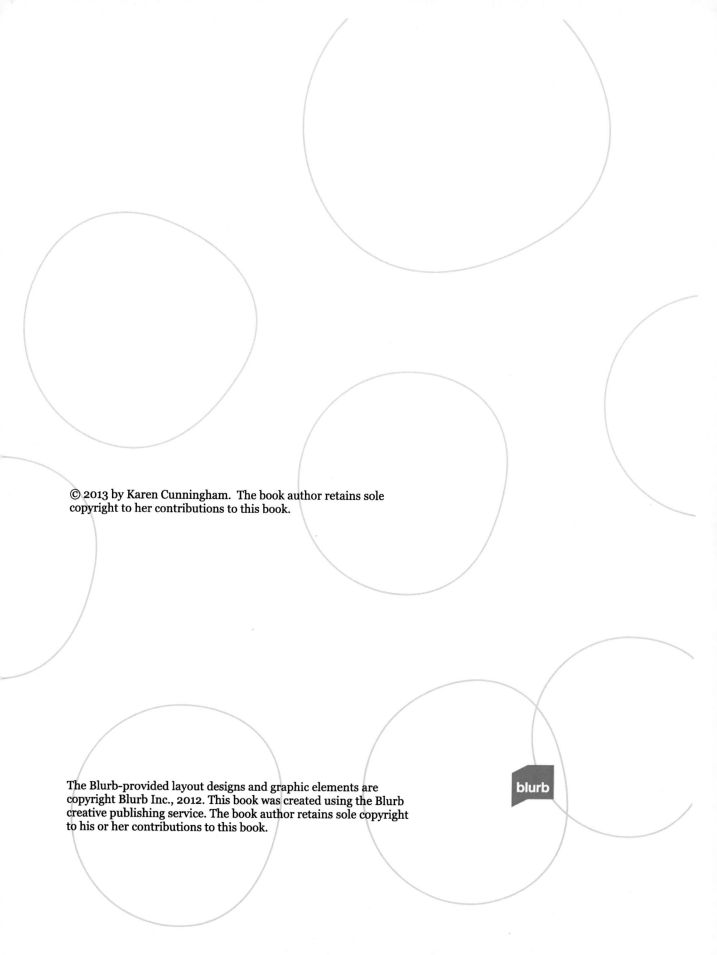

blurb

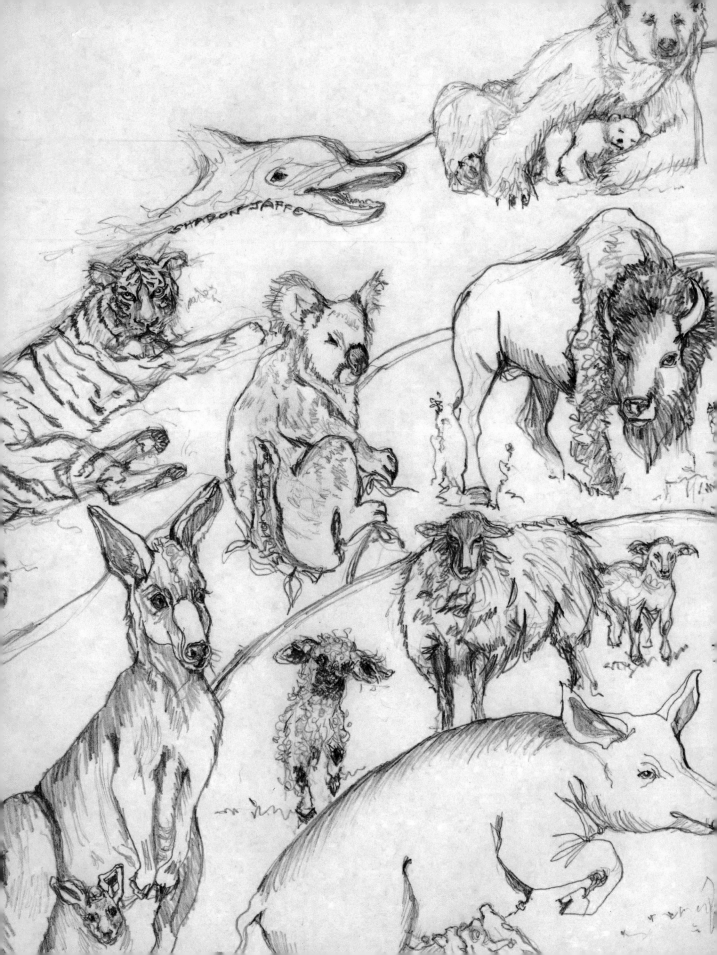

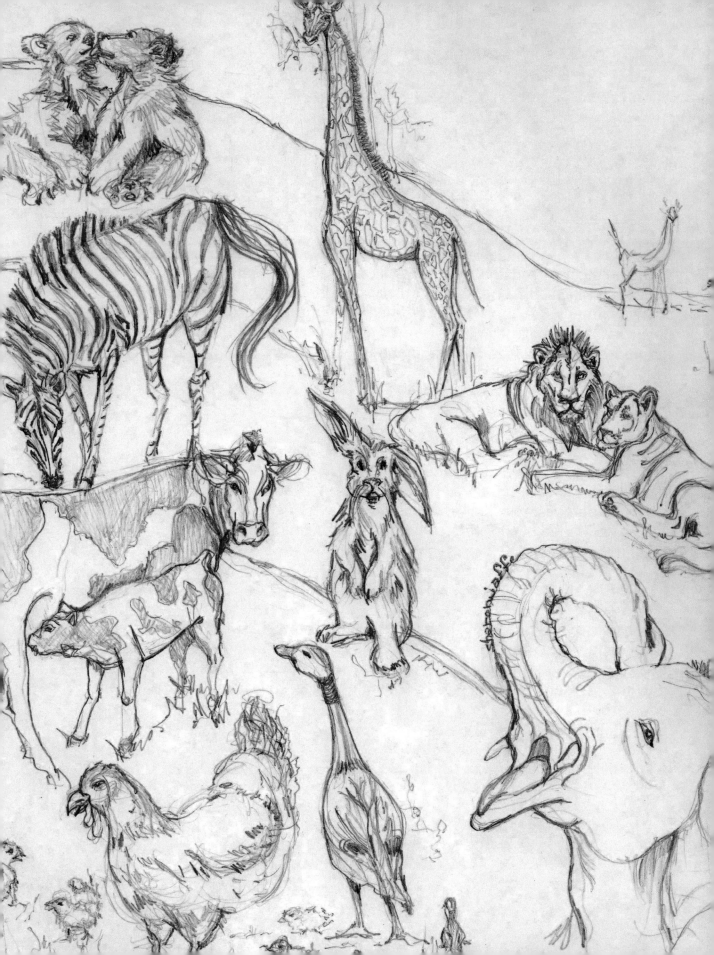

FOR THE ANIMALS

Along my Plant Based Journey that also removed gluten and sugar, I also learned so much about our food industry and the sadness involved in the use of farm animals. The more I have learned – the more determined I am to help people realize that eating plants is not only a much better and healing choice for our health, but it is the only humane way to eat. The Meat and Dairy Industry have so much to be ashamed of.

FOR OUR PLANET

With the combination of big agriculture and the relentless invasion of the GMO squad – what we can do for our planet is support neither. To think that the chemical companies that gave us the likes of some of the most noxious chemicals and pest resistant pesticides are now trying to get us to believe that they are now food benefactors, is akin to believing in Santa Claus as an adult – we all need to do our homework.

FOR YOUR HEALTH

A Plant Based Diet is simply the best choice for your health – your cholesterol will plummet and you will have more energy than you thought possible. It is medically proven that eating a plant based diet can reverse Type 2 Diabetes and quiet so many other disease states including Autoimmune diseases – I am living proof of that.

For the animals
For our planet
For your health

Starting a revolution one plate at a time

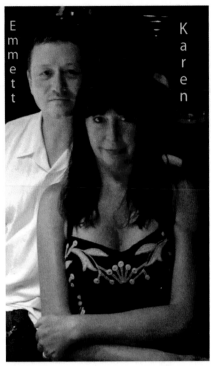

Emmett

Karen

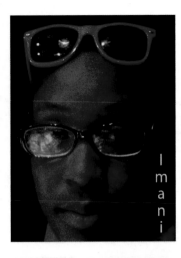

Imani

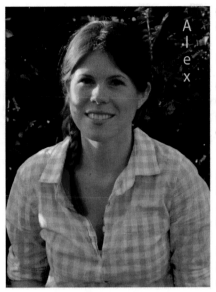

Alex

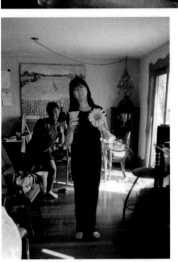

healthy

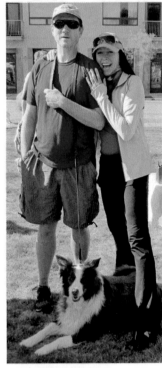

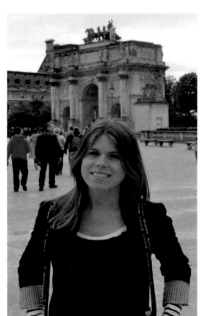

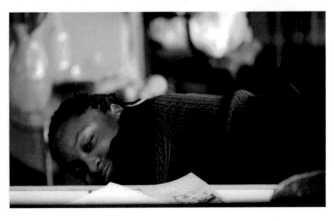

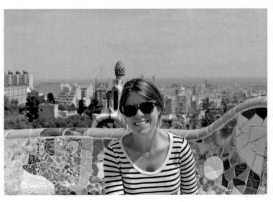

eat sleep drink relax exercise meditate love laugh share joy live

364 Days of Healthy Eating

(because nobody is perfect)

Volume 1   by Karen Cunningham

Acknowledgements:

I must acknowledge my Mother and Father first. Tongue in cheek here when I say they did not like to cook. OK, my Father did but with memories of salted oranges and strawberry jam omelettes still stuck in my head since I was nine, it is no wonder I ended up with a burning passion for wonderful food.

This journey of eating healthy food followed by cooking healthfully started at a young age. As a vegetarian child, it grew difficult to eat in a meat and potatoes household. My mother still says I was a royal pain to feed, but remarks at my contentment with beans, carrots, and mashed potatoes.

Even as a young woman, I thoroughly enjoyed the idea of elaborate dinner parties with friends. For some part of my adulthood, chicken and fish were a regular part of my repertoire – but eating animals never fully appealed to me and the more I became plant oriented, the better I felt about my relationship with food.

For the last 15 years I have been cooking like a crazy woman, researching all things healthy and discovering exotic ingredients. For this book, I went through thousands of my old files looking for recipes that could be adapted to my new way of eating. So many people have asked me "What on earth do you eat? Not only do you have a plant-based diet, but you are gluten free and use no added sugar!"

So, I started documenting my recipes, photographing them and writing everything down. Thankfully my best supporter in the world, my super hubby Emmett, became my biggest fan and has been completely by my side throughout this journey. And to my son, Daniel, now you know how to eat well! Thanks for letting me experiment on you too.

Now over to our vegan Thanksgiving dinner last year (2012). My dear friend Imani McElroy (a new Medical Student at UCLA and the Editor of this book) said, "Hey you should write a book," and without missing a beat I said "YES!". That was how it all began.

I have been cooking for my friends for many years and now it was seriously game on at a professional level. A huge thanks here to so many friends who willingly allowed me experiment on them and gave me recipes and inspiration- Imani, Leanne, Sharon, Laurie, Victoria, Danette, Aura, Kwanua, Bev - you all know who you are.

To bring credibility to this publication, my trusty assistant Cynthia Gubbins searched the Internet for vegan registered dieticians and we were incredibly lucky to find the fabulous Alexandra Caspero, who joined our team and has added her professional spin on many things from oils to recipe breakdowns and so much more.

Tom Seawell - my dear friend and photographer extraordinaire, thank you so much for the stunning cover photo - in short, you rock! To see Tom's work go to- www.tomseawell.com

A huge thanks to Danette Davis for allowing us to shoot our cover photo in her beautiful home and for loaning me so many of her beautiful plates and linens for the photographs. She has also been a good ear and a great sense of inspiration – she is responsible for the Jicama Tacos Recipe! And to her daughter, Madison Davis, for serving as an extra pair of editing eyes.

Sharon Jaffe, my wonderful friend and an amazingly talented artist took my direction to reflect respect for our animals and our earth and translated my Book Statement, "For the Animals – For our Planet – For your Health", into the stunning Frontis pages of the book.

And finally, and this is not directly related to the book, a huge thank you to Dr. Victor Prieto, Don Kemp, Chris, Sarah and the staff at St. Francis Memorial Hospital – you saved my life when I was diagnosed with an autoimmune disorder and set me on this path, I would not be here without you all! And to Dr. David Curtis, who told me that I was an "army of one", I hope I have you as a huge supporter now, and thank you for your support of this project.

This book is a testament to using food as medicine and to how utilize visually appealing plant-based meals to appeal to even the most carnivorous of my friends. Tom and Ron - how about that non-chicken, chicken ey? I think you both raved on for quite a bit.

I hope you find delight in every recipe and photograph in this book.

This has been an incredible journey 365 recipes later – we have 364 Days of Healthy Eating (because nobody is perfect) – Volume One!

OUR TEAM:

Karen Cunningham B.S. MFA
Recipes, Cooking, Art Direction, Photos, Photo Styling

Alexandra Caspero RD CLT
Recipe Analysis, Recipe Contributor, Nutritional Guides

Imani McElroy (Medical Student Charles R. Drew/UCLA)
Book Designer and Editor

Contributing Photographers
Tom Seawell www.tomseawell.com (http://www.tomseawell.com)
Cover Photograph

Contributing Artist
Sharon Jaffe
Frontis Artwork

Contributing Author
Dr. Kelly Martin B.S. Pharm.D.
Vegan Protein Information

INTRODUCTION

For whatever reason brought you here, I am glad you came. Maybe you are looking for a more compassionate way of eating, you have health concerns requiring dietary changes, simply want a healthier lifestyle; or perhaps you have moral objections to the corporate food chains' agricultural practices and the thought of eating genetically modified food makes your skin creep - or any combination of these reasons - Welcome!

I have compiled an entire year's worth of healthy recipes that I hope will tantalize your senses and nourish your body and spirit —all the while, noting that one can still enjoy wonderful treats without guilt.

Watching the incredible reactions that I received when posting pictures of something scrumptious online, compelled me to entice you into healthy eating by including photographs of absolutely every recipe included.

Each recipe has been thoroughly tested by my Team and analyzed by vegan RD Alex Caspero. With each recipe, please assume that I only use Gluten Free, Vegan, Organic and non-GMO ingredients. When selecting your ingredients, do try to choose as many organic products as you can to ensure your diet is as pure as possible.

Cheers to you and your new healthy lifestyle!

- Karen

Table of Contents

Table of Contents

Table of Contents

Table of Contents

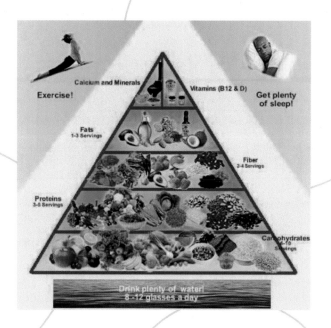

Recipe Legend:

(E) - Easy
(NCF) - Not Cleanse Friendly
(Q) - Quick
(R) - Raw
(X) - Expert
($) - Costs $2 or less per serving

EVOO - Extra Virgin Olive Oil

Measurement Conversions:

Unit	Fl. Oz.	Fl. Conversion	mL	Dry Oz.	lbs	grams
1 tsp	1/6 fl. oz.	1/3 Tbsp	5	1/2 dry oz.		15
1 Tbsp	1/2 fl. oz.	3 Tbsp	15	2 dry oz.		60
1/8 cup	1 fl. oz.	2 Tbsp	30	3 dry oz.		90
1/4 cup	2 fl. oz.	4 Tbsp	59	3.5 dry oz.		105
1/3 cup	2 3/4 fl. oz.	1/4 cup + 4 tsp	79			
1/2 cup	4 fl. oz.	8 Tbsp	118	4 dry oz.	1/4	125
2/3 cup	5 1/3 fl. oz.	10 2/3 Tbsp	158			
3/4 cup	6 fl. oz.	12 Tbsp	177	6 dry oz.		180
1 cup	8 fl. oz.	1/2 pint	237	8 dry oz.	1/2	250
1 pint	16 fl. oz.	2 cup	474	20 dry oz.	1.25	610
1 qt	32 fl. oz.	2 pint	948	40 dry oz.	2.5	1220
1 liter	34 fl. oz.	1 qt + 1/4 cup	1007			
1 gallon	128 fl. oz.	4 qt	3792			

Oven Conversions:

Gas Mark	Farenheit	Celsius
1/4	225	110
1/2	250	130
1	275	140
2	300	150
3	325	170
4	350	180
5	375	190
6	400	200
7	425	220
8	450	230
9	475	240

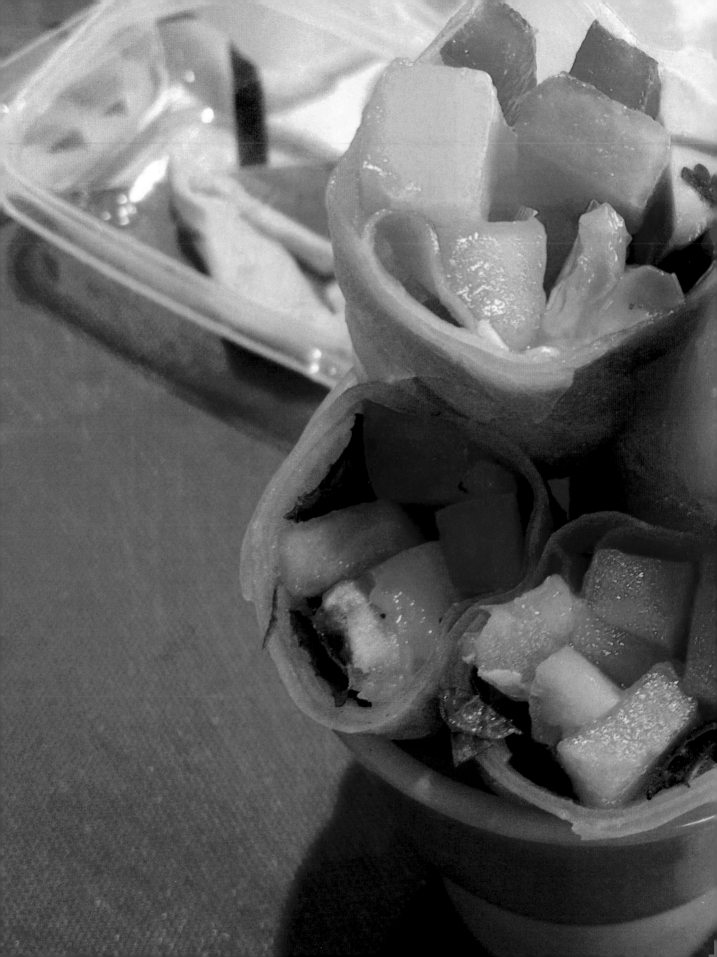

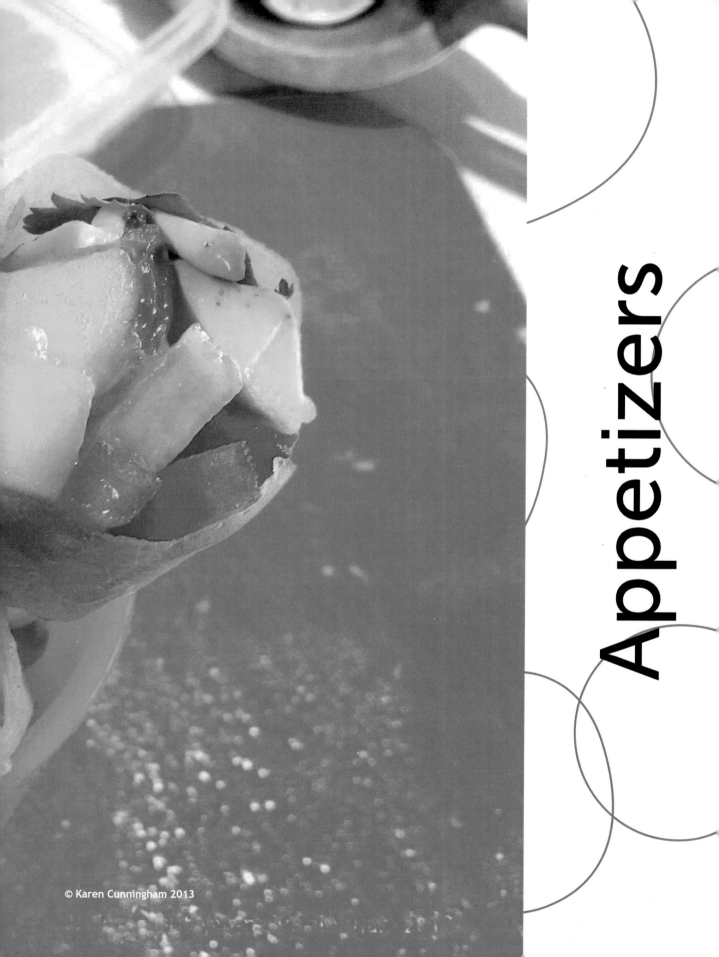

Appetizers

© Karen Cunningham 2013

Curried Beets with Coconut, Peas and Pine Nuts (Q)(E)($)
Servings: 4
Per serving*: 332 Calories, 22.4g Fat, 39g Carbs, 8g Fiber, 8g Protein

*including ½ cup green peas and omitted the garbanzo beans

Ingredients:

1 cup coconut milk
1 cup vegetable stock
roasted or boiled beets – 8 beets
garbanzo beans – optional
fresh green peas – a handful or so
1 Tbsp EVOO
1 tsp mustard seeds
1 tsp cumin seeds
1 Tbsp curry powder (less if you have a spicy blend)
2 Tbsp toasted pine nuts
2 tsp turmeric
3 Tbsp unsweetened desiccated coconut

Directions:

Boil or roast the beets with their skins on and whole. Allow to cool and then skins will peel off easily.

Chop the boiled beets into 1 inch squares

Heat oil in pan and add the seasoning - mustard seeds, cumin seeds, and curry.

When mustard seeds start to wiggle around, add the chopped beetroot, green peas, turmeric and salt

Saute them for a couple of minutes

Add the grated coconut milk and vegetable stock and fry for one more minute.

Just before serving sprinkle on the coconut (or leave it until it is individually served and then add the pine nuts.

Adjust salt and chilies to taste. Garnish with coriander.

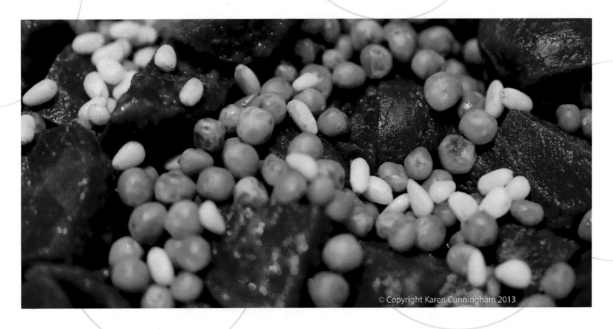

Tropical Fruit and Avocado Spring Rolls (Q)(R)($)

Per Wrap: 108 Calories, 4g Fat, 16g Carbohydrates, 3.6 Fiber, 1.6g Protein

Ingredients:

As much as you like – sliced thinly
red bell pepper
avocado
grapefruit
mango
papaya
mint
cilantro
lime

Dipping Sauce
3 Tbsp mirin
1 Tbsp Bragg's Liquid Aminos
1 tsp sesame oil
1 tsp fresh grated ginger or 1/2 tsp powdered
1 tsp lime
1 Tbsp apple cider vinegar

Directions:

Soak rice paper wrappers* in hot water for a couple of minutes and then gently remove to your working surface for assembly.

*available from most Asian markets and larger supermarkets

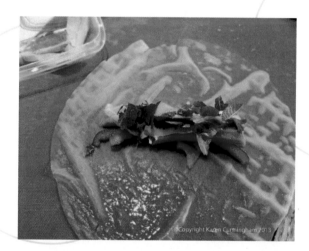

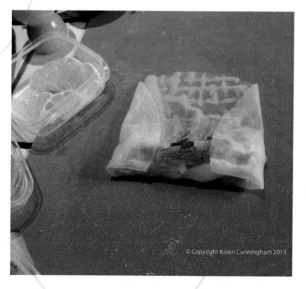

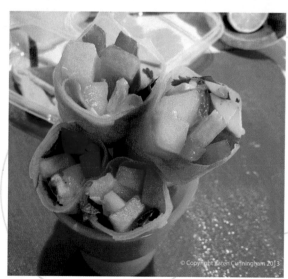

Millet Cakes (E)($)

Serves: 8-10 as single cakes
Per 1 cake: 203 Calories, 5.3g Fat, 31.5g Carbs, 7.6g Fiber, 8g Protein

Ingredients:

3/4 cup uncooked dry millet
1 cup cooked garbanzo beans
1 Tbsp chia seeds
1 Tbsp coconut oil - plus more for cooking cakes
1 medium red bell pepper - diced
1 scallion - finely chopped
2 cloves garlic - minced
1/2 tsp mineral salt
1 tsp ground cumin
1/2 tsp ground coriander

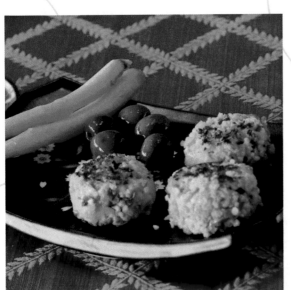

Directions:

Add millet to a medium saucepan with 1 1/2 cups of water. If it gets too dry – add more water about 1-2 Tbsp at a time.

Cook on medium heat until the water is just absorbed. It should be like quinoa is when cooked. It only just holds together, but quickly breaks apart with a fork. You want this consistency for the cakes.

As millet cooks, heat 1 tablespoon of coconut oil in a separate skillet.

Add red pepper and scallion and cook over medium heat for about 4 minutes.

Add minced garlic and cook for another minute.

Set aside.

Once millet has cooked add everything together and mix well – almost, but not quite mashing.

Use the same saute pan as used for the red peppers (no need to wash).

Heat additional tsp of coconut oil (if needed) in the pan.

Meanwhile, measure out 1/3 cup amounts of millet mixture and roll in the palm of your hands before pressing into patties.

Add patties to hot saute pan and cook over medium-high heat for about 3 minutes per side, or until crispy and lightly browned on the outside.

Repeat this step to cook the remaining patties.

Papaya Caviar (Q)(E)(R)($)

Serves: 2

Per serving: 41 Calories, 1.5g Fat, 6.7g Carbs, 0.9g Fiber, 1g Protein

Ingredients:

1 cup sliced cucumber rounds
½ cup sliced papaya
2 Tbsp papaya seeds
¼ cup coconut yoghurt

Directions:

Halve a papaya and scoop out all the seeds, removing any remaining membrane.

Set in a small bowl, and season liberally with sea salt.

Allow this to sit together for at least an hour, so that the seeds can absorb some salt.

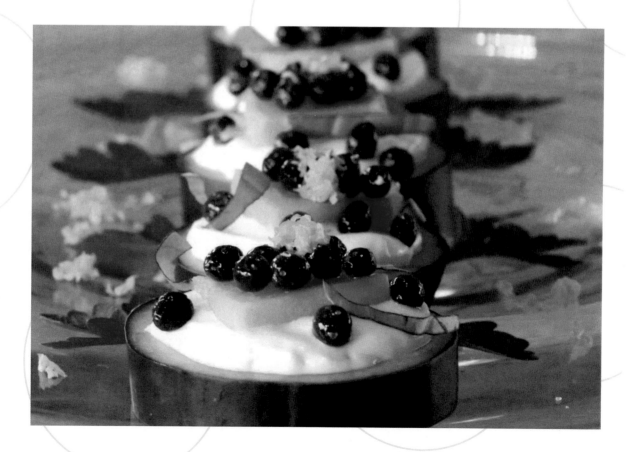

Apricot Cashew Cheese Dates (E)(R)

Serves: 4
Per serving: 549 Calories, 34.1g Fat, 59.2g Carbs, 7.4g Fiber, 11.5g Protein

Ingredients:

1 1/2 cups raw cashews
2 1/2 Tbsp fresh squeezed lemon juice
2 Tbsp coconut oil
10 dried apricots
sea salt (to taste)
1/4 cup chopped raw almonds (toast them for an extra special treat)
20 Medjool dates - pits removed

Directions:

Place the cashews in a bowl of room temperature water (enough to cover) and let them soak for 6 hours or overnight.

Place the cashews, lemon juice, coconut oil, apricots and sea salt in a food processor and blend until very smooth.

Add sea salt to taste.

Place a large spoonful of the cashew cheese inside each date.

Top with the chopped almonds and drizzle each date with a little raw honey. Serve.

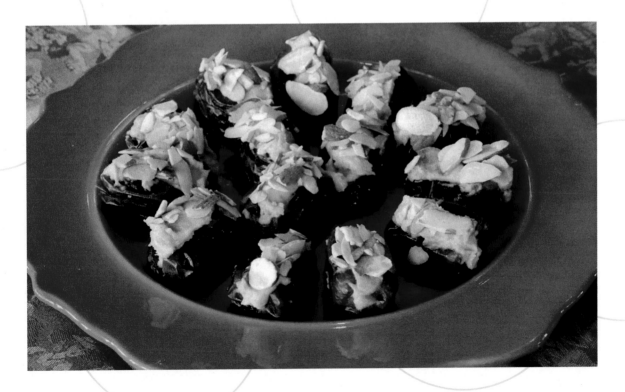

Not Tuna "Nori" Rolls

Serves 3-4
Per serving: 160 Calories, 10.5g Fat, 11.9g Carbs, 3.3g Fiber, 6.9g Protein

Ingredients:

1 1/2 cups sunflower seeds, raw and soaked
1/2 cup dill weed - chopped
1/2 sweet onion - chopped
2 celery ribs -chopped
1 tomato - coarsely chopped
3 -4 Tbsp lemon juice
1/2 jalapeno pepper – finely chopped
1 tsp mineral salt
1 tsp EVOO
fresh ground black pepper, to taste
1/2 cup bell pepper, chopped into matchsticks
(optional)
1/2 cup cucumber, peeled and chopped into
matchsticks (optional)
6 sheets nori, or lettuce

Directions:

Place sunflower seeds, dill, onion, celery, tomato, lemon juice, salt, olive oil, and pepper to taste in food processor and pulse until chopped but a little bit chunky.

Spread the mixture evenly over each nori sheet.

(Optional: place a few pepper or cucumber matchsticks on the mixture before rolling.).

Roll sheets up and slice into 1 1/2 inches pieces.

Serve on a bed of lettuce.

*Wrap on the Left: Avocado, sprouts and cucumber
*Wrap on the Right: mixed bell peppers, zucchini, avocado

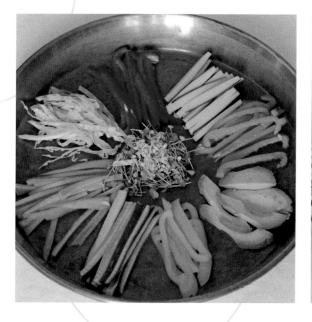
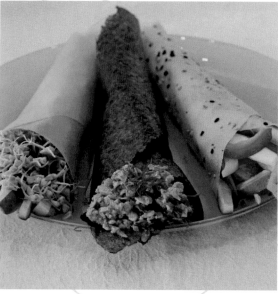

Beet Garbanzo Frittata ($)

Serves: 4

Per serving: 518 Calories, 15.3g Fat, 80.2g Carbs, 17.3g Fiber, 18.3g Protein

Ingredients:

1 medium onion - chopped
1 medium potato - peeled
3 large beets – peeled
3 carrots – peeled
1 ½ cups cooked garbanzo beans
½ cup GF flour
3 Tbsp EVOO
½ tsp mineral salt

Directions:

In a medium sized non-stick pan, saute the onion in 1 Tbsp of the EVOO until soft over medium heat.

Add remaining ingredients and press down fairly firmly using a flexible spatula.

Cook undisturbed for about 10 minutes.

Remove from heat and then heat broiler to high.

Place pan under broiler until the tops browns.

Remove, let cool for about one minute then slice and serve with your favorite green.

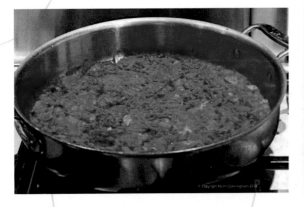
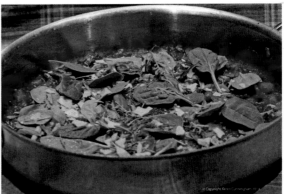

Moroccan Garbanzo Burgers
Makes 8 patties
Per patty: 235 Calories, 5g Fat, 39g Carbs, 10.2g Fiber, 10.8g Protein

Ingredients:

2 cups cooked garbanzo beans
1/2 large red onion - chopped
2 cloves garlic - chopped
small bunch flat leaf parsley
1 Tbsp ras el hanout (see page 371)
1 Tbsp gluten free flour
14 dried apricots
1 Tbsp fresh mango
½ tsp cayenne pepper
¼ tsp mineral salt and cracked pepper
1 Tbsp peanut oil

Mango or Apricot Sauce
Simply blend mango or apricot with a pinch of
mineral salt and a touch of cayenne pepper.

Directions:

In a food processor chop garbanzo, red onion and
garlic until crumbly then place into a medium sized
bowl.

Chop the remaining ingredients until they are a small
crumbly texture.

Mix all ingredients and form into small patties.

Refrigerate for a couple of hours (they hold together
better when cold).

Lightly grease a griddle with the peanut oil and turn
to medium heat.

Cook each patty until browned on each side

Serve with herbed yoghurt sauce (see page 214) and
fresh mango or apricot sauce and a large green salad.

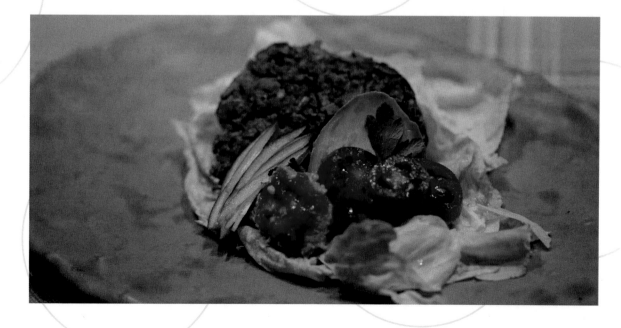

Parsnip Remoulade (R)

Serves: 4
Per serving: 175 Calories, 9.8g Fat, 21.5g Carbs, 6g Fiber, 2.2g Protein

Ingredients:

16 oz parsnips – peeled and ribboned – either with vegetable peeler or mandolin
2 Tbsp apple cider vinegar
1 Tbsp tahini paste
2 Tbsp EVOO
1 ½ Tbsp chopped roasted pistachio nuts
¼ tsp ground black pepper

Directions:

Peel and shave the parsnips into ribbons – place into a large bowl.

Toss parsnips with vinegar and salt – let sit for 10 minutes and then drain.

Squeeze out as much extra liquid as possible.

Transfer to a smaller bowl and combine the extra ingredients, except for the pistachios.

Plate and serve immediately with the pistachios sprinkle don top.

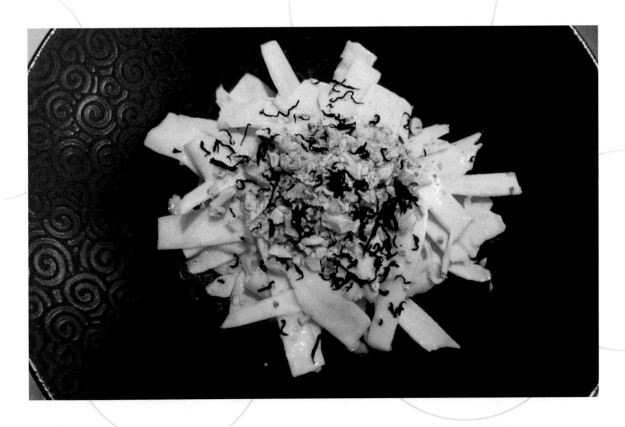

Chili Poblanos ($)(E)

Serves: 6
Per chili: 122 Calories, 2.2g Fat, 27.1g Carbs, 3.5g Fiber, 1.8g Protein

Ingredients

6 medium poblano chilies – slit lengthwise and seeds gently removed
3 large plantains
1 red onion – finely chopped
½ red bell pepper – cut six thin slices and dice the rest
1 Tbsp EVOO

Directions

Preheat oven to 350 degrees.

On a high heat barbecue, cook the unpeeled plantains until completely blackened on all sides. Remove from heat

Meanwhile sauté on medium heat, the pepper (minus the six thin strips) with the onion until slightly golden in the EVOO – remove from heat

When the plantains are cool enough to handle, remove the skins and chop into small pieces or mash gently

Mix in the onion pepper mixture and fill the chilies

Bake the chilies for about 35 minutes until the peppers are soft

Enjoy with your favorite toppings – cashew cheese (see page 243) or cashew sour crème (see page 238) are great.

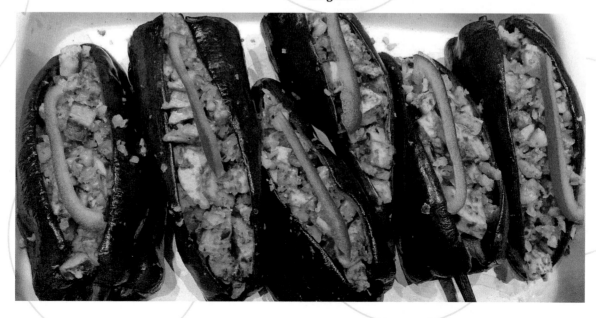

Dates with Walnuts (Q)(E)

Serves: 6

Per serving: 72 Calories, 2.4g Fat, 12.8g Carbs, 1.6g Fiber, 1.4g Protein

Ingredients:

12 medjool dates – pitted
12 walnut halves

Directions:

Make a lengthwise slit in the date and remove the seed.
Place a walnut half in each piece
Arrange on a serving plate

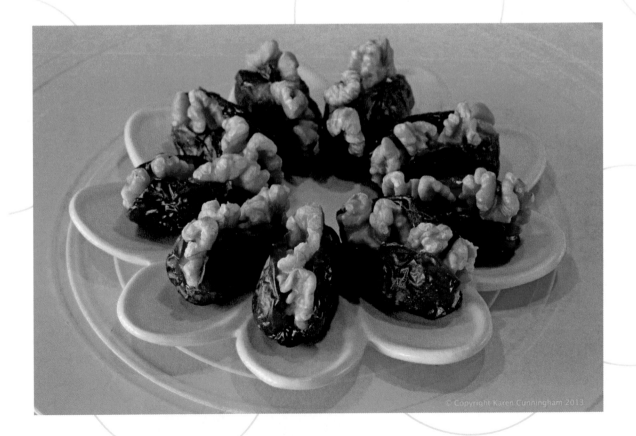

© Copyright Karen Cunningham 2013

Eggplant Caviar (E)

Serves: 4

Per serving: 199 calories, 14.1g Fat, 19.4g Carbs, 9.2g Fiber, 3.6g Protein

Ingredients:

2 pounds smallish eggplants - halved
EVOO for brushing, plus 2 ounces
2 shallots - minced
4 cloves garlic - minced
1 pound tomatoes - peeled and chopped
2 tablespoons lemon juice
mineral salt and freshly ground black pepper

Directions:

Preheat oven to 350 degrees F.

Brush eggplant with olive oil and roast eggplants, cut side down at 350 degrees for 30 minutes or until soft.

Saute the garlic and shallots in 2 ounces olive oil over low heat until they are translucent and aromatic.

After the eggplant has cooled, remove the pulp from the skins, and place in a food processor and process until smooth.

Place mixture in a bowl and add remaining ingredients along with garlic and shallots.

Season, to taste, with salt and pepper and serve with crackers or vegetables or as a pasta topping

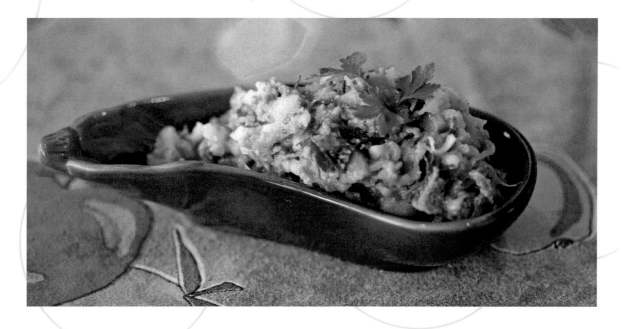

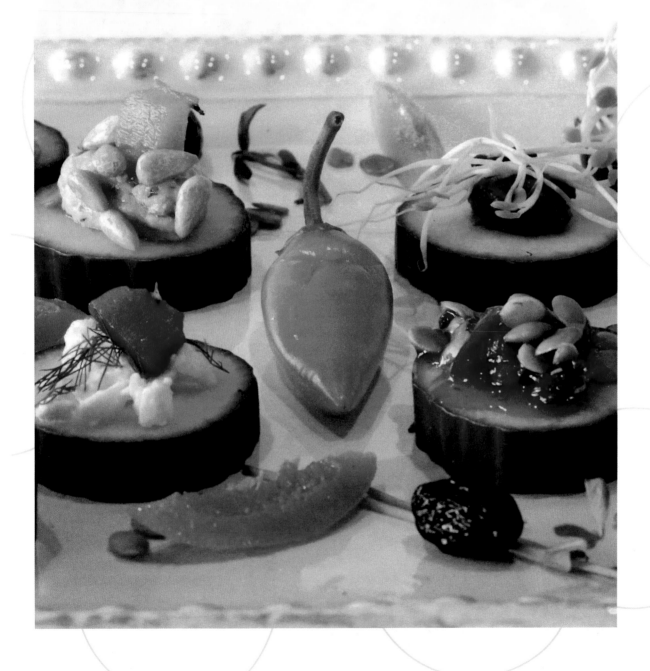

Cucumber Appetizers (Q)(E)($)

Top Left - Topped with hummus pine nuts and yellow bell pepper.

Top Right - Topped with beet hummus and clover sprouts.

Bottom Left - Topped with macadamia nut cheese, fresh dill and red bell pepper.

Bottom Right - Topped with sundried tomatoes in EVOO and pumpkin seeds.

NOTE:
Scattered on the plate are salt cured olives, preserved lemon and pea sprouts.

Buckwheat Pancakes ($)(E)

Serves: 5
Per serving : 135 Calories, 7.6g Fat, 15g Carbs, 1.9g Fiber, 3g Protein

Ingredients:

1/2 cup buckwheat flour
1/2 cup GF all purpose flour
1 tsp baking powder (non aluminum)
1/2 tsp salt
1 - 1/3 cups coconut milk

Directions:

Blend and then heat griddle with coconut or grapeseed oil and drop pancakes on hot griddle - we used about a tsp size each

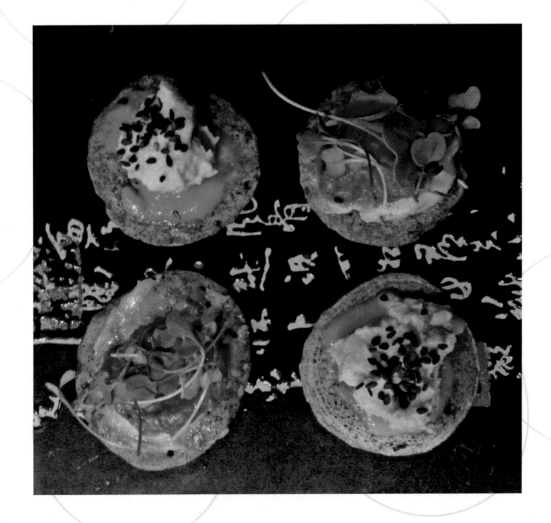

Shishito Storm Peppers (Q)(E)($)
Per serving: 131 Calories, 5g Fat, 21g Carbs, 3.4g Fiber, 4.5g Protein

Ingredients:

1/2 pound shishito peppers - washed and thoroughly dried
1 tsp grapeseed oil
1/4 – ½ tsp togarashi (see page 370)
mineral salt

Directions:

Heat an indoor grill pan or outdoor grill to medium high (about 375°F to 425°F).

Place the peppers in a medium bowl, add the oil, and toss to coat; set aside.

When the grill is ready, place the peppers on the grill in a single layer, making sure they're not touching.

Grill the peppers uncovered, turning them occasionally, until they start to char and blister, about 6 to 8 minutes total.

Return the peppers to the bowl, toss immediately with the togarashi and mineral salt, and serve.

** You could also add a squeeze of lemon

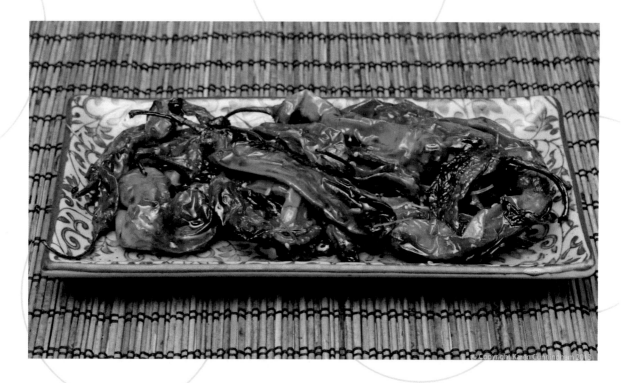

Vegetable Spring Rolls (Q)(E)($)

Serves: 4

1 spring roll: 203 Calories, 4.2g Fat, 31.7g Carbs, 13.2g Fiber, 8g Protein

Ingredients;

4 large rice paper wrappers
2 Tbsp black sesame seeds
4 whole Napa cabbage leaves
4 oz block firm marinated tempeh or tofu, cut into 4-by 1/2-inch strips
1/3 cup bean sprouts
1/2 sheet nori, sliced into 1/2-inch strips
1 medium carrot - julienned into 4 inch strips
1 small jicama – julienned into 4 inch strips
1 medium cucumber - julienned into 4-inch strips
2 spring onions - sliced lengthwise into 4 inch strips
1/2 small bell pepper - sliced into 4 inch matchsticks
4 small sprigs of fresh mint, basil and cilantro

Directions:

Soak 2 wrappers at a time in a bowl of cool water for 2 to 3 minutes or until they are soft and pliable.

Remove one wrapper and place onto a smooth surface.

Avoiding the outer 2 inches, sprinkle 1/2 Tbsp of black sesame seeds onto the wrapper.

Place one cabbage leaf and a few strips of each remaining ingredient onto the wrapper slightly left or right of center of wrap.

Fold each wrap and set aside

Serve with almond ginger dipping sauce (see page 196).

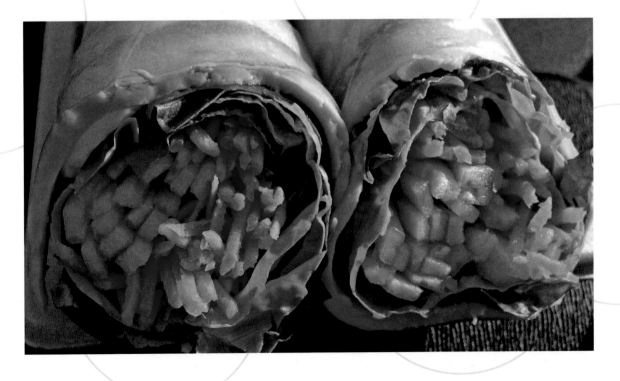

Grilled Tofu with Asian Inspired Dip ($)

Serves: 2

Per serving (½ recipe): 343 Calories, 30.6g Fat, 7.1g Carbs, 1.9g Fiber, 13.8g Protein

Ingredients:

8oz super firm tofu
1/2 cup of asian inspired marinade (see page for recipe)
1 Tbsp grapeseed oil
2 Tbsp lemon grass – finely diced

Directions:

Cut the tofu in half.

Heat the griddle to fairly hot.

Add the oil and gently sauté the lemon grass until it is soft – about a minute.

Make a sideways slit in the tofu and press the lemongrass into each piece.

Place the tofu on the griddle and cook until it is well browned on each side.

Serve with the asian inspired marinade (see page 210).

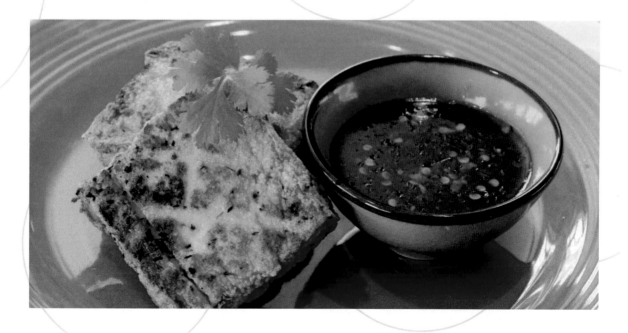

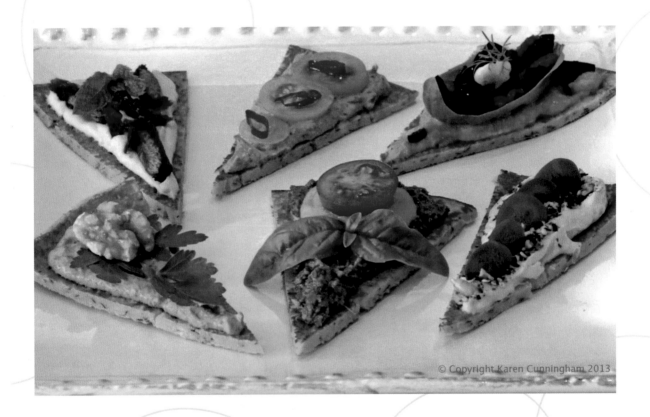

Besan Appetizers (see page 296 for besan recipe)

Top Left - Besan with Sour Cashew Crème with Peaches and Mint

Top Middle - Besan with Super Nu and Zhug with tomatoes and Chili

Top Right - Besan with Almond Cheese with Basil, Tomato and Olive

Bottom Left - Besan with Sour Cashew Crème with Zhug, Parsley and Walnuts

Bottom Middle - Besan with Zhug with Almond Cheese, Tomato and Basil

Bottom Right - Besan with Sour Cashew Crème with Super Nu and Salt Cured Olives

Buffalo Bites (NCF)
Makes 12 bites
Per serving (2 bites): 145 Calories, 21.8g Fat, 6.8g Carbs, 1.8g Fiber, 6g Protein

Ingredients:

16 oz. extra-firm tofu
1/2 cup buffalo bites sauce (see page 219)
1 Tbsp grapeseed oil
1 tsp liquid smoke
1/4 cup garbanzo flour or almond meal
2 Tbsp nutritional yeast
1/4 tsp black pepper
1 tsp garlic powder
1 tsp onion powder

Directions:

Drain the tofu the wrap in a clean kitchen towel and place between two cutting boards. Put a heavy frying pan or pile of cookbooks on top.

Press the tofu overnight to drain as much liquid as you can.

Cut the tofu into 12 finger like pieces, using the short side as your length.

Make small holes all over the strips to help the tofu absorb the marinade.

Whisk the Buffalo Bite sauce, oil, and liquid smoke together.

Set 2/3 of it aside in the refrigerator until serving.

Brush the tofu with the remaining marinade, covering each side evenly – if there is any sauce left just pour over the tofu

Cover and marinate 10 – 12 hours in the refrigerator

Preheat the oven to 350F

Line a cookie sheet with parchment paper.

Mix the remaining ingredients together in a shallow bowl

Roll each piece of tofu in the breading, making sure it sticks to each side evenly and arrange on the cookie sheet.

Bake for 15 minutes, then flip all the pieces over. Bake another 20 minutes, until the sticks are crispy.

Gently toss in the remaining sauce

Skewer and serve with ranch dressing (see page 218) and celery and carrot sticks

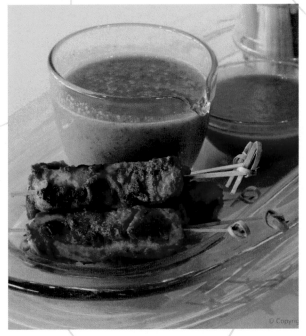

Cucumber Avocado Ceviche (R)($)(Q)(E)

Per serving: 195 Calories, 15g Fat, 16g Carbs, 9.5g Fiber, 1.6g Protein

Ingredients:

14 oz small crunchy Persian or pickling cucumbers
2 avocados
2 Serrano chilies
1 small head of garlic
1 small bunch of cilantro – stems removed
1/4 cup parsley – chopped
2 Tbsp EVOO
¼ tsp mineral salt
¼ cup lime juice
Optional Extra – top with a few tablespoons of
chopped bell pepper – we used yellow

Directions:

Cut one of the avocados into ¾ inch square pieces,
place in a medium mixing bowl and drizzle with 2 tsp
of the lime juice.

Cut the cucumbers into similar sized pieces and add to
the avocados then place in the refrigerator to keep
cool.

Place the second avocado and the remaining
ingredients into a blender and process until smooth.

Pour over the avocado and cucumber mix and serve
within a couple of hours.

NOTE
This will not hold up well for many hours and cannot
be frozen

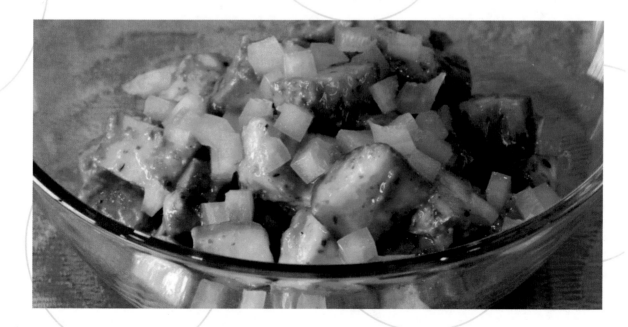

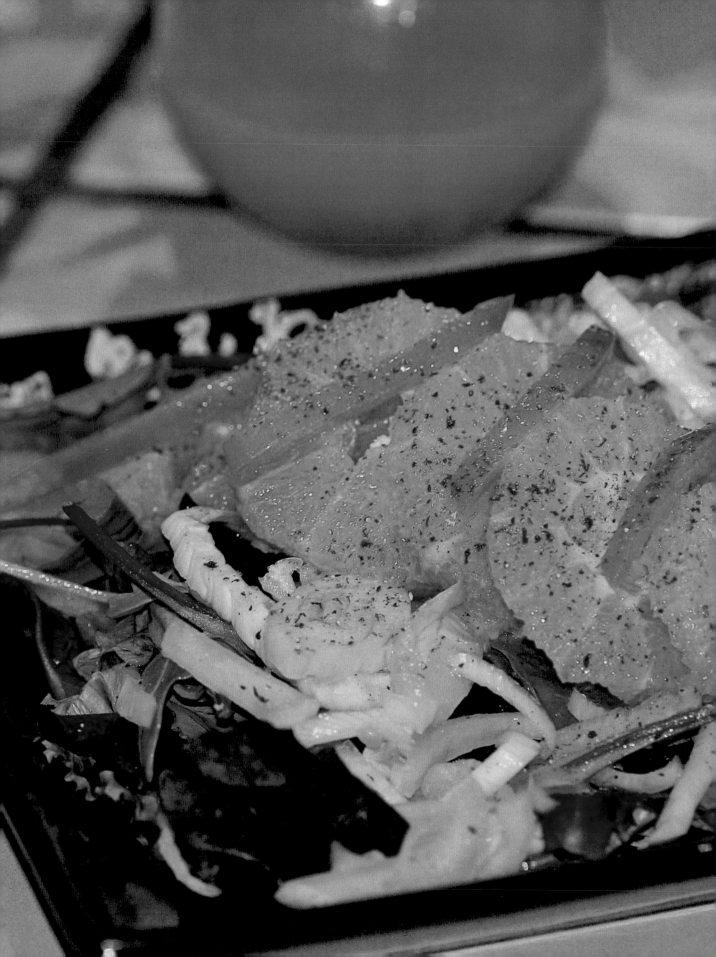

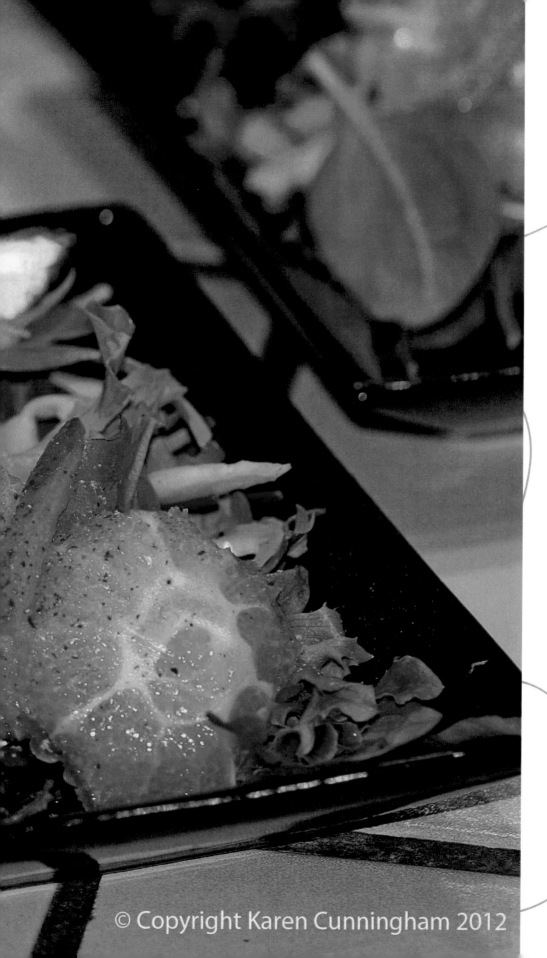

Salads

Kale with Peanut Sauce* (Q)(E)($)(R)
Serves: 2
Per serving: 308 Calories, 23g Fat, 10g Carbs, 4g Fiber, 12.6g Protein

*see page for peanut sauce recipe

Ingredients:

1 bunch kale - finely chopped
1/4 cup natural peanut butter
1 Tbsp EVOO
1 Tbsp Bragg's Liquid Aminos
1/2 tsp coriander
1/4 tsp chili powder
1/4 tsp cumin
1 onion - chopped
1 garlic clove
1/4 cup vegetable broth or water

Directions:

Sauté the onion and garlic in the EVOO on low heat until the onion becomes translucent.

Throw everything else in the skillet and gently sauté for just a few minutes until the kale has just wilted.

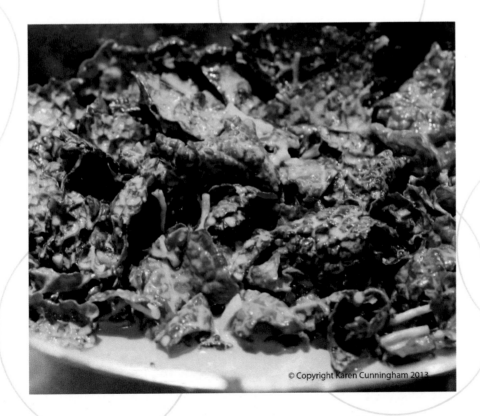

© Copyright Karen Cunningham 2013

Asian Cole Slaw (R)(Q)($)(E)

Serves: 8
Per serving: 230 Calories, 18g Fat, 14.7g Carbs, 4.6g Fiber, 5.7g Protein

Ingredients:

5 Tbsp raw almond butter (or peanut butter)
2 Tbsp EVOO
2 Tbsp peanut oil
1 tsp sesame oil
5 Tbsp lemon juice
3 Tbsp Bragg's Liquid Aminos or tamari sauce
2 tsp maple syrup
1 1/2 Tbsp garlic - minced
2 Tbsp ginger root - minced
5 cups green cabbage - thinly sliced
2 cup red cabbage - thinly sliced
2 cups Napa cabbage - shredded
2 large carrots - julienned
2 yellow or red bell peppers - thinly sliced
5 stalks green onions - chopped on an angle
3/4 cup fresh cilantro - chopped
1/2 cup mixed seeds for extra crunch and nutrition –
try a mix of flax, sesame.

Directions:

In a bowl, whisk together oil, vinegar, almond butter, Tamari sauce, dates, garlic, and ginger.

In a separate large bowl, mix the green cabbage, red cabbage, Napa cabbage, carrots, bell peppers, green onions, and cilantro.

Toss salad with almond butter mixture before serving.

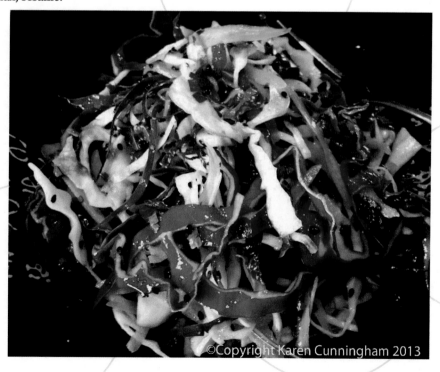

©Copyright Karen Cunningham 2013

Carrot Ginger Salad (Q)($)(E)(R)

Serves: 4
Per serving: 204 Calories, 19g Fat, 2.3g Sat Fat, 6.2g Carbs, 3g Fiber, 3g Protein, 116% of
DV Vitamin A

Ingredients:

2 medium carrots - peeled and julienned
1 cup baby spinach leaves
2 Tbsp pine nuts -toasted
2 Tbsp sesame seeds – mix all colors for extra appeal
1 Tbsp flax seeds whole
1 Tbsp flax seeds ground
1 Tbsp sesame oil
1 Tbsp Wildwood zesty garlic aioli
2 Tbsp apple cider vinegar
2 Tbsp grape seed oil
1 tsp freshly grated ginger
salt & pepper to taste

Note:
I like an additional squeeze of fresh lime

Directions:

Mix carrot and spinach – chill well

In a separate bowl whisk all other ingredients and
taste – adjust to suit your taste and then mix with
carrot and spinach and serve immediately.

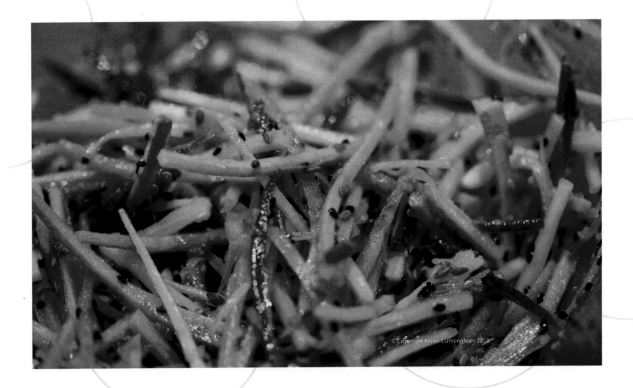

Quinoa Salad with Roasted Peppers and Tomato ($)(E)
Serves: 4
Per serving: 20 Calories, 2.9g Fat, 43.1g Carbs, 5.5g Fiber, 8.1g Protein

Ingredients:

1 cup uncooked quinoa- any color, or mixed
1 cup roasted pepper sauce
1/2 cup finely chopped sundried tomatoes
1/4 cup unsulphured raisins
2 Tbsp chopped parsley
2 roasted bell peppers - sliced into strips (see page 334)
1 1/2 cups halved small sweet tomatoes.

Directions:

Bring about six cups of water to the boil and add the quinoa, boil on medium heat for about 15 minutes. *

Remove from heat and rinse with cold water in the lined or small holed colander .

Allow to drain for 5 minutes.

Slice the roasted peppers

Chop the sundried tomatoes

Halve the small tomatoes

Roughly chop the parsley

Pour quinoa into a serving bowl and mix the roasted pepper tomato sauce through it gently until the quinoa takes on a fairly uniform pink color.

Then add all other ingredients except the little tomatoes.

Finish the dish with the halved tomatoes and some extra parsley. This is equally delicious, hot cold or at room temperature

Add some spice if you like things hot.

*Note:
Quinoa should still be a little crunchy as you don't want mush. It is a curly grain and when it is cooked it appears to have a little tail on it.

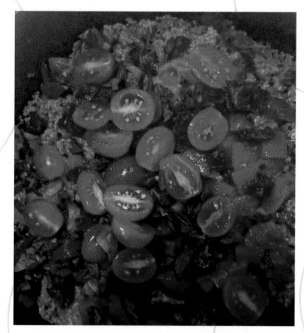

Grilled Fennel with Orange, Almonds and Mint Salad ($)(Q) (E)

Serves: 4

Per serving: 251 Calories, 15.7g Fat, 28.1g Carbs, 7.9g Fiber, 4.3g Protein

Ingredients:

2 bulbs fennel - sliced into 1/2-inch thick slices
3 oranges - peeled and segmented,
1 orange juiced and zested - only zest half of orange
2 tsp dry mustard powder
1/4 cup EVOO
3 Tbsp sliced almonds - toasted
2 Tbsp fresh mint leaves - chopped
Salt and freshly ground pepper

Directions:

Heat grill to high.

Brush the fennel with EVOO and season with salt and pepper, to taste.

Grill for 3 to 4 minutes per side or until slightly charred and almost cooked through.

Place fennel on a platter and scatter orange segments over the top.

Whisk together the orange juice, zest, mustard, and EVOO in a small bowl.

Season with salt and pepper, to taste.

Drizzle vinaigrette over the salad.

Sprinkle with almonds and mint and serve.

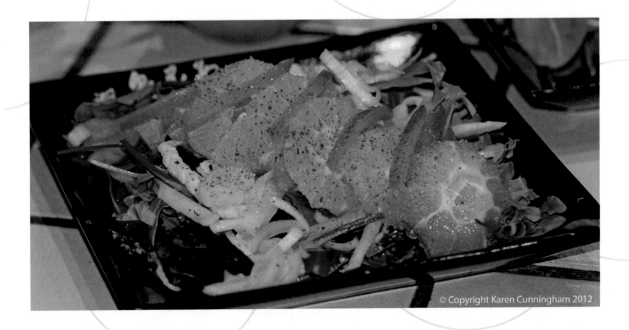

© Copyright Karen Cunningham 2012

Cabbage Salad (Cole Slaw) (Q)($)(E)(R)

Serves: 6
Per serving: 114 Calories, 6.5g Fat, 14.3g Carbs, 3.4g Fiber, 1.6g Protein

Ingredients:

1/2 small red cabbage - grated
3 or 4 carrots - grated
1 apple - grated
1/2 bunch fresh parsley leaves - finely minced(remove the thick stems)
1 or 2 two spring onions - chopped
Juice of one orange
Juice of one lemon
1 tsp sesame oil
2 Tbsp EVOO
1 date blended with enough water to make a syrup
1 Tbsp toasted sesame seeds
salt and pepper to taste

Directions:

Toss all together .

Note:
Will keep several days in the refrigerator

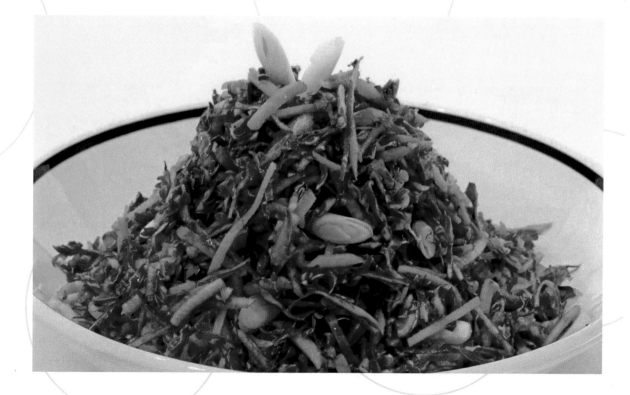

Almost Nicoise Salad ($)(E)(NCF)

Serves: 4 - 6
Per Serving: 230 calories, 14g Fat, 25g Carbohydrates, 6g Fiber, 3.6g Protein

Ingredients:

1 lb small golden or mixed colored potatoes - steamed until cooked al dente
1/2 lb green beans - steamed for just a minute or two and then run through a cold water bath to avoid continued cooking
1 small shallot – finely diced
3 Tbsp EVOO
1 Tbsp apple cider vinegar
1/2 cup brine cured green olives pitted
1/2 cup olives of choice brine cured
parsley to taste - chopped
dill weed to taste - chopped
fresh round black pepper
salt to taste or a squeeze of lemon juice
1 Tbsp capers

Directions:

Halve baby potatoes and arrange in a shallow dish with chopped green beans, olives and capers

Heat 1 Tbsp EVOO in a small pan and add the shallots to slowly soften over low heat. Add the shallot mixture and the rest of the EVOO to the potatoes...Sprinkle with pepper and chopped parsley as you wish and enjoy.

Note: Potatoes are a starchy vegetable and should be consumed in small amounts only – you can adjust this recipe and add lots of different veggies for a change of pace.

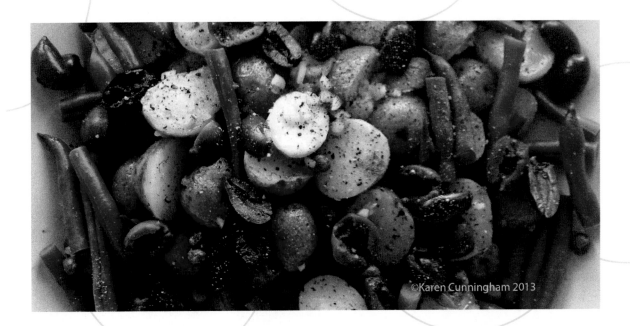
©Karen Cunningham 2013

Tabbouleh Salad (Q)($)(E)(R)
Serves: 6
Per serving: 251 Calories, 4g Fat, 46g Carbs, 5g Fiber

Ingredients:

1 cup finely chopped cauliflower*
1/3 cup EVOO
1/3 cup lemon juice
1/2 cup green onions - chopped
1 cup fresh parsley - chopped
1/4 cup fresh mint - chopped
2 tomatoes - chopped**
1/2 medium cucumber - peeled, seeded and chopped
1/4 tsp salt

*Take a piece of cauliflower that looks about the size of 1 cup and gently chop it in a food processor or blender on low speed until it resembles bread crumbs.

**Do not refrigerate tomatoes as they lose all flavor

Directions:

Add oil, lemon juice, onions, parsley, mint, and cucumber; toss to combine.

Season to taste with salt and black pepper.

Cover, and refrigerate for at least 1 hour.

Add chopped tomatoes just before serving.

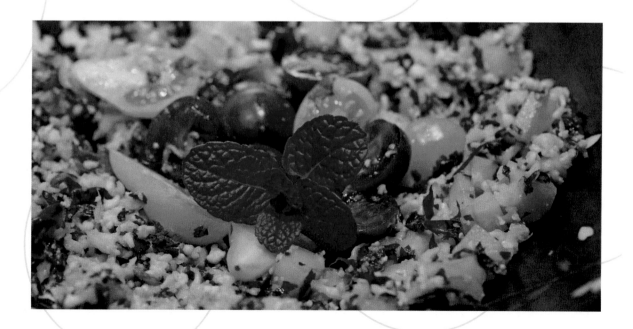

Apple, Kale, Walnut and Cranberry Salad (Q)($)(E)(R)
Serves 2
Per serving: 296 Calories, 20.6g Fat (all healthy fats from walnuts and tahini), 26g Carbs, 6g Fiber, 10.2g Protein

Ingredients:

SALAD
1 large green apple unreeled, but cored and cut into pieces
3 stalks kale - de-ribbed and sliced very thinly
1/2 cup walnuts (or pecans)
2 Tbsp unsweetened dried cranberries
1/2 stalk celery - sliced thinly

DRESSING

1 Tbsp lemon or lime juice, freshly squeezed
2 garlic cloves, peeled
1/2 tsp dry mustard powder
1 tsp sesame paste (Tahini) or 2 Tbsp of sesame seeds
2 tsp light-colored miso (or salt to taste)
2 Tbsp water
additional lemon juice, salt, and freshly ground black pepper to taste

Directions:

DRESSING
Combine ingredients in a small blender

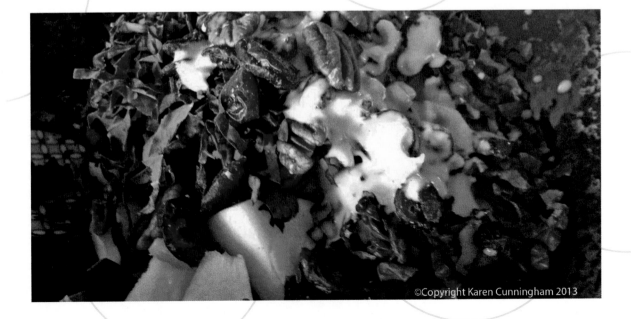
©Copyright Karen Cunningham 2013

Golden Beet, Orange and Mango Salad (Q)($)(E)(R)

Per serving: 171 Calories, 4g Fat, 34 Carbs, 5.7g Fiber, 3.4g Protein

Ingredients:

golden beets
1 mango - peeled, chopped
1 orange - sliced (tangerine works well too)
EVOO
1/4 cup orange juice
1 Tbsp apple cider vinegar

Directions:

Grabs some beets and leave them whole and steam them until a skewer goes through them quite easily.

Depending on the size of your beets, this could be up to an hour. Let them cool once cooked. This could be something you do a day or two ahead of when you want the salad.

Peel your beets once cooked and chop into sizes that appeal to you.

Add one chopped slightly under ripe peeled mango and some orange segments from two oranges or tangerines.

Drizzle with EVOO or as I did in this recipe, tangerine infused EVOO and add apple cider vinegar and orange juice.

Toss together and garnish with some additional orange slices.

NOTE:
To really pack a punch on the flavor meter I sprinkle smoked paprika over the top.

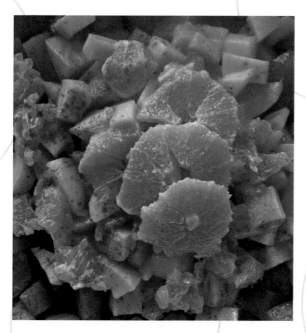

Citrus Salad (R)(E)($)(Q)

Serves: 2
Per serving (1/2 recipe): 131 Calories, 4.3g Fat, 23.8g Carbs, 3.6g Fiber, 1.9g Protein

Ingredients:

1 orange – peeled and sliced
1 tangerine – peeled and sliced
2 Tbsp pomegranate seeds
2 Tbsp unsweetened desiccated coconut
1 tsp orange flower water
1 tsp EVOO
2 Tbsp lemon juice
lemon slices for garnish
pinch mineral salt

Directions:

Mix orange flower water, lemon juice, EVOO and salt together.

Arrange sliced citrus on platter and drizzle with the dressing.

Sprinkle with coconut and pomegranate seeds.

NOTE:
You could also sprinkle this with a little cayenne pepper or cinnamon

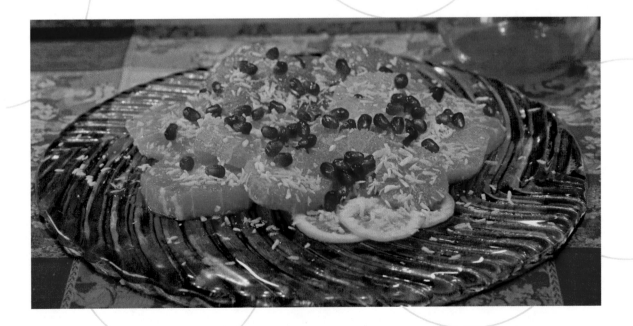

Mango Avocado Salad (R)(Q)($)(E)

Serves: 2-3
Per serving (1/3 recipe): 175 Calories, 11.9g Fat, 19g Carbs, 6.3g Fiber, 2g Protein

Ingredients:

1 ripe mango – peeled and chopped
1 avocado – peeled, seeded and chopped
½ red bell pepper – finely diced
1 Tbsp spring onions – chopped (white parts only)
1 Tbsp cilantro – chopped
1 tsp EVOO
2 Tbsp lemon juice

Directions:

Mix and enjoy.

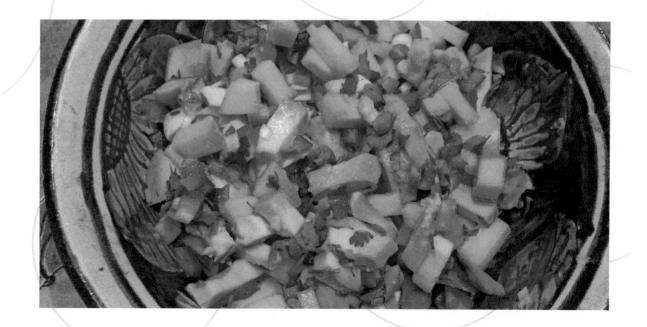

Garbanzo Pesto Salad (E)($)

Serves: 4
Per serving: 186 Calories, 6g Fat, 22.6g Carbs, 5.5g Fiber, 8.4g Protein

Ingredients:

2 cups cooked garbanzo beans
3 Tbsp of your favorite pesto
1 tomato – chopped
2 Tbsp parsley – chopped
2 Tbsp lemon or lime juice

Directions:

Mix and enjoy.

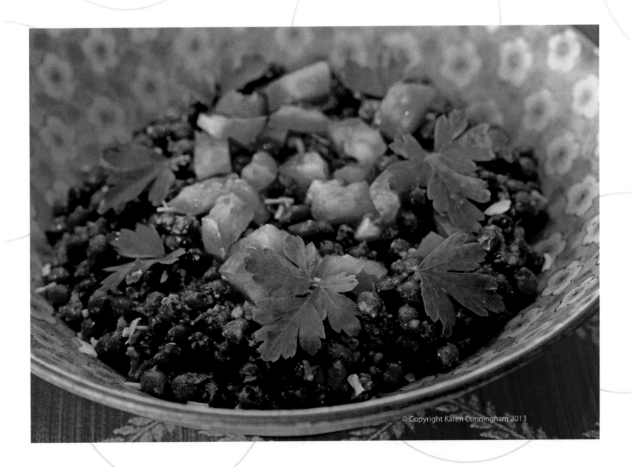

© Copyright Karen Cunningham 2013

Beet Cabbage Salad (Q)(R)($)(E)
Per serving: 54 Calories, 0.4g Fat, 12.2g Carbs, 2.8g Fiber, 1.7g Protein

Ingredients:

3 medium red beets - grated
1/4 small red cabbage - shredded
1 medium green apple - peeled and grated or julienned
1/2 cup parsley - chopped
1/4 cup cilantro - chopped
1 tsp dry mustard
1 inch piece of fresh ginger - peeled and chopped finely
3 cloves garlic - crushed
1 Tbsp lemon or lime juice
1/4 tsp salt (helps the veggies sweat out their juices)
ground black pepper to taste
cracked black or white pepper to taste

Directions:

Mix all ingredients together and wait about an hour for the flavors to marry.

** Did you notice this is a fat free salad?
Serve with a cup of split green pea soup, 1/2 an avocado with 1/2 tsp pomegranate concentrate (Carlo brand - no sugar) 1/2 cup brown, or black rice.

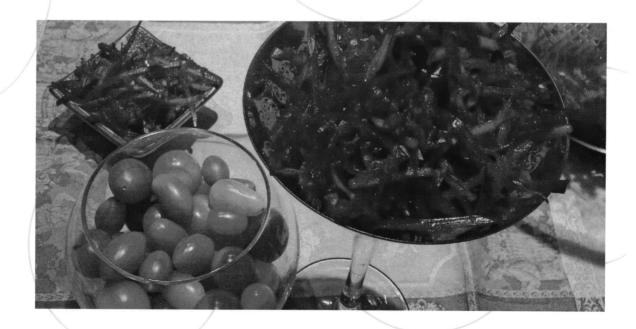

Grilled Fruit Salad (E)

Serves: 6
Per serving*: 173 Calories, 6.8g Fat, 29.8g Carbs, 4.3g Fiber, 2.8g Protein

*Analyzed without dressing, with pine nut parmesan

Ingredients:

1 iceberg lettuce – outer leaves removed and lettuce quartered
1 pineapple – peeled –cored and cut into ¾ inch rings
2 firm mangos – peeled and cut into large slices
1 small firm papaya – peeled – seeded and cut into ¾ inch rings
½ cup brazil nut parmesan or pine nut parmesan (see page 235 for brazil nut parmesan recipe or page 234 for pine nut parmesan)

*Depicted below is the mango habañero sauce (see page 193).

Directions:

Thread fruit onto skewers and grill on hot griddle for a few minutes.

Serve with your favorite sauces.

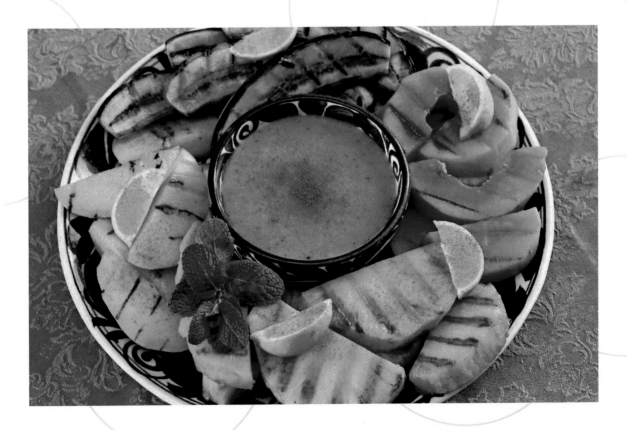

Asian Style Kale Salad (R)(Q)(E)($)
Per serving: 86 Calories, 5.7g Fat, 8g Carbs, 1.6g Fiber, 3g Protein

Ingredients:

1 lb kale - destemmed and thinly chopped
1 Tbsp white sesame seeds – lightly toasted
¼ tsp mineral salt
1 Tbsp EVOO
2 cloves garlic – crushed
1 ½ Tbsp lemon juice
1 Tbsp tamari
1 Tbsp sesame oil
crushed red pepper flakes for garnish – optional
1 scallion – thinly sliced – as garnish

Directions:

In a large bowl toss the kale with the salt and EVOO and gently massage the oil into the kale to soften it.

Add the garlic, tamari, lemon juice and sesame oil and toss well.

Place into a serving bowl and dress with the sesame seeds, onion and red peppers.

*This salad is great with a side of cooked grains such as buckwheat, rice, quinoa or millet.

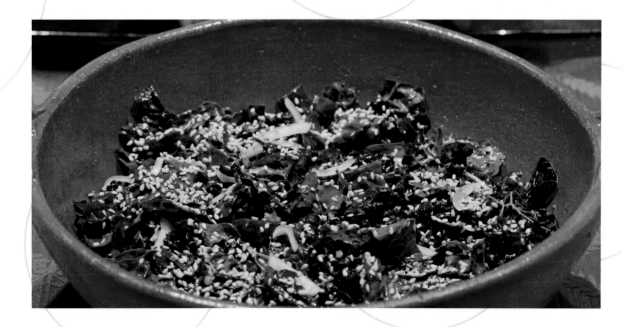

Apple, Fennel and Pistachio Salad (R)(Q)($)(E)
Per serving: 140 Calories, 8g Fat, 13.5g Carbs, 4.2g Fiber, 4.4g Protein

Ingredients:

1 medium sized fennel bulb, or 2 small bulbs – thinly sliced
1/2 small Granny Smith apple – peeled and thinly sliced
1/2 small red onion - thinly sliced
½ sliced and seeded Jalapeno or Serrano pepper – thinly sliced
2 Tbsp lemon juice
1 tsp EVOO
½ cup of shelled pistachios - coarsely chopped
½ cup fennel fronds - coarsely chopped
½ cup parsley - coarsely chopped
mineral salt and pepper to taste

Directions:

Mix everything together.

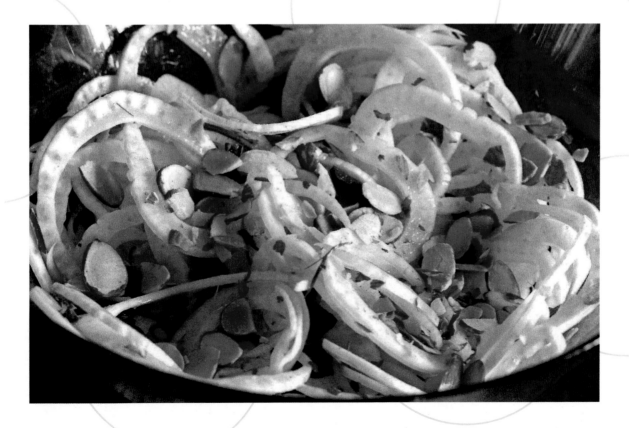

Carrot Coriander Salad (R)(Q)($)(E)

Serves: 2

Per serving: 123 Calories, 7.2g Fat, 14.6g Carbs, 3.7g Fiber, 1.5g Protein

Ingredients:

3 carrots – peeled and sliced on a mandolin on thin. If you do not have a mandolin, you can simply use a vegetable peeler to make thin ribbons of carrot
1 small red onion – sliced into thin ribbons
2 Tbsp cilantro – chopped fine
1 tsp coriander seeds – fresh ground over the top of your salad
1 tsp orange zest
1 Tbsp orange juice
1 Tbsp EVOO
Optional – 1 – 2 tsp sesame seeds

Directions:

Mix the orange zest, orange juice and EVOO together.

Layer the vegetables on a plate and drizzle with the dressing.

Grate the coriander over the top.

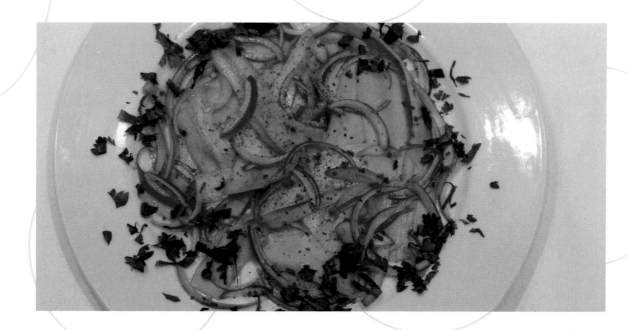

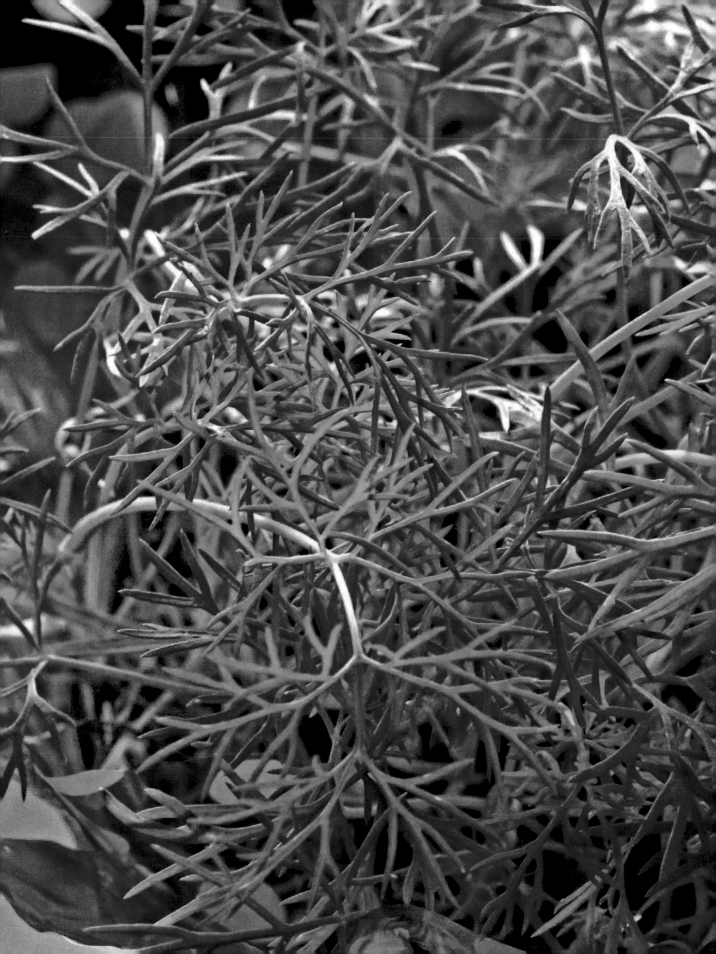

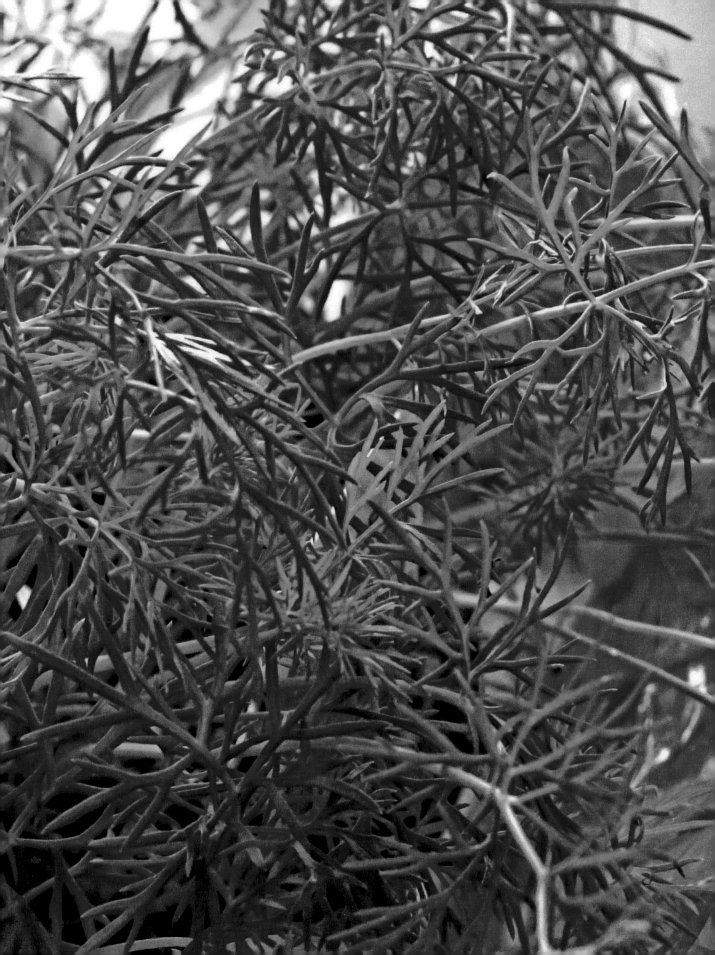

Cucumber Dill Avocado Salad (Q)(E)($)
Serves: 1 main, 2 side
Per serving (1/2 recipe): 326 Calories, 12.1g Fat, 47.3g Carbs, 10.2g Fiber, 8.5g Protein

Ingredients:

1 cup cooked millet
1 Persian cucumber – chopped
1 spring onion – finely sliced
1 small tomato – chopped
½ stick celery - chopped
2 Tbsp lemon juice
1 tsp apple cider vinegar
1 Tbsp simple cashew crème (see page 239)
½ avocado – chopped
1 tsp flax seeds
2 Tbsp parsley – chopped
1 Tbsp fresh dill – chopped or 1 tsp dried dill
¼ tsp mineral salt
Fresh ground pepper
Fresh sprouts to top – optional

Directions:

Mix and enjoy – adjust seasonings to your taste.

NOTE:
Let this sit for 30 minutes or more to infuse the flavor of the dill.

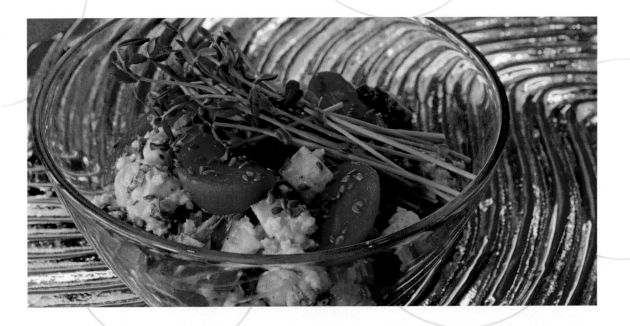

Grilled Peach Salad (Q)(E)($)

Serves: 4

Per serving: 341 Calories, 29.8g Fat, 19.4g Carbs, 6.1g Fiber, 5.6g Protein

Ingredients:

4 firm peaches - halved
4 cups mixed salad greens
2 cups baby tomatoes
1 cup Pecans – lightly toasted
2 scallions – thinly sliced
1 tsp fresh dill – thinly sliced
2 Tbsp brazil nut parmesan (see page 235) or pine nut
parmesan (see page 234)
2 Tbsp EVOO
1 Tbsp lemon juice
1 Tbsp lime juice

Directions:

On a hot, slightly greased griddle (use Grape seed oil) grill the peach cut side down until slightly charred.

Remove from heat and place cut side up on a plate.

When they cool quarter them.

Arrange the greens on a platter and then arrange the remaining ingredients on top adding the EVOO and juices at the last minute.

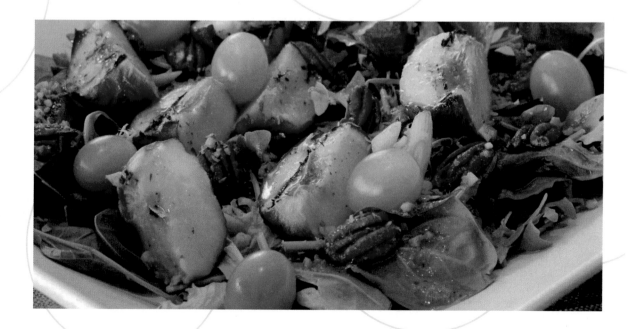

Japanese Seaweed Salad (Q)(R)($)

Serves: 4

Per serving: 77 Calories, 4.6g Fat, 6.9g Carbs, 3g Fiber, 2.3g Protein

Ingredients:

3/4 ounce dried wakame seaweed (whole or cut)
3 Tbsp apple cider vinegar
1 Tbsp tamari sauce
1 Tbsp sesame oil
1 tsp date purée (see page 304)
red pepper flakes
1 tsp ginger - finely grated
1/2 tsp garlic - minced
2 scallions - thinly sliced
1/4 cup carrot- shredded
2 Tbsp fresh cilantro - chopped
1 Tbsp sesame seeds – toasted – leave untoasted for a pure raw experience

Directions:

Soak seaweed in warm water to cover, 5 minutes.

Drain, rinse then squeeze out excess water.

If wakame is uncut, cut into 1/2-inch-wide strips.

Stir together vinegar, tamari sauce, sesame oil, date purée, pepper flakes, ginger, and garlic in a bowl until date is well combined.

Add the seaweed, scallions, carrots, and cilantro, tossing to combine well.

Sprinkle salad with sesame seeds.

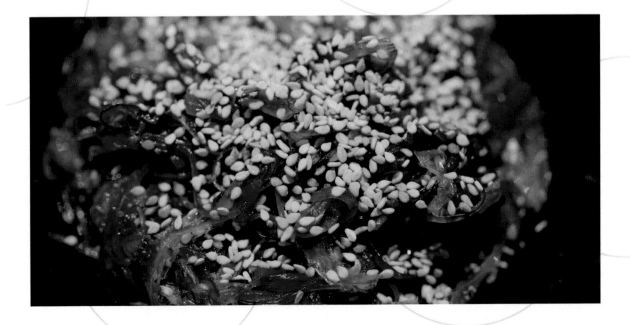

Sea Vegetable Salad (R)(Q)(E)
Serves: 6
Per serving: 181 Calories, 11.7g Fat, 19g Carbs, 4.5g Fiber, 4.2g Protein

Ingredients:

12 oz Kelp (I use Sea Tangle Brand from Amazon) –
rinse and cut into small lengths of about 2 inches –
Kelp is chewy and long pieces are not easy to eat
3 carrots – julienned
3 Tbsp cilantro or parsley – chopped
2 spring onions – sliced diagonally
1 orange bell pepper – thinly sliced
1 cup Napa cabbage – thinly sliced
1 cup pea sprouts
1 avocado – peeled, deseeded and sliced

DRESSING
2 Tbsp EVOO
2 tsp sesame oil
1 Tbsp apple cider vinegar
1 Tbsp orange juice
½ tsp ground black pepper
Mix in a shaker cup or blender

OPTIONAL
1 Tbsp sesame seeds
1 tsp red pepper flakes

Directions:

place all ingredients except for avocado and pea
sprouts into a large serving bowl and add the
dressing.

Just before serving add the avocado and pea sprouts.

DRESSING
Mix well and let sit for 10 minutes (or not)

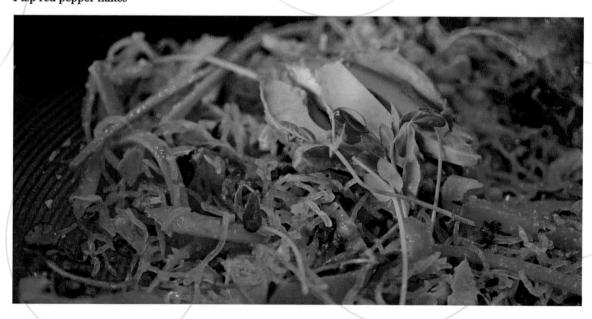

Asian Salad (R)(Q)($)(E)

Serves: 2

Per serving: 408 Calories, 14.7g Fat, 51g Carbs, 13.3g Fiber, 19.7g Protein

Ingredients:

1 cup white cabbage – chopped
1 cup orange bell pepper - chopped
1 cup sprouted mung beans
1 cup cucumber – chopped
¼ cup spring onion - finely chopped
2 Tbsp black sesame seeds – white will do
1 Tbsp EVOO
1 tsp sesame oil
¼ tsp mineral salt
1 Tbsp orange juice
1 Tbsp lemon juice

Directions:

Mix and enjoy!

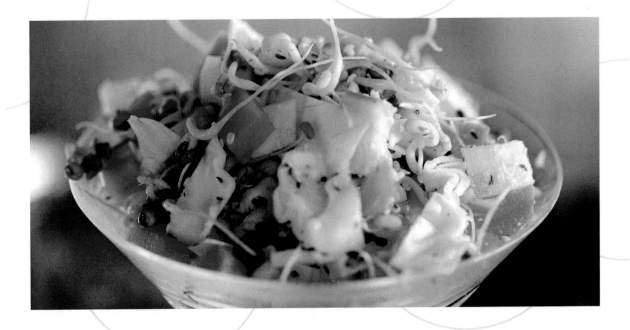

Amaranth Tabbouleh Salad(Q)($)

Serves: 6

Per serving: 170 Calories, 11.5g Fat, 15.2g Carbs, 5.6g Fiber, 4.6g protein

Ingredients:

1 cup amaranth (you will need a fine meshed sieve for this as the grain is very small)
8 cups loosely packed parsley leaves - chopped
1 cup chopped fresh mint (preferably spearmint)
3 scallions - finely chopped
2 Persian cucumbers – unpeeled and finely chopped
1/4 cup celery leaves - chopped
1 medium tomato - finely chopped
4 radishes - finely chopped
1/4 cup fresh lemon juice
1/3 cup EVOO
mineral salt and freshly ground pepper to taste

Directions:

Cook the amaranth in a large pot of boiling water for about 20-25 minutes – then drain and allow to cool.

Transfer to a large bowl, then stir in the remaining ingredients - season to taste.

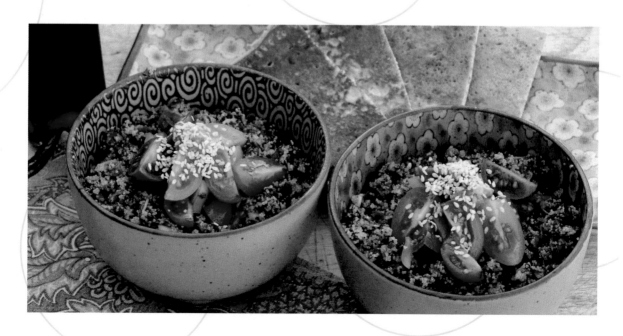

Blood Orange Spinach Salad (R)(Q)(E)

Serves: 2
Per serving (1/4 recipe): 308 Calories, 24.8g Fat, 16.7g Carbs, 3.6g Fiber, 10.2g Protein

Ingredients:

3 cups baby spinach
1 cup sprouts – alfalfa, pea etc
2 small oranges – peeled and sliced into rings
1 cup raw pumpkin seeds
½ cup salt cured olives
2 Tbsp EVOO
1 tsp tamari
2 Tbsp orange juice
¼ cup juice sweetened cranberries
cracked black pepper to taste

Directions:

Mix and Enjoy

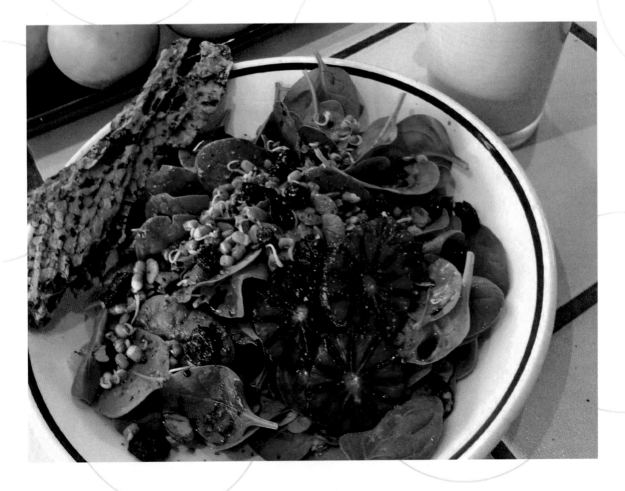

Spinach Pea Shoot Salad (Q)(R)(E)($)

Serves: 3-4
Per serving: 238 Calories, 22g Fat, 7g Carbs, 3g Fiber, 7g Protein

Ingredients:

2 cups baby spinach
½ cup walnut halves
¼ cup toasted pumpkin seeds – untoasted for true
raw experience
1 cup pea shoots
¼ cup red onion – sliced finely
½ cup salt cured olives
2 Tbsp EVOO
2 Tbsp lemon juice
mineral salt and pepper to taste

Directions:

Mix and enjoy.

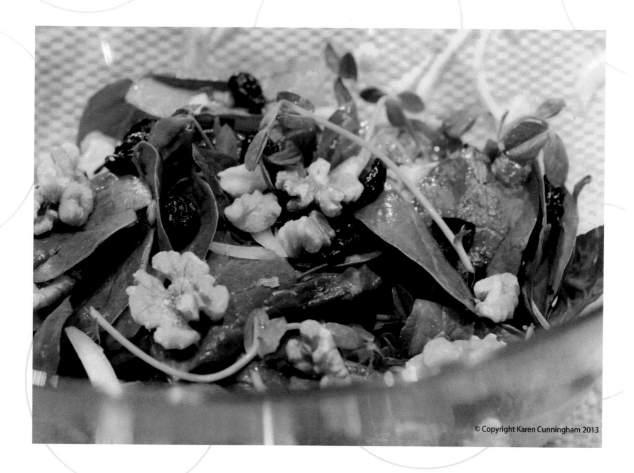

Quinoa with Tomato Salad (Q)(E)($)

Serves: 4

Per serving: 273 Calories, 5.8g Fat, 45g Carbs, 4.7g Fiber, 7.4g Protein

Ingredients:

2 cups cooked quinoa – we use black quinoa, but any will be just fine
2 Tbsp sundried tomatoes – julienned
4 Tbsp parsley – chopped
4 Tbsp – roasted red or yellow bell peppers - we used both
1 avocado – peeled, deseeded and chopped
1 cup pea sprouts

DRESSING
½ cup orange juice
¼ cup lemon juice
2 Tbsp EVOO
pinch of salt
Cracked black pepper to taste – optional

Directions:

Mix gently.

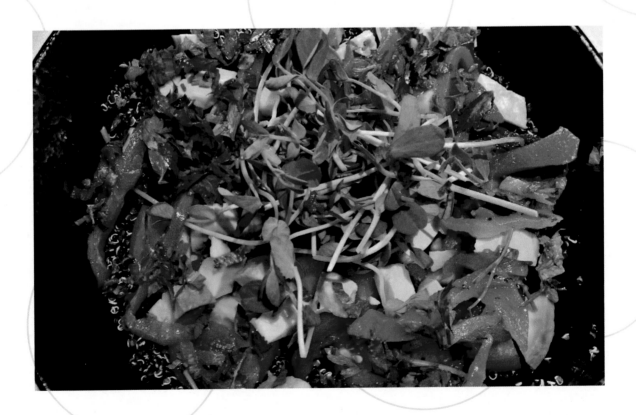

Green Papaya Salad (R)(Q)($)

Serves: 4

Per serving: 134 Calories, 7g Fat, 16g Carbs, 3.5g Fiber, 3g Protein

Ingredients:

1 small green papaya
2 cups bean sprouts
3 spring onions - cut into long matchstick-like pieces
1 zucchini – cut into thin strips
1/2 cup fresh basil - leaves left whole or chopped
handful of fresh coriander
1 red chili - sliced, seeds removed (reduce or omit, to taste)
optional: 1/2 cup roasted peanuts or cashews

DRESSING
2 Tbsp grapeseed or peanut oil
2 Tbsp tamari sauce
3 Tbsp lime juice
1/8 to 1/4 tsp. chili flakes or cayenne pepper, to taste

Directions:

Mix all Dressing ingredients together in a cup. Set aside.

Use a sharp knife to peel the green papaya, then slice it in half and use a spoon to scrape out the seeds.

Using the largest grater you have, grate the papaya, or you can use a potato peeler to create thin, ribbon-like strips.

Place in a large bowl.

Mix all ingredients together – taste and adjust seasonings

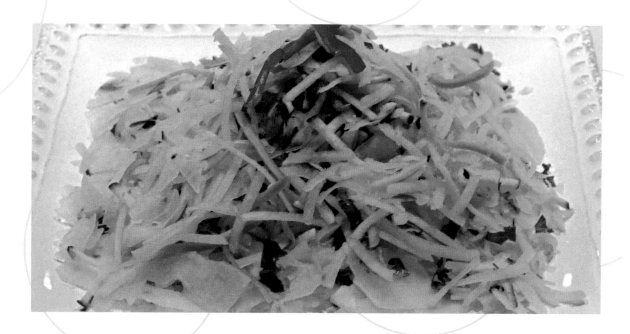

Roasted Beets and Kale Salad (E)($)

Serves: 6
Per serving: 266 calories, 20g fat, 17g Carbs, 4g Fiber, 7.1g Protein

Ingredients:

3 large beets
1 Tbsp EVOO
mineral salt and ground black pepper to taste
3 cups baby kale
1/2 cup chopped walnuts
1/4 cup dried cherries
2 Tbsp golden raisins - optional
1 – 2 Tbsp lemon juice
1 Tbsp dry mustard
2 cloves garlic - minced
2 tsp apple cider vinegar
2 Tbsp EVOO

Directions:

Preheat oven to 350 degrees F (175 degrees C). Line a baking sheet with aluminum foil.

Trim roots and stems from beets. Coat beets with 1 tablespoon olive oil and sprinkle with salt and black pepper. Place beets onto prepared baking sheet.

Roast beets for 30 minutes; turn beets over and continue roasting until tender, 30 minutes to 1 hour more. Let beets cool. Peel skins from beets and cut into 1-inch cubes. Toss cooked beets with kale, walnuts, dried cherries, and golden raisins in a large salad bowl.

Whisk lemon juice, mustard, garlic, and cider vinegar in a bowl. Slowly drizzle 2 Tbsp olive oil into apple cider mixture, whisking constantly, until dressing is combined. Pour dressing over salad and toss to coat. Refrigerate at least 1 hour for flavors to blend before serving.

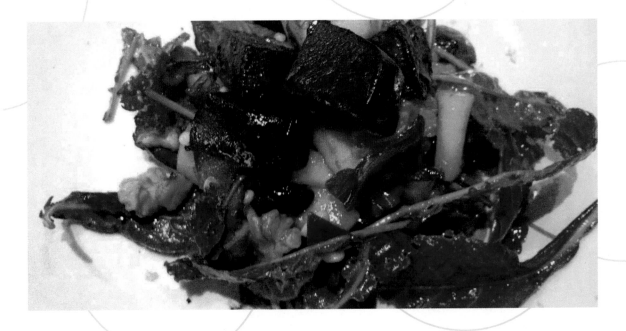

Kale Salad with Tomatoes and Basil and Parsley Dressing (E) (Q)($)(R)

Per serving: 202 Calories, 14g Fat, 17.3g Carbs, 4.3g Fiber, 4.9g Protein

Ingredients:

1/2 bunch of Kale (Ribs removed and diced finely)
Chopped tomatoes of your choice and amount.

DRESSING
1/2 bunch basil - stems removed
1/2 bunch parsley with stems
2 cloves garlic
juice from 1 orange
juice from 1 lemon
juice from 1 lime
2-3 Tbsp Extra virgin olive oil
salt and pepper to taste

Directions:

Place all of the dressing ingredients into a high speed blender and combine until very smooth.

Taste and adjust seasonings to suit.

If the citrus is a little too much for you, add 1/2 tsp maple syrup to mellow the flavor.

Now toss the kale into individual salad bowls, add chopped tomatoes and add the dressing and toss.

NOTE
Factoid - Kale is one of the highest nutrient dense foods available. Adding citrus makes the iron content more available.

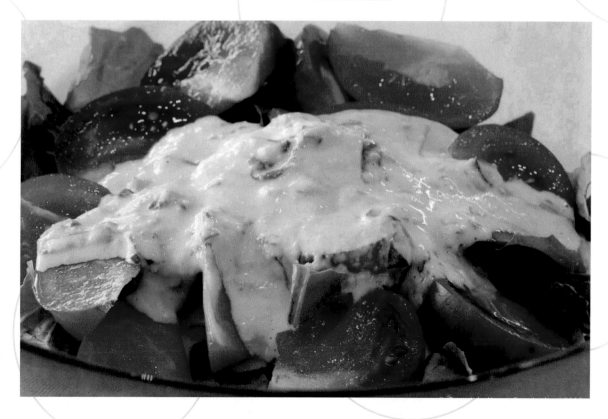

White Bean Salad (Q)(E)($) - Contributed by Alex Caspero

Serves: 4
Per serving: 208 Calories, 11.8g Fat, 20g Carbs, 6g Fiber, 6.9g Protein

Ingredients:

2 cups cooked Cannelini beans - rinsed and drained
1 cup cherry tomatoes - halved
1 cup celery - finely chopped
¼ cup parsley - chopped
⅓ cup lemon juice
3 Tbsp EVOO
1 tsp dried sage

Directions:

Mix all ingredients together in a bowl except for the tomatoes.

Place in the fridge to marinate for 30 minutes

Remove from fridge

Add chopped tomatoes and serve.

NOTE:
Cannot be frozen.

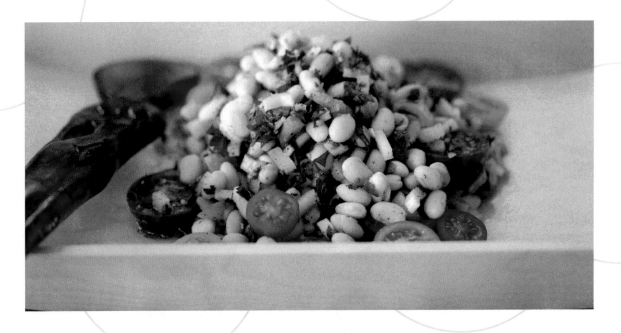

Millet Salad (E)($)

Serves: 6
Per serving: 392 Calories, 2.7g Fat, 74g Carbs, 14.5g Fiber, 19.5g Protein

Ingredients:

1 cup millet, well rinsed uncooked
2 1/2-3 cups water
1 cups cooked black beans
1 cup cooked kidney beans
2 large tomatoes - chopped
1 small red bell pepper - diced
1 medium cucumber - seeds removed and diced
1 medium onion - diced
2 Tbsp parsley - chopped
2 Tbsp chopped cilantro
1 cup fresh corn – sliced off the cob

DRESSING
1/3 cup water
3 Tbsp lemon juice
1 Tbsp Apple Cider vinegar
2 tsp fresh garlic - minced
1 tsp mineral salt (optional)
1/8 tsp cayenne pepper
1/4 tsp black pepper
1 tsp cumin

Directions:

Cook the millet in 2 cups of water until water is absorbed, about 30 minutes - adding more hot water if needed.

Fluff with fork and allow to steam and cool.

In a large bowl, combine millet, black beans, tomatoes, pepper, cucumber and onion.

Mix all dressing ingredients until well blended and pour over the salad, tossing to blend.

Cover and refrigerate until the salad is well chilled.

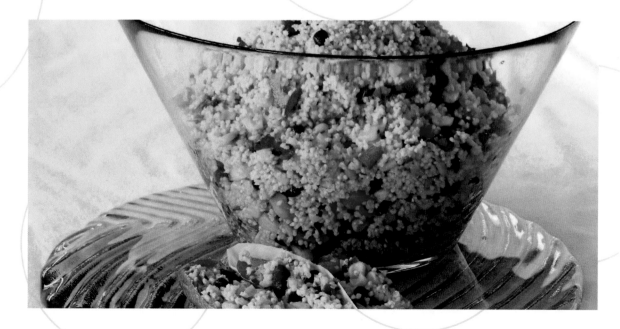

Cucumber French Lentil Salad (E)($)

Serves: 6
Per serving: 19.2 Calories, 7.7g Fat, 22.5g Carbs, 10.7g Fiber, 9g Protein

Ingredients:

1 cup french green lentils (because they cook quick)
1 bay leaf
3 cups water
3 Tbsp EVOO
2 Tbsp apple cider vinegar
2 cloves garlic – minced
2 tsp dry mustard
½ tsp dry dill
3 celery stalks – finely diced
1 cup chopped cucumber
½ cup finely diced fennel bulb
½ cup finely diced white onion
¼ cup finely diced yellow bell pepper

Directions:

Boil lentils in the 3 cups water with the bay leaf until done – about 20 minutes.

Drain, remove and cool.

Toss all other ingredients together in a serving bowl and then gently fold in the cooked lentils.

Season with salt and pepper if desires.

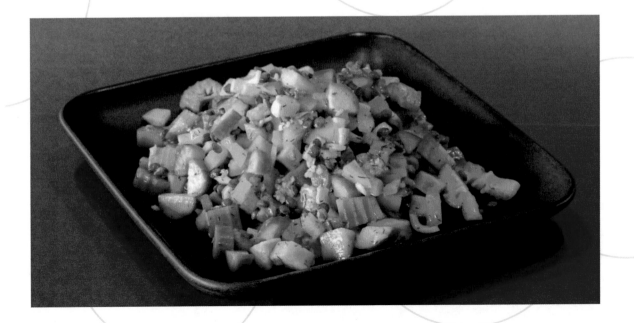

Tomato Cucumber Dill Relish (Q)(E)($)(R)

Serves: 4

Per serving: 41 Calories, 0.6g Fat, 8.9g Carbs, 1.9g Fiber, 1.9g Protein

Ingredients:

2 cups diced peeled seeded cucumber (about 2)
1 pounds plum tomatoes (about 12 large) - seeded, chopped
1/4 cup chopped fresh dill
1/8 cup white vinegar
2 tsp coarse kosher salt
Additional fresh dill sprigs for garnish

Directions:

Mix and enjoy!

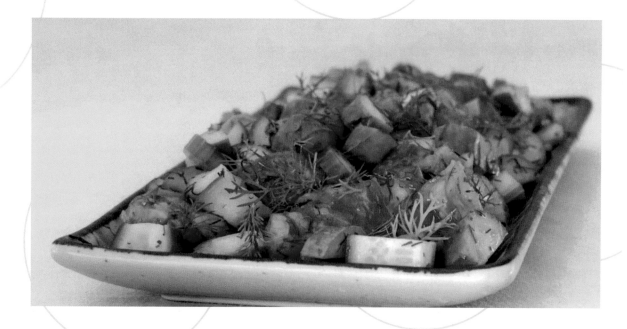

Tomato Salad with Basil Garlic Dressing (R)(Q)(E)($)
Per serving (1/2 serving): 263 Calories, 25.7g Fat, 10g Carbs, 3.2g Fiber, 2.6g Protein

Ingredients:

DRESSING:
1 cup basil leaves with
1 tsp lemon zest
2 Tbsp lemon juice
¼ cup EVOO
¼ tsp mineral salt

Directions:

Simply slice 4 tomatoes and lay them on a serving platter.

Sprinkle with black pepper.

Toss a few basil leaves over the top.

Serve tomatoes with a dollop of the sauce and a ½ tsp Macadamia nut feta or other dairy free cheese.

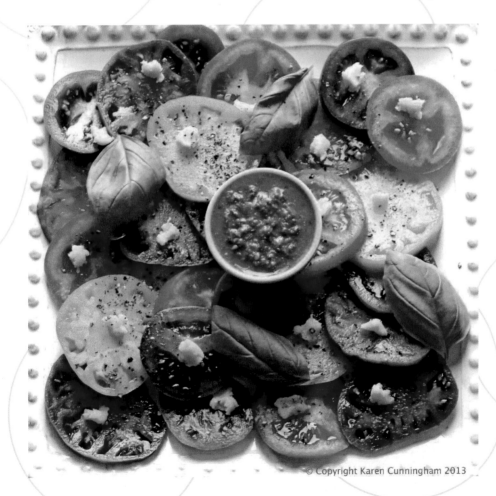

© Copyright Karen Cunningham 2013

Celery Leaves and Spinach Salad (R)(Q)(E)($)- Contributed by Alex Caspero

Serves: 4

Per serving: 77 Calories, 7.4g Fat, 2.6g Carbs, 1.2g Fiber, 1.2g Protein

Ingredients:

1 Tbsp minced shallot
1/2 Tbsp apple cider vinegar
1 tsp grainy Dijon mustard
2 Tbsp extra-virgin olive oil
pinch salt/pepper to taste
3 cups baby spinach leaves
1 cup arugula leaves
1 cup loosely packed celery leaves

Directions:

Whisk together vinegar, mustard, and shallot.

Slowly add olive oil and whisk until combined.

Season to taste with salt pepper.

Toss with spinach, arugula, celery leaves.

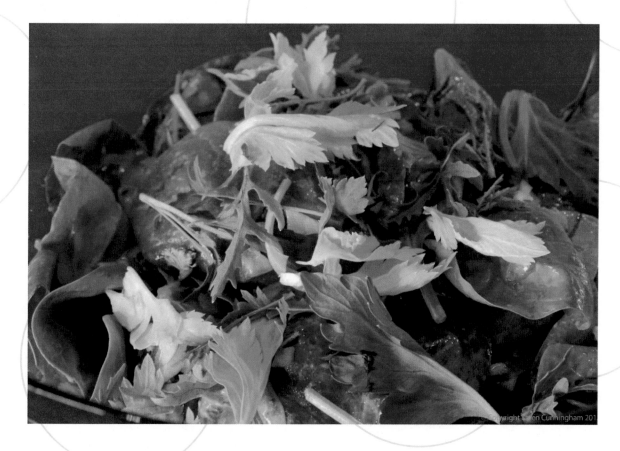

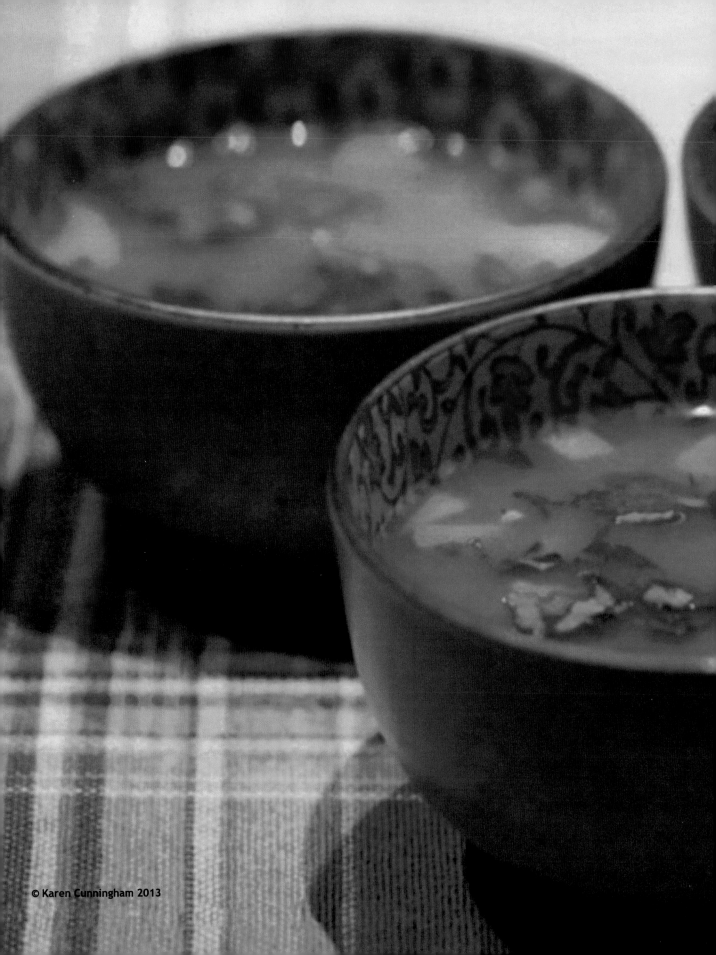

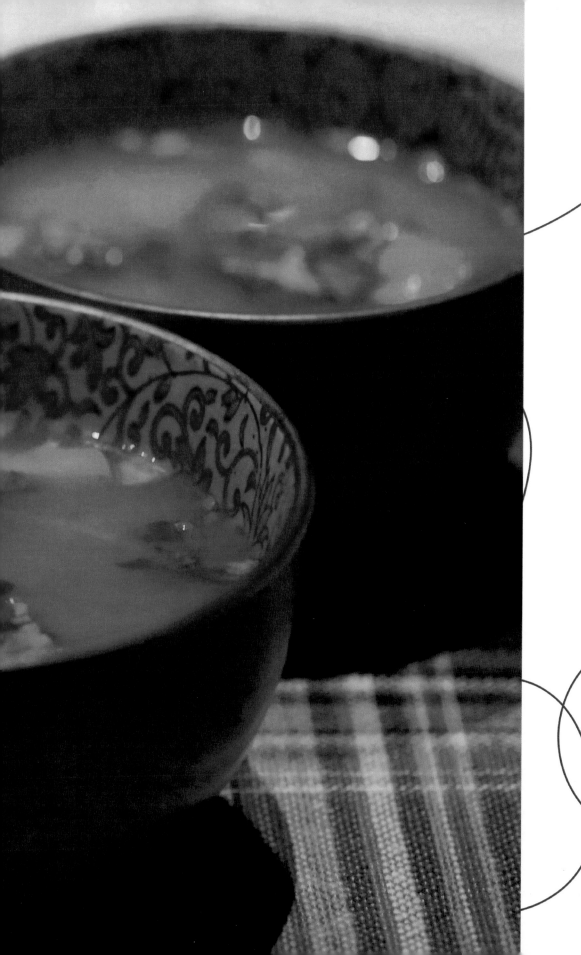

Soups

Borscht (E)($)

Serves 6 - 8
Per serving: 231 Calories, 6g Fat, 37g Carbs, 7.2g Fiber, 9.7g Protein

Ingredients:

2 Tbsp EVOO
1 large onion - finely chopped
3 carrots - peeled and grated
3 cups shredded green cabbage
5 red beets (beetroot) - peeled and grated – wear
gloves unless you want stained hands for days ☺
1 stick celery - diced
2 green apples – peeled cored and chopped into ½"
pieces
2 large potatoes - peeled and grated
½ cup tomato paste
6 cloves garlic - minced
8 cups vegetable broth
2 fresh bay leaves
1/2 tsp cracked black pepper
1 tsp paprika (sweet)
Grated zest of half small orange
Juice from 1 small orange
1 Tbsp lemon juice
vegan sour crème for the top of each bowl - optional
(see page 238)

Directions:

Sauté the onions and carrots in the EVOO on low heat
until the onion is softened (4-6 minutes).

Add the cabbage, beets, and celery and sauté for about
15 minutes.

Stir in the apples, potatoes, tomato paste, garlic,
broth, bay leaves, and pepper.

Bring to a boil.

Lower heat, cover, and simmer for 20 minutes.

Add the paprika, orange and lemon juice. Add salt and
pepper to taste.

NOTE:
Try it hot with vegan sour crème. This soup was
originally served cold, but I like it hot.

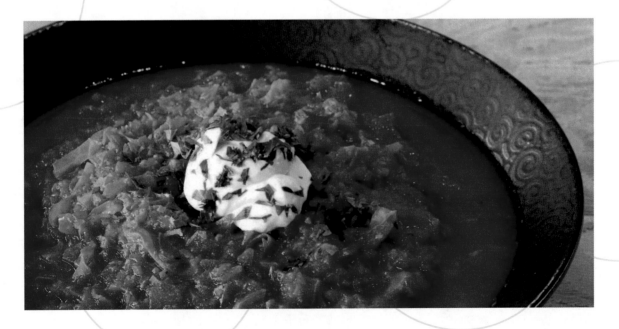

Kale Soup (R)(Q)(E)($)

Serves 6

Per Serving: 211 Calories, 16g Fat, 13g Carbs, 4.2g Fiber, 7.2g Protein

Ingredients:

1 bunch of Kale – remove the woody stems
1/4 cup broccoli pieces
1/4 cup other mild green veggies
1 whole peeled carrot - roughly chopped
2 cups small tomatoes (preferably yellow or orange to keep the soup green) – canned can be used instead
small pinch of dried rosemary (or leaves from a 1 inch sprig of fresh)
1/2 avocado
1/3 cup of fresh basil leaves
1/4 cup raw pine nuts
1/4 cup raw almonds
1/2 cup raw pumpkin seeds
1/4 cup red or sweet onion finely chopped
1/4 cup carrots - chopped
1 jalapeno pepper with seeds (see note) - chopped
1 Tbsp lemon or lime juice
2 Tbsp walnut pesto (see page 177)
2 Tbsp light miso (or garbanzo miso)
2 cloves garlic
2 cups of filtered water

Note: Jalapeno peppers can vary in heat from a 2 – 10 do check the heat of your jalapeno before adding it to the soup. If in doubt leave it out and add chopped jalapeno at the end to your taste

Directions:

Blend all together until resembling a cream based soup.

Taste and add seasoning to suit.

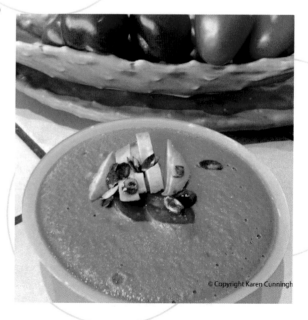

© Copyright Karen Cunningh

Minestrone Soup (E)(Q)($)

Serves: 6 -8

Per serving: 339 Calories, 8g Fat, 46.9g Carbs, 15.5g Fiber, 20.7g Protein

Ingredients:

8 cups vegetable stock
2 Tbsp EVOO – maybe more for serving
1 large brown onion – chopped
3 cloves garlic – chopped finely
2 Tbsp tomato paste
4 carrots – peeled and sliced 1/4" pieces
2 stalks celery - sliced 1/4" pieces
I sweet potato - thinly sliced
1 cup rice pasta
1/2 savoy cabbage
1 cup cooked red lentils
6 sprigs thyme
2 cups cooked white cannelini beans
2 cups baby spinach

Directions:

In a soup pot heat the oil on medium heat and saute the onion for about 5 minutes, stirring occasionally.

Add carrots, celery and sweet potato and stir another two minutes.

Add the remaining ingredients except for the spinach and bring to the boil.

Simmer until the pasta is cooked.

Add the spinach.

Remove from heat and serve.

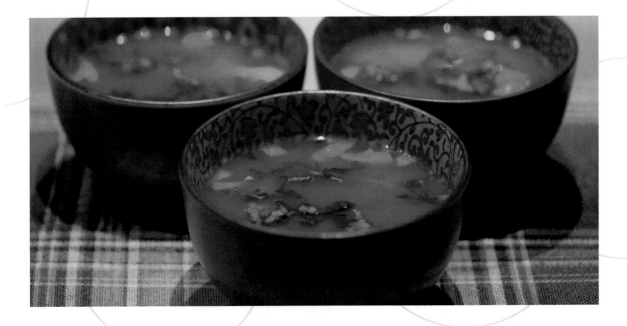

Roasted Tomato Soup (E)($)

Serves: 6

Per serving: 123 Calories 6.5g Fat, 10.4g Carbs, 2.5g Fiber, 6.8g Protein

Ingredients:

2 lbs of your favorite tomatoes – halved
1 red onion – roughly chopped
1/2 tsp dried rosemary +1 sprig rosemary (optional)
1 tsp thyme
¼ tsp dried sage
2 Tbsp EVOO
1 Tbsp miso paste
6 cups vegetable broth
1 pitted date

Options
1 Tbsp Pine nuts per serve
¼ cup cooked garbanzo beans – per person for a
more complete meal

Directions:

Heat oven to 350 degrees.

Sprinkle the tomatoes, cut side up with the herbs and
spices, except for the rosemary sprig.

On a covered cookie sheet, place the tomatoes cut side
down with the onions and drizzle with the EVOO. Add
the sprig of rosemary to the baking pan. Roast for 35-
40 minutes or so until the onions are a little brown
and the tomatoes a little shriveled looking. Remove
from the oven and cool until the tomatoes can be
safely handled.

Pinch up on the tomato to remove the skins and
discard the skins.

Heat the vegetable broth in a soup pan, add the date,
tomatoes, onions and any juices from the pan and
cook for about ten minutes. Add the miso at the end.
Adjust seasonings to your taste.

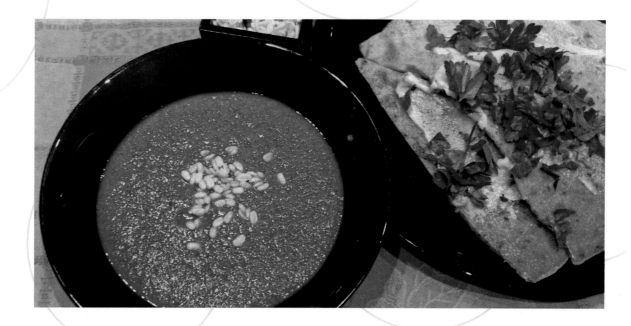

Split Pea Soup (Q)(E)($)
Serves 4-6
Per serving: 473 Calories, 3.4g Fat, 79g Carbs, 28.4g Fiber, 32.8g Protein

Ingredients:

3 cups green split peas
9 cups vegetable stock
1 medium-size yellow onion - chopped
2 small sweet potatoes
3 garlic cloves - chopped
2 carrots – small dice ½ inch maximum
2 celery stalks - diced
2 tsp dried rosemary
½ tsp ground mustard
1 tsp smoked paprika
½ tsp ground white (or black) pepper
1 Tbsp lemon juice
mineral salt and pepper – to taste

Directions:

Fill a large soup pot with filtered water and add the split peas, bring to the boil and simmer gently for about 20 minutes.

Add the vegetables and herbs and spices and cook another 20 minutes or so until the vegetables are soft. Adjust spices

Serve in individual bowls and top with a little chopped tomato or quinoa and cilantro.

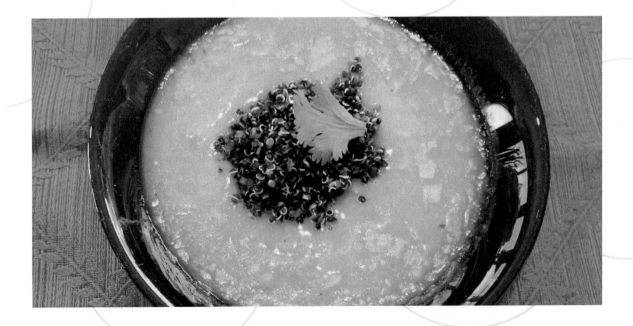

Tomato Mushroom Soup (E)(Q)($)

Serves: 6
Per serving: 126 Calories, 6.5g Fat, 10.7g Carbs, 2.1g Fiber, 7.4g Protein

Ingredients:

6 oz sliced mushrooms – oyster – white crimini – brown –Your choice
2 Tbsp EVOO
2 leeks – halves lengthwise and sliced thin
¼ tsp mineral salt and ground black pepper – or to taste
2 garlic cloves - minced
1/2 tsp fennel seeds
1 bay leaf
1 Tbsp tomato paste
1 pound tomatoes – finely chopped
1 Tbsp miso paste
6 cups vegetable broth

Directions:

In a large pot, heat oil over medium. Add leeks; season with salt and pepper and cook for 5 minutes or until tender.

Add garlic, porcini, and chopped mushrooms, season with salt and pepper, and cook for 5 minutes or until mushrooms just begin to brown.

Add tomatoes, fennel seeds, bay leaves, miso and tomato paste, and cook for 3 minutes. Add broth.

Reduce heat to low and simmer for 30 minutes.

Discard bay leaves before serving.

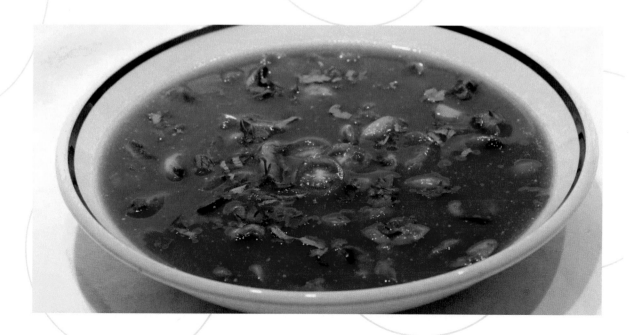

Wild Rice Soup (E)($)

Serves: 6
Per serving: 305 Calories, 19.8g Fat, 24.7g Carbs, 4g Fiber, 9.9g Protein

Ingredients

1 + 1/2 cups Wild Rice or Brown
1 cup Carrots - diced
2 stalks Celery - diced
1 large Yellow Onion - diced
2 tsp Thyme
1 Tbsp EVOO
4 cloves garlic - minced
¼ tsp mineral salt and fresh Black Pepper
6 cups vegetable broth
1 Bay Leaf
¼ tsp Cinnamon
Pinch of Nutmeg
14 ounces Coconut Milk

Directions

Start the rice cooking according to package directions in a separate pot from the soup.

Meanwhile in a large soup pot sauté the carrots, celery, onion and thyme in EVOO on medium-low heat. Season well with salt and pepper. When the vegetables begin to soften add garlic and mix every few minutes until vegetables look almost cooked (al dente).

Add broth, bay leaf, cinnamon and nutmeg. Season with salt and Black Pepper. Simmer for 10 minutes. Add most of the coconut milk. Simmer for ten minutes.

When rice is cooked stir into the soup. Taste and re-season if needed. Remove bay leaf before serving. Drizzle with remaining coconut milk

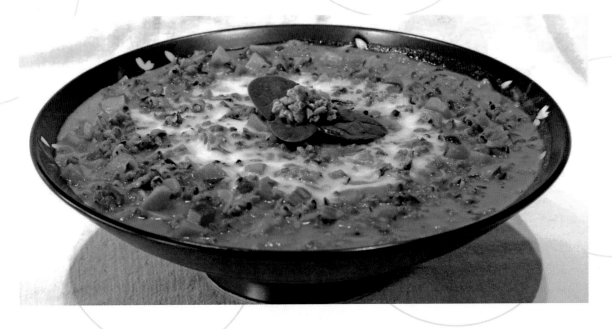

Curried Carrot Soup (E)($)(Q)

Serves: 4

Per serving: 224 Calories, 11.3g Fat, 29.9g Carbs, 8g Fiber, 4.4g Protein

Ingredients:

8 cups carrot - grated
2 Tbsp EVOO
2 large leeks light green and white parts only - sliced thinly
1 tsp curry powder (or to taste)
1/4 cup roasted shelled pistachios, chopped
4 cups water

Directions:

Heat oil in large pot over medium heat

Add carrots and leeks.

Cover and cook for about 15 minutes, stirring occasionally until vegetables are tender and some have started to brown a little.

Stir in curry powder and cook for 30 seconds.

Add water and bring to a simmer.

Remove from heat and blend.

Taste and adjust seasonings or add a dash of salt

Serve with the pistachios.

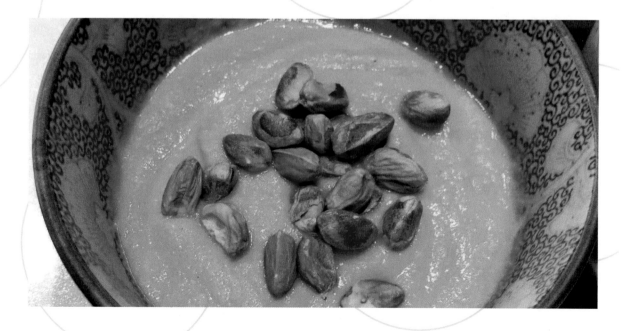

Roasted Beet and Cumin Soup(E)($)

Serves: 6
Per serving: 180 Calories, 10.7g Fat, 20.3g Carbs, 3.9g Fiber, 3.6g Protein

Ingredients:

6 red beets (about 3 medium)
2 Tbsp EVOO
1 leek (white and pale green parts only) - chopped
1 small onion - thinly sliced
2 celery stalk - chopped
1 Tbsp roasted cumin
1 tsp grated ginger
1/4 tsp ground allspice
1/2 tsp ground white pepper
2 cups water (or more as you wish)
2 small bay leaf
2 fresh thyme sprigs
2 fresh parsley sprig
1/4 cup sour crème (see page 238)

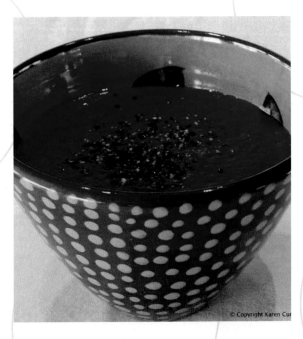
© Copyright Karen Cur

Directions:

Preheat oven to 350°F.

Wrap beets in foil and roast until tender when pierced with fork, about 1 hour. Cool.

Peel beets and cut beets into 1/2-inch pieces.

Heat oil in heavy medium saucepan over medium-high heat.

Add leek, onion, and celery and cook until beginning to brown, stirring frequently, about 13 minutes.

Stir in ginger, allspice, white pepper, and 1/2-inch beet pieces.

Cook until vegetables begin to stick to bottom of pot, stirring frequently, about 7 minutes.

Add 2 cups water, bay leaf, thyme sprig, and parsley sprig.

Bring to boil. Reduce heat to low, cover, and simmer until vegetables are very tender, about 25 minutes.

Remove bay leaf, thyme sprig, and parsley sprig.

Cool soup slightly.

Working in batches, purée soup in blender with sour crème.

Season to taste with salt and pepper.

NOTE:
Can be made 1 day ahead. Cool slightly, cover, and refrigerate.

Gently rewarm soup (do not boil). Divide between 2 bowls. Garnish each with sour crème. Sprinkle with reserved beet cubes.

Ethiopian Spicy Tomato Lentil Stew (E)($)

Per serving (¼ serving): 266 Calories, 4.4g Fat, 43.6g Carbs, 19g Fiber, 14.8g Protein

Ingredients:

1 cup brown lentils
4 cups water
1 large yellow onion - diced
2 carrots - peeled and diced
4 cloves garlic - minced
2 Tbsp fresh ginger - grated
2 Tbsp peanut oil
10 plum tomatoes - chopped
1/2 cup tomato paste
1 cup vegetable stock
1 cup frozen green peas

SPICE BLEND

2 tsp ground cumin
2 tsp Hungarian paprika
1 tsp ground fenugreek
1/2 tsp dried thyme
1/4 tsp ground cardamom
1/4 tsp ground coriander
1/8 tsp ground allspice
1/8 tsp ground cloves
1/8 tsp ground cinnamon
1/8 tsp cayenne pepper
1/2 tsp mineral salt

Directions:

Boil the lentils for about 45 minutes or until tender. Remove from heat and drain.

In a medium pot, sauté the onions and carrots in the oil until just soft.

Add the garlic, ginger and spice blend. Sauté 5 more minutes.

Add the tomatoes and cook 5 more minutes.

Add tomato paste, mix well, then add the vegetable stock.

Add the cooked lentils and bring to the boil.

Serve with rice or Injera bread (see page 298).

NOTE:
Can be frozen.

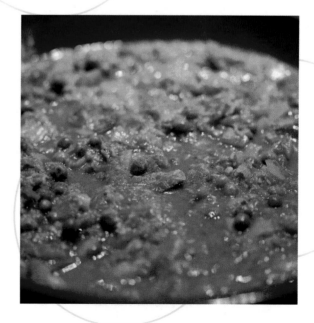

Brazilian Fejioada ($)

Serves: 6
Per serving: 518 Calories, 5.4g Fat, 96g Carbs, 15g Fiber, 21.7g Protein

Ingredients:

5 1/2 cups cooked black beans
3 cups vegetable stock
1 Tbsp grapeseed oil
1 large yellow onion - diced
2 medium red bell peppers - diced
1 large tomato - diced
4 garlic cloves - minced
1 canned chipotle pepper (more if you like it hot)-
chopped
2 cups sweet potatoes - peeled and diced (or butternut
squash)
2 tsp fresh or dried thyme leaves
2 tsp fresh parsley
1 tsp mineral salt
3 cups cooked brown rice

Directions:

In a large saucepan, heat the oil to medium.

Add the onion, bell peppers, tomato, garlic, and chipotle peppers and saute for 8 to 10 minutes.

Add the beans, stock, sweet potatoes, and thyme and cook for 25 to 30 minutes over medium heat, stirring occasionally.

Stir in the parsley and salt and cook for 5 to 10 minutes more.

Spoon the rice into bowls and ladle the feijoada over the top.

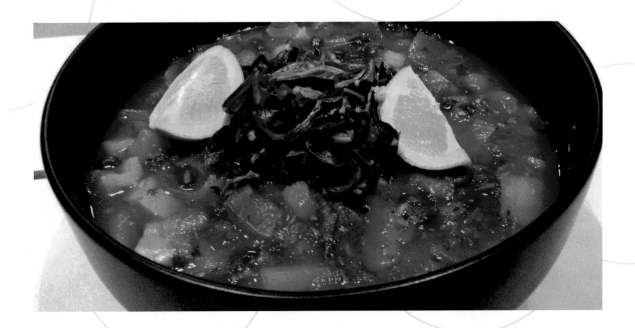

Thai Coconut Soup (E)($)

Serves 6:
Per serving: 228 Calories, 19.9g Fat, 10.6g Carbs, 2.8g Fiber, 5.9g Protein

Ingredients:

2 cups coconut milk
3 cups vegetable stock
4 stalks lemongrass - *bruised then cut into 2" pieces
or 2 Tbsp prepared lemongrass
3-4 kaffir lime leaves (or young lemon or lime leaves)
– torn or 3" piece of ginger - sliced thinly
1 medium onion, quartered
3-4 Thai bird's eye chilies - sliced into larger pieces
1 cup button mushrooms –quartered
2 cups white cabbage – chopped into 1" pieces
½ cup shredded kale
1 small date – chopped finely
¼ tsp cracked pepper
3 Tbsp lime juice
2 Tbsp Bragg's Amino acids or tamari sauce
4 Tbsp minced cilantro

Directions:

In a stock pot bring the vegetable stock to a boil. Add ginger, lemongrass, kaffir lime leaves, onion and date. Simmer 5 minutes on low heat.

Add coconut milk, chilies, and Bragg's sauce. Simmer 5 more minutes.

Add mushrooms and heat through.

Add kale

Remove the pot from heat and add lime juice and cilantro.

Serve with steamed rice or coconut Jasmine rice.

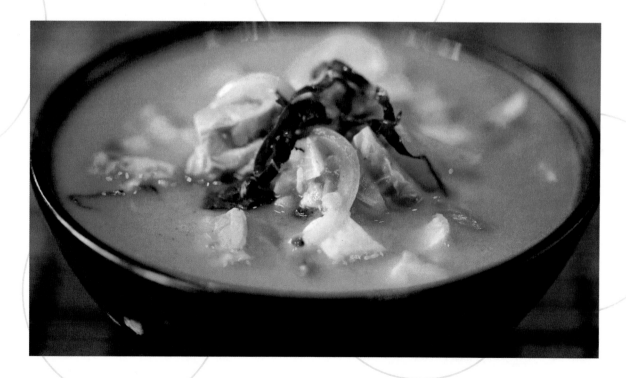

Avocado Apple Soup (R)(Q)($)

Per serving: 189 Calories, 14.4g Fat, 17.1g Carbs, 5.6g Fiber, 1g Protein

Ingredients:

1 avocado - chopped
2 medium apples - peeled and chopped
1 Tbsp onion - chopped
handful arugula leaves
2 Tbsp EVOO
2 cups water - for blending

Garnish:
minced onion
salt and pepper to taste
red pepper flakes

Directions:

Blend.

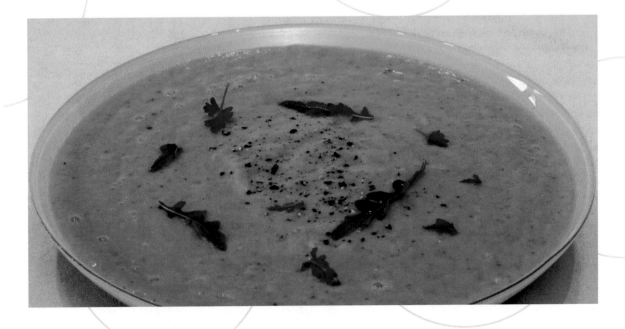

Spicy Lentil Tomato Soup (E)($)

Serves: 4

Per serving: 266 Calories, 4.4g Fat, 43.6g Carbs, 19g Fiber, 14.8g Protein

Ingredients:

1 cup brown lentils
4 cups water
1 tsp dried ground ginger (or 1" piece of fresh ginger - grated)
1 tsp cinnamon
1 jalapeno, deseeded and roughly chopped
1 small bay leaf
1 sweet potato – peeled and chopped into 2 inch chunks
1 cup sliced green beans
1 stalk celery - diced
1 red pepper - diced
1 Tbsp EVOO
2 tsp ground coriander
1 tsp turmeric
2 cups water
3 cups chopped tomatoes – with skins and seeds

Directions:

Place lentils and water in a saucepan. Bring to a boil, and add the ginger, cinnamon, jalapeno, and bay leaf.

Reduce heat, and simmer the lentils for 30 minutes or until cooked – may be less time.

Meantime, steam your sweet potato pieces for 10 minutes (or until tender). Remove from heat and mash. Set aside.

In a medium skillet add EVOO, and add your green beans, celery, red pepper, and seasonings. Saute on low heat until all the vegetables are tender. Remove from heat. Set aside.

Once your lentils are done, remove bay leaf and add lentils and 3 cups crushed tomatoes to a large soup pot. Add your mashed sweet potato, and all vegetables.

Mix well and bring to a boil.

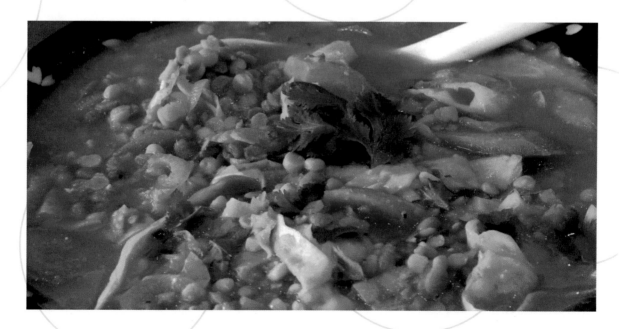

Carrot Ginger Soup (R)($)(E)(Q)
Serves 6
Per serving: 114 Calories, 5.2g Fat, 17.2g Carbs, 6g Fiber, 1.7g Protein

Ingredients:
10 carrots – scrubbed not peeled if organic
1 green apple – cored
1 avocado – peeled and seeded
3 Tbsp lemon juice
¼ tsp mineral salt
1 tsp fresh ginger (1/2 tsp dry)
¼ tsp allspice
½ tsp ground coriander
2 cups water

Directions:

Blend to a creamy purée.

Heat to 116 degrees in your dehydrator or on the lowest setting on your stove until just warm – do not bring to the boil or this becomes a cooked and not raw soup.

Enjoy with any nuts or seeds you like.

NOTE:
Cannot be frozen.

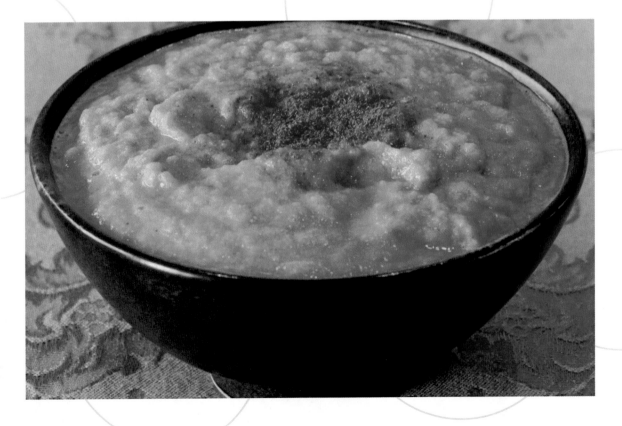

Roasted Cauliflower Curry Soup(E)($) - Contributed by Alex Caspero

Serves: 2
Per serving: 144 Calories, 10.1g Fat, 12.2g Carbs, 4.5g Fiber, 4.8g Protein

Ingredients:

1 head cauliflower
2 yukon gold potatoes (optional)
1/2 onion
2 shallots
curry powder

Directions:

Roast cauliflower, potatoes, onion and shallots with curry powder until tender.

Simmer in vegetable broth or unsweetened non-dairy milk for 15 minutes.

purée with immersion or high powered blender until creamy.

Top with sunflower seeds, warmed in a non-greased skillet, and cilantro.

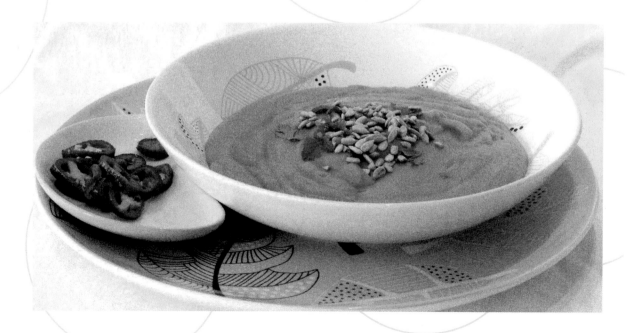

Creamy Cauliflower Asparagus Soup (E)($)

Serves: 7
Per serving: 217 Calories, 19g Fat, 9.6g Carbs, 3.8g Fiber, 5.7g Protein

Ingredients:

3 cups cauliflower – roughly chopped into 2 inch pieces
18 spears asparagus – woody ends removed and chopped into 3rds
3 Tbsp EVOO
1 cup onion - chopped
3 cups vegetable stock
2 cloves garlic - minced
¼ tsp mineral salt
1 1/2 cups almond milk
½ tsp dried basil
1 tsp dried chives
1 tsp ground cumin
fresh ground black pepper to taste

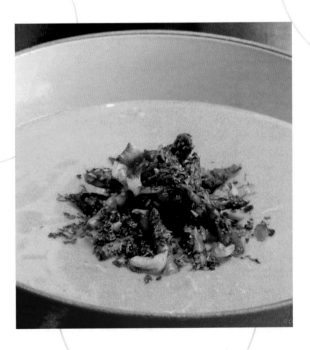

Directions:

In a large soup pot over medium heat

Add 2 Tbsp of the EVOO and onion and sauté until onion starts to brown – stirring occasionally.

Add the salt, cauliflower and 6 spears of the asparagus – sauté about 6 minutes.

Add the garlic and sauté for another two minutes.

Add the vegetable stock and bring to the boil – simmer about 5-10 minutes – you can turn the heat down once the mix starts to boil.

Remove from heat and let stand.

In a separate medium pan:
Add the 1 Tbsp EVOO

Add the remaining asparagus and a pinch of mineral salt and sauté for about 2 minutes.

Turn off heat and remove from burner. Set aside.

In a blender or food processor, or with a hand blender – blend the cauliflower asparagus mixture until creamy.

Add the almond milk and blend until mixed.

Return to the soup pot and bring to a simmer on medium heat.

As soon as the soup starts to simmer add the spices and the sautéed asparagus – serve.

Alkalizing Avocado Soup(E)(Q)

Serves: 4
Per serving: 100 Calories, 7.6g Fat, 8.3g Carbs, 4.4g Fiber, 2.2g Protein

Ingredients:

1 avocado – peeled, seeded and chopped
1 medium sized English cucumber – peeled & chopped
2 stalks celery - chopped
2 cups baby spinach
handful of baby kale
1/4 cup fresh parsley
¼ cup fresh basil
1/2 cup fresh cilantro
2 Tbsp lemon juice
½ inch piece of fresh ginger – squeeze with garlic press to get juice
1 1/2 cups filtered water
1/4 tsp Mineral sea salt, or to taste
1 tsp dulse flakes

Directions:

Blend all ingredients except for the salt and dulse which are gently stirred in at the end.

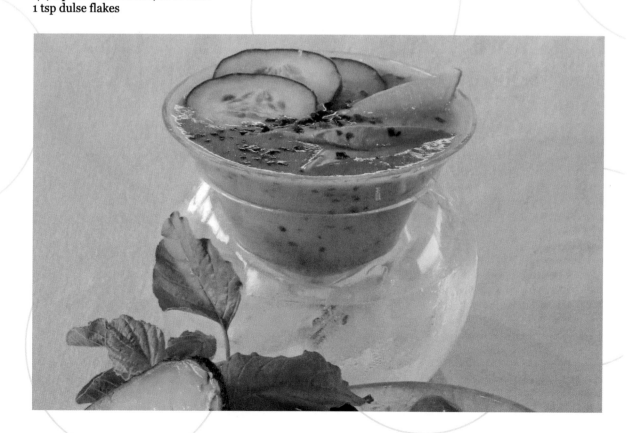

Watercress Soup (E)

Serves: 4
Per serving: 219 Calories, 13.2g Fat, 18.4g Carbs, 7.3g Fiber, 9.8g Protein

Ingredients:

1 onion - chopped
1 tsp coconut oil
2 cups green peas
1 cup raw slivered almonds
4 cups water
1/4 tsp salt
3 bunches (about six cups) watercress - roots removed

Directions:

Saute onion in coconut oil over medium heat in a soup pot over medium heat until onion is soft, then add the peas, salt and water and bring to the boil.

Turn heat to low and simmer peas and onions for 2 minutes.

Turn off the heat and add the watercress - let it wilt in the pot for about one minute.

Transfer soup to a high speed blender. Add the almonds and purée.

Note: Keep cooking process to an absolute minimum to preserve the nutrients and the beautiful vibrant green color.

Serve in bowls with your favorite toppings. We used toasted almonds and Saffron coconut

SAFFRON COCONUT
Saffron coconut - take a pinch of saffron and mix it with 1 Tbsp hot water.

Then add the saffron mix to 2 cups of unsweetened desiccated coconut.

Mix thoroughly and then dry the mixture on a tray in the oven on warm.

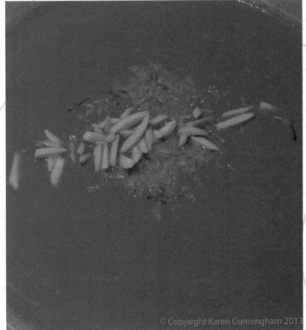

Celebration Hot Pot (E)

Serves: 4

Per serving: 405 Calories, 11.7g Fat, 59.5g Carbs, 12.9g Fiber, 23.7g Protein

Ingredients:

1 tsp grapeseed oil
1/2 tsp sesame oil (see note)
1 Tbsp ginger-root, peeled and minced
4 cloves garlic - minced
12 cups water
1/2 Tbsp wakame or other seaweed
1 1/2 cups carrots - cut into matchsticks
1 1/2 ounces dried shiitake mushrooms (see note)
1 1/2 cups frozen shelled edamame
5 ounces buckwheat soba noodles, uncooked (see note)
1 lb. baby bok choy, cut into 1/2-inch slices
6 to 8 Tbsp mellow white miso (see note)
1 tsp prepared wasabi (optional or to taste)
2 cups dashi (see page 307)

NOTE:
Soak dried shiitake overnight before using or if you are in a hurry pour boiling water over them and let sit 30 minutes or so.

Make sure your Buckwheat noodles are pure buckwheat and GF.

There are lots of different Miso pastes. The light ones have a very mellow flavor

Directions:

Heat grapeseed oil in a large wok or soup pot over medium heat.

Saute garlic for about a minute until fragrant.

Add 8 cups water and 2 cups dashi.

2 Tbsp Light Miso

Add fresh vegetables.

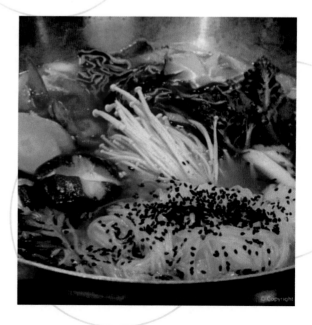

Crème of Mushroom Soup (E)

Serves: 4
Per serving: 64 Calories, 4.3g Fat, 5.5g Carbs, 2.1g Fiber, 2.3g Protein

Ingredients:

2 cups cauliflower florets (small pieces)
1⅔ cup unsweetened almond milk
1 tsp onion powder
¼ tsp mineral salt
Freshly ground pepper - to taste
1 Tbsp EVOO
1½ cups white mushrooms – sliced
½ yellow onion – small dice

Directions:

Place cauliflower, milk, onion powder, salt and pepper in a small saucepan. Cover and bring to a boil over medium heat.

Reduce heat to low and simmer for 7-8 minutes, until cauliflower is softened. Then, purée the mix and set aside

Meanwhile, add oil, mushrooms and onion to a medium-sized saucepan. Heat over high heat until onions are translucent and beginning to brown, about 5 minutes or so. Reserve a few pieces of the mushroom for garnishing your plate.

Add puréed cauliflower mixture to sautéed mushrooms. Bring to a boil, cover and simmer for 10 minutes, until thickened.
Serve immediately.

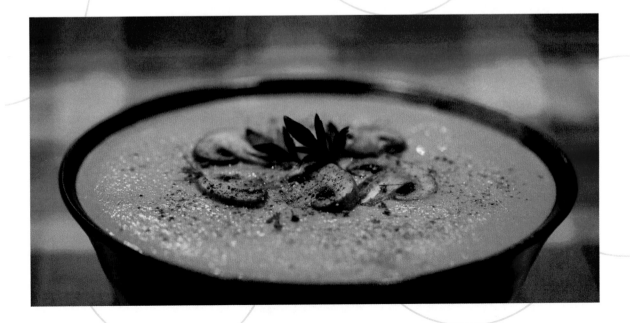

Miso Wonder Soup (E)

Serves: 4

Per serving: 169 Calories, 7.8g Fat, 22.3g Carbs, 4.5g Fiber, 11.3g Protein

Ingredients:

4 cups vegetable stock (I used the Alkalizing broth - see page 305)
2 Tbsp miso
1 Tbsp sesame oil
1 package Kelp noodles (chop them a bit or you will be slurping them forever)
1 red bell pepper
1 cup mushrooms – sliced
1 small onion - chopped into large pieces
1 carrot - sliced
1 zucchini - sliced
½ cup dried seaweed-hijiki or other
1 stick celery - sliced
sweet potato - thinly sliced
1 cup pea shoots- drop in right at the end
sesame seeds

Directions:

Bring to just below boiling and enjoy.

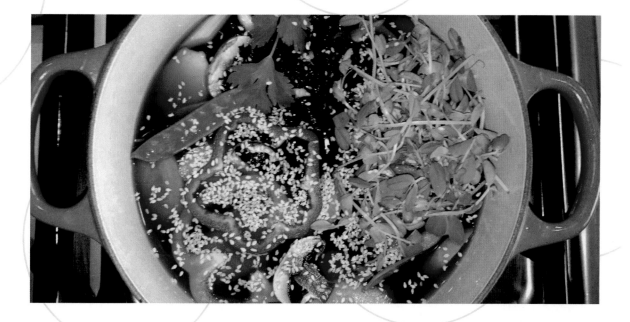

87

Raw Tomato and Pepper Soup (Q)(E)($)(R)

Serves: 4
Per serving: 50 Calories, 1.3g Fat, 8.2g Carbs, 2.9g Fiber, 2.7g Protein

Ingredients:

1 organic red pepper - cored, deseeded and chopped
3 medium tomatoes
½ celery stalk
1 cup unsweetened almond milk
¼ cup sweet onion - chopped
1 Tbsp nutritional yeast
3/4 tsp. Mineral salt
1 small garlic clove
1 Tbsp fresh lemon juice

For garnish:
Chopped red and yellow bell peppers and sliced avocado.

Directions:

Blend all ingredients in the blender and serve just warm with the garnish vegetables on top.

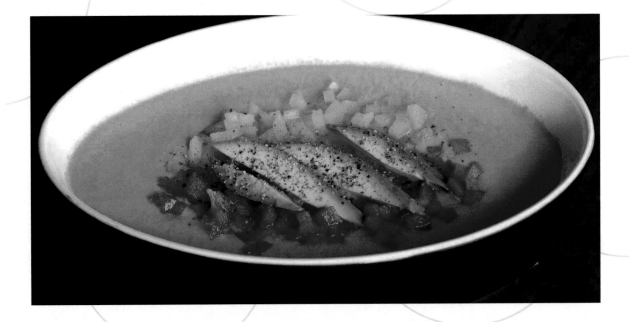

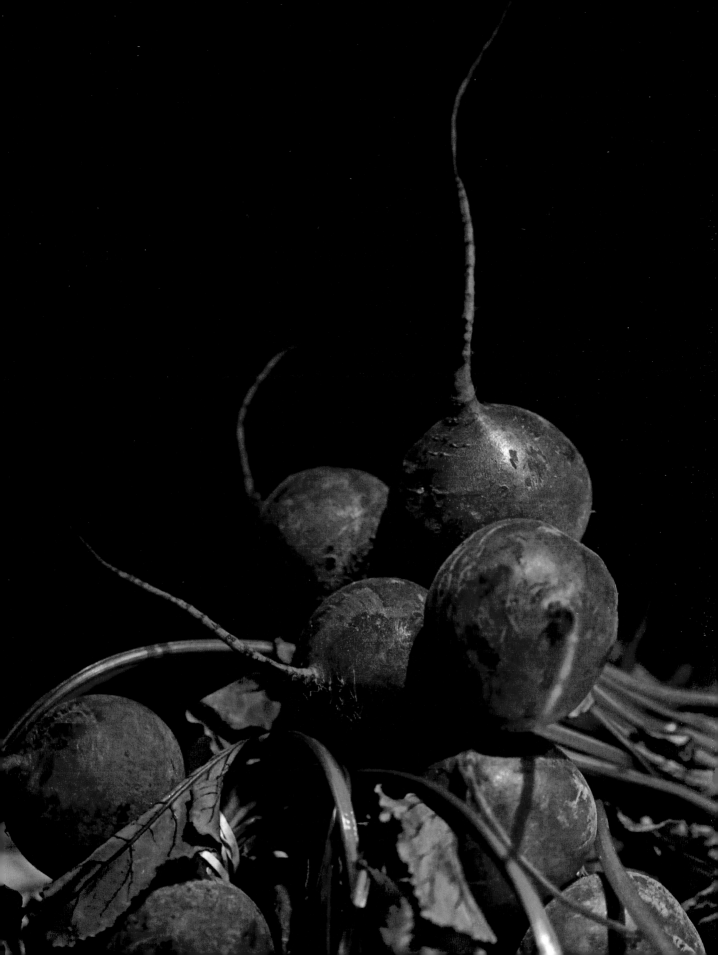

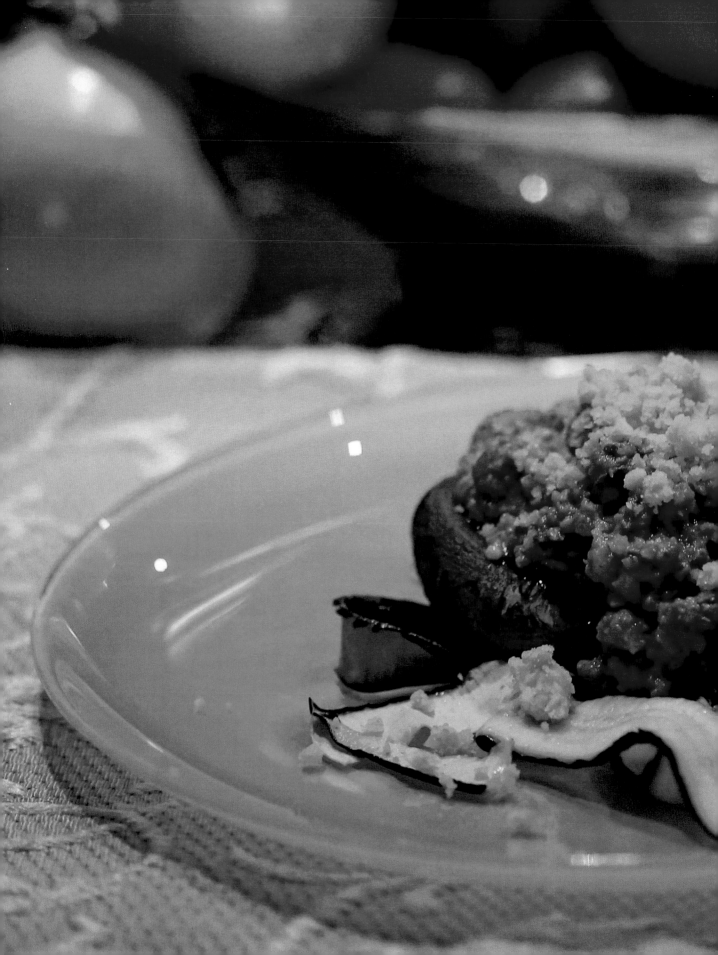

Mains

Mujadarra (E)($)

Serves: 6
Per Serving: 319 Calories, 8g Fat, 1g Sat Fat, 50g Carbs, 11.6g Fiber, 20% of DV of Iron

Ingredients:

1 cup green lentils (or brown)
1 cup brown basmati rice
3 onions chopped small dice
1 red bell pepper chopped small dice
3 cloves crushed garlic
3 Tbsp EVOO
3 1/2 cups water
1 tsp cinnamon
1 tsp turmeric
1/2 tsp allspice
1 tsp cumin powder
1/4-1/2 tsp black pepper
1 tsp salt (to taste)
3 3/4 cups water

Directions:

Saute onions med heat in 3 Tbsp oil until soft and brown, this takes about 40 minutes for the onions to caramelize.

Midway through browning process, add chopped garlic and red bell peppers.

Meanwhile cook lentils and rice separately, rinse and drain and keep aside until the onion mixture is ready – keep warm.

Mix everything together except for half of the onion mix, which is ladled over the top of the final dish.

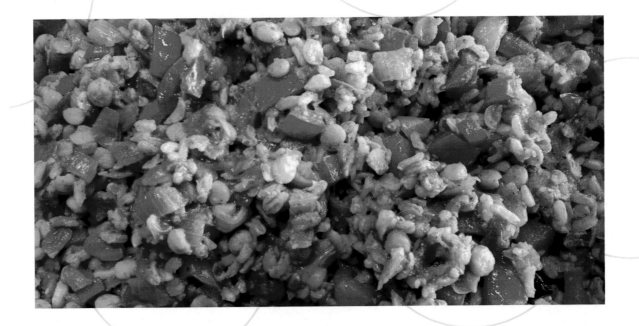

Baked Sweet Potatoes with Roasted Macadamia Nuts and Coconut (E)

Serves: 6

Per Serving: 324 Calories, 18g Fat, 8g Sat. Fat, 40g Carbs, 7g Fiber, 4g Protein

Ingredients:

2 1/2 pounds orange-fleshed sweet potatoes
1/3 cup coconut milk
1 Tbsp fresh ginger - grated
1 Tbsp maple syrup
1/2 tsp fine-grain sea salt
1/3 cup raw, unsweetened grated coconut
2 Tbsp EVOO
1/3 cup toasted macadamia nuts, chopped

Directions:

Preheat your oven to 350 degrees, a rack in the upper third.

Oil 6 ramekins or a single medium-sized casserole dish.

Wrap each sweet potato in foil, pierce numerous times with the tines of a fork and place in the oven for somewhere between an hour and an hour and a half, until each is baked through. Times vary greatly depending on the size of your sweet potatoes - in the end you should be able to cut through the center flesh as if it were soft butter.

Remove the potatoes from the oven, let them cool for a few minutes, and cut each sweet potato in half. Scrape the flesh into a medium mixing bowl. You should have about three cups of sweet potatoes.

In a large bowl mash the sweet potatoes with the coconut milk. If my sweet potatoes are on the fibrous side, I take a hand blender to them for a minute or so (alternately you could use a food processor).

Stir in the ginger, maple syrup and salt.

Let it sit for a few minutes, stir again and taste - adjust the seasoning if you need to - this is your chance to get the right amount of salt and ginger in the sweet potatoes before they go in the oven.

Spoon the sweet potato mixture into individual baking dishes (or single larger baking dish), sprinkle with coconut, drizzle with EVOO and bake uncovered until warm and the coconut golden roughly 30 - 40 minutes.

Remove and sprinkle with the toasted macadamia nuts.

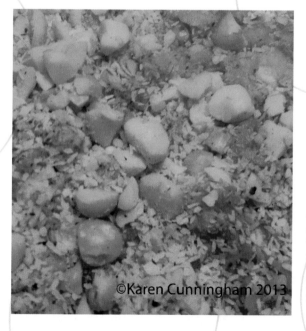
©Karen Cunningham 2013

93

Vegetarian Chili ($)(E)

Serves: 8
Per serving: 258 Calories, 4g Fat, 0.5g Sat. Fat., 50g, Carbs, 13g Fiber, 16g Protein

Ingredients*:

1 Tbsp Vegetable Oil (grapeseed, EVOO or sunflower)
1 large carrot - diced
1 medium Onion - chopped
4 cloves of garlic – minced
1 large sweet bell pepper (capsicum) – chopped
1 green, yellow or orange bell pepper – chopped (I sometimes use two red peppers)
1 Jalapeno (fresh or canned) diced – adjust to suit your taste
1-2 tsp chili powder (be careful they all have different degrees of heat)
1 tsp ground cumin
1 cup cooked Kidney beans (red or white)
1 cup cooked pinto beans
1 cup cooked garbanzo beans
1 360 g (13 oz) can organic tomatoes
1/2 tsp freshly ground pepper
2 Tbsp (or more) chopped parsley
1/2 cup finely diced kale or
1/2 cup loosely chopped spinach
1/2 cup chopped cilantro

* if you can make this from scratch – all the better
* If using canned beans – rinse thoroughly to remove some sodium

Directions:

In a large (non-aluminum) soup pot, heat oil over low heat and sauté onion and carrot and all peppers until vegetables are very soft (about 10 minutes). Lid is on and you stir occasionally

Then remove the lid and add the garlic chili powder, cumin and cook an additional 2 – 3 minutes – stirring occasionally.

Add beans, tomatoes and simmer another 10 minutes.

Add ground pepper.

Serve in bowls topped with a couple of slices of avocado and chopped parsley or cilantro.

Options:
Serve over brown rice, brown rice past or cooked buckwheat or quinoa

1 Tbsp of cashew cheese (see page 243) really makes this a gourmet's delight

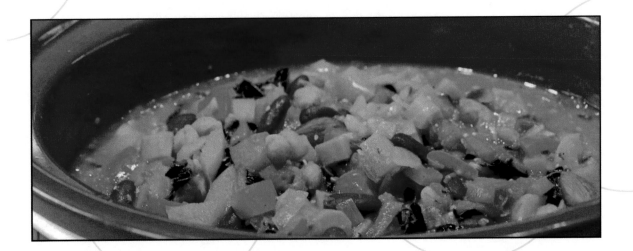

"Lobio" - Georgia Kidney Bean Salad (Q)($)(E)

Serves: 4
Per serving: 211 Calories, 10.3g Fat, 23g Carbs, 6g Fiber, 9.4g Protein

Ingredients:

1 can cooked kidney beans or 4 oz dried kidney beans
1 onion, peeled and finely chopped
2 sprigs of cilantro
1 sprig of parsley
1/2 generous cup of shelled walnuts
3 garlic cloves, peeled
1/8 tsp red pepper (optional)
1/4 tsp of cinnamon
Pinch of ground cloves
1/2 tsp pomegranate juice concentrate (use tamarind or cranberry as substitute). Use more if desired

Directions:

FOR DRY BEANS: Soak the beans overnight covered with water. The next day, drain and rinse them. Place in a large pot and cover with fresh water. Add 1/2 tsp of salt. Bring the water to a boil and simmer until the beans are tender, about 1 hour. Drain.
-Or-
FOR CANNED BEANS: Heat beans to the boil, remove from the heat.

While the beans are still warm (canned or fresh), stir in the chopped onion.

Finely chop the cilantro, parsley, walnuts, garlic and hot pepper. Add to the beans.

In a small cup mix together the cinnamon, cloves, the remaining 1/4-tsp of salt; stir into the bean mixture.

Pour in enough pomegranate juice to moisten the beans and mix well.

Allow the beans to cool to room temperature, then serve liberally garnished with pomegranate seeds, fresh parsley, cilantro and walnuts for presentation.

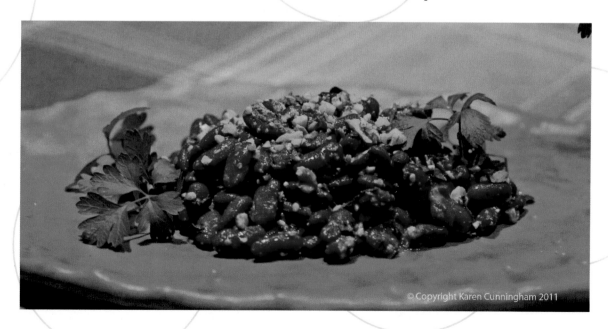

Cuban Black Beans (E)($)
Serves: 6
Per Serving: Calories: 366, Fat: 9g , Sat. Fat: 1.4g, Carbs: 74g, Fiber: 14g , Protein: 18g ,
Vitamin A: 88%, Vitamin C 95%, Iron 29% , Calcium 12%

Ingredients:

1 1 lb bag dried black beans
3 cups vegetable stock
2 onions, diced
1 carrot, chopped finely
1 head garlic, chopped finely
1 green bell pepper, diced
1 red bell pepper, diced
1 Tbsp tomato paste or 1 large tomato, diced
3 Tbsp EVOO
2 Tbsp red wine vinegar
1-2 tsp Bragg's Liquid Aminos
2 tsp Spanish paprika
1 tsp cumin
1 tsp dried oregano
1 dried bay leaf

Directions:

Soak beans overnight, rinse well and place in a crock pot.

Saute the onions, carrot, garlic and peppers until soft and just starting to change color – then add all ingredients to the crock pot.

Cook for about 8 hours

Note:
Make sure that the beans are covered with the stock and you may want to check periodically that there is enough liquid in the pot so the beans are not dry

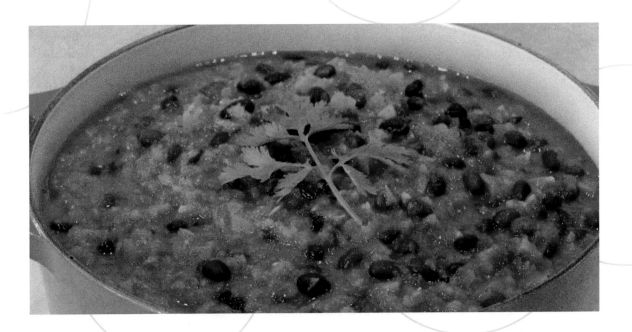

Jicama Mushroom Tacos ($) - Inspired by Danette Davis
Serves: 2
Per serving: 207 Calories, 14g Fat, 18g Carbs, 6g Fiber, 6.8g Protein

Ingredients:

1 x 4 inch round Jicama – peeled and sliced thin (this is the hardest part of this recipe.*
8 oz mushrooms – sliced
1 small red onion – finely diced
¼ tsp mineral salt
1 Tbsp EVOO
6 Tbsp salsa – of your choice or sliced tomatoes
4 Tbsp avocado – mashed with
2 tsp lime juice
½ cup lettuce – shredded
extra lime juice for drizzling on finished tacos
2 Tbsp cashew sour crème (see page 238)

*Use a mandolin to make really thin slices.

Directions:

Sauté the mushrooms and onion over medium high heat, until browned

Fill tacos with lettuce, mushroom mix and salsa or tomatoes and mashed avocado.
Drizzle a little cashew sour crème over each one and enjoy!

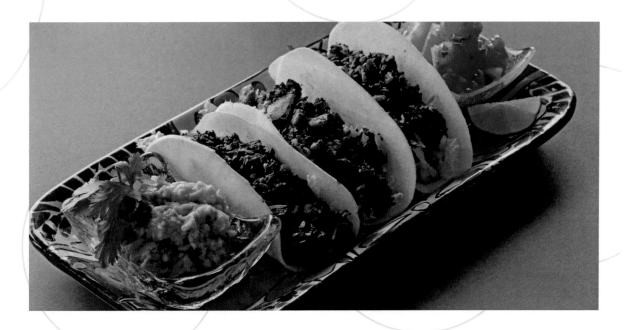

Lentils with Pomegranate (E)($)
Serves: 4
Per serving: 531 Calories, 16.8g Fat, 86.6g Carbs, 24.1g Fiber, 23.1g Protein

Ingredients:

1 1/2 cups of dry lentils – your choice
1 whole pomegranate
1 onion finely chopped
4 cloves garlic - minced
3 Tbsp olive
salt and pepper to taste
2 cups chopped green vegetables – chard, kale etc
5 sprigs parsley chopped
3 sprigs fresh mint – chopped
2 Tbsp toasted pine nuts
2 Tbsp toasted walnuts
grated zest of one lemon, plus
2 Tbsp lemon juice (zest the lemon before juicing the lemon)
3 Tbsp pomegranate concentrate – unsweetened syrup can be found in most Middle Eastern markets.

Directions:

Place lentils in a pot and cover with water. Add about 1/2 tsp salt.

Bring to the boil and let simmer gentle until cooked – will depend on your lentil 10-30 minutes.

Remove from heat and drain lentils, reserving the liquid.

While lentils are boiling chop the onion and garlic and sauté gently in the EVOO until onions are translucent. Be careful not to brown, this will overpower the pomegranate and will not have the desired flavor.

In a heatproof serving dish, layer the chopped greens, including the mint and parsley.

Ladle in the cooked lentils and the other ingredients, leaving some pomegranate and pine nuts for garnish.

Stir very gently and add the extra pomegranate and pine nuts

Dollop almond or cashew crème over the top in each individual bowl as you wish. (See page 239 for cashew crème recipe)

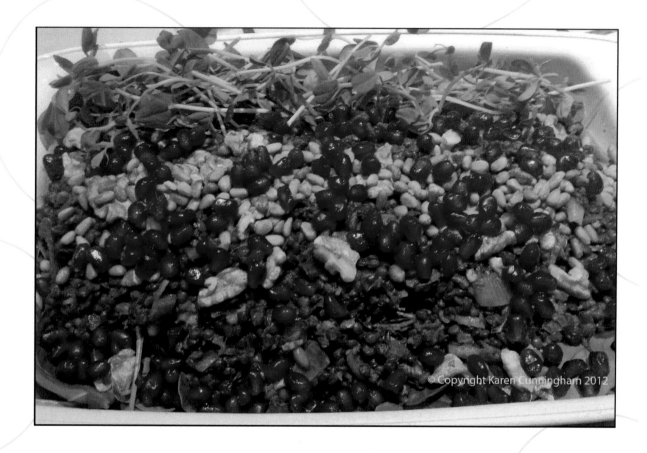

Mushroom Tempeh Stroganoff (E)($)

Per Serving, 6: 388 calories, 11.7g fat, 48.6g Carbs, 11.7g fiber, 27.6g protein

Ingredients:

12 oz tempeh cubed
8 oz small portobella, brown or white mushrooms –
quartered
1 large red or orange pepper - seeded and chopped
2 small Anaheim or other mild flavored chili - seeded
and chopped
1 large red or yellow onion – diced 1/2 inch pieces
2 Tbsp EVOO
2 cups vegetable stock
2 Tbsp tomato paste
1 1/2 Tbsp smoked or sweet paprika
12 oz cooked white beans – cannelini, white kidney
1/2 cup water
2 Tbsp lemon juice
1 Tbsp Nutritional Yeast*
1 cup green peas – fresh is best
Salt and Fresh ground pepper to taste
Cayenne pepper if you like things a little hotter*

Garnish with :
fresh parsley - chopped
cashew crème (see page 239)

*NOT baking yeast and this does not add yeast to your
gut– it is a baking item that adds a wonderful cheese
like flavor to food

**Cayenne is great for cleansing
the blood

Directions:

Heat 1 Tbsp EVOO in a medium sized skillet (about 12
ins) on medium heat
Add cubed Tempeh and brown on all sides – about 5-
10 minutes. Remove
Tempeh to a plate.

Add the remainder of the EVOO and sauté the onions
until soft and just starting
to brown. Then add the peppers - sauté for another
two minutes, before adding
the mushrooms...Turn up the heat a little and keep
stirring the mixture until the
mushrooms start to give off a little moisture.

Add the tomato paste, vegetable stock and paprika
and stir well to combine, once
mixture starts to simmer – turn heat to low again and
let the mixture simmer.

In the meantime, purée the drained white beans in a
blender with 1/2 cup of water - blend until
smooth.

Add puréed bean mixture to the mushrooms and stir

Add the Nutritional Yeast and lemon juice and mix
well together.

Turn heat to low and let your dinner simmer in one
pan until the sauce starts to thicken – or you are ready
to eat.

Just before serving add the green peas and the
tempeh

Adjust seasonings and enjoy over a cup of cooked
quinoa or brown rice with a spoonful of savory cashew
crème.

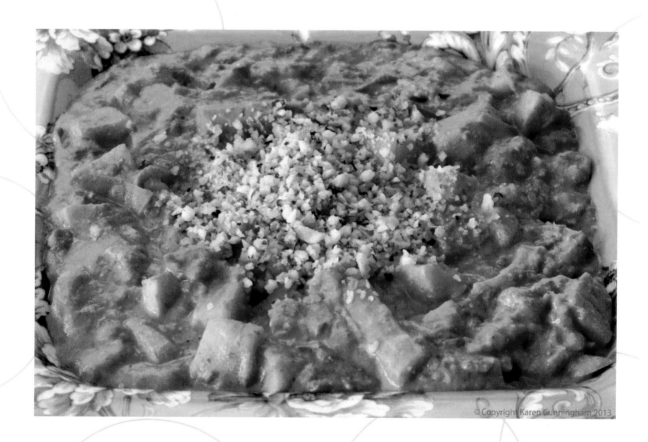

© Copyright Karen Cunningham 2013

Mushroom Lasagne (X)($)
Serves: 8
Per serving: 450 Calories, 29g Fat, 43.9g Carbs, 4.8g Fiber, 10.2g Protein

Ingredients:

1 Tbsp EVOO
2 cups thinly sliced leek
8 garlic cloves - thinly sliced
3/8 tsp salt - divided
7 cups sliced cremini mushrooms (about 1 1/2 pounds) - divided
4 cups sliced shiitake mushroom caps (about 1 pound)
2/3 cup unsweetened cranberry juice
1 Tbsp fresh thyme - chopped
1 Tbsp fresh oregano - chopped
1 Tbsp fresh sage - chopped
3 Tbsp white truffle oil
1 tsp black pepper, divided
2 1/2 cups almond milk
1 bay leaf
2 Tbsp coconut butter or more EVOO
3 1/2 Tbsp garbanzo flour
1/8 tsp ground nutmeg
3 cups cashew cheese (see page 243)
1/4 cup chopped fresh flat-leaf parsley
1 Tbsp grated lemon rind
Coconut oil cooking spray
8 ounces brown rice lasagna noodles – cooked to the directions and then laid on a flat tray – slightly oiled and covered to avoid drying out
1 cup brazil nut parmesan cheese (see page 235)

Directions:

Heat olive oil in a large Dutch oven over medium-high heat. Add leek, garlic, and 1/4 tsp salt; sauté 2 minutes. Add 4 cups cremini mushrooms and shiitake mushrooms; sauté 10 minutes or until mushrooms release moisture and begin to brown. Stir in wine; cook 3 minutes or until liquid almost evaporates, stirring frequently. Remove from heat; stir in thyme, oregano, sage, truffle oil, and 1/2 tsp pepper.

Combine milk and bay leaf in a heavy saucepan; cook over medium-high heat to 180° or until tiny bubbles form around edge (do not boil). Remove from heat; cover and let stand 10 minutes. Remove bay leaf

Melt coconut butter in saucepan over medium heat. Add remaining 3 cups cremini mushrooms; sauté 4 minutes or until tender. Add flour, stirring with a whisk until blended. Cook 1 minute, stirring constantly; gradually add milk. Bring to a boil; reduce heat, and simmer 8 minutes or until thick. Stir in remaining 1/8 tsp salt, 1/4 tsp pepper, and nutmeg.

Preheat oven to 350°.

Combine cashew cheese, parsley, lemon rind, and remaining 1/4 tsp black pepper in a bowl. Spread 1/2 cup milk mixture in bottom of an 11 x 7-inch glass or ceramic baking dish coated with cooking spray. Arrange 3 noodles over sauce; top with 2 cups mushroom mixture. Sprinkle with 1/4 cup cashew cheese and 1/4 cup Parmesan. Arrange 3 noodles over cheese. Top with 1 cup cashew mixture. Repeat layers once with 3 noodles, 2 cups mushroom mixture, 1/4 cup mozzarella, 1/4 cup Parmesan, 3 noodles, and 1 cup ricotta (dish will be very full); spread remaining sauce over top. Cover with foil; place baking dish on a baking sheet. Bake at 350° for 30 minutes. Remove from oven; increase oven temperature to 450°. Uncover the lasagna, and sprinkle with remaining 1/2 cup cashew cheese and remaining 1/2 cup Parmesan; bake an additional 10 minutes or until golden brown.

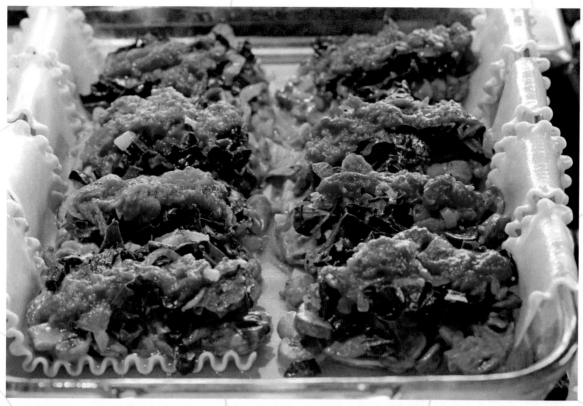

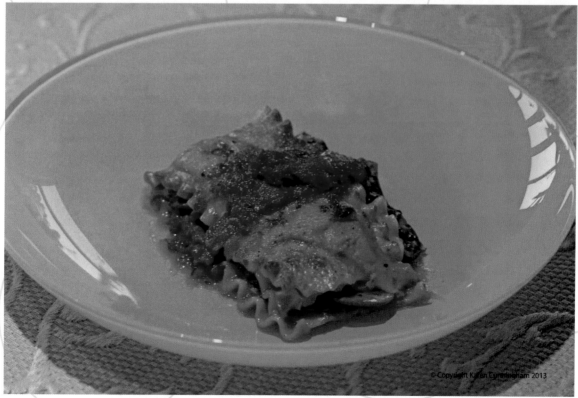

Walnut Mushroom Bolognese

Serves 6
Per Serving*: 121 Calories, 5.9g Fat, 13.4g Carbs, 4.7g Fiber, 5g Protein
*Analyzed without parmesan topping.

Ingredients;

SAUCE:
2 pints grape or cherry tomatoes - sliced lengthwise
1 garlic clove - finely minced
1 Tbsp EVOO
1/2 tsp apple cider vinegar
1/2 tsp sea salt
1/2 tsp dried oregano
1/4 tsp crushed red pepper flakes
4-5 sun-dried tomatoes packed in EVOO
(recommended: Mediterranean Organic)
1/2 pound cremini mushrooms
3/4 cup soaked walnuts
1 tsp fresh thyme leaves
1 tsp sea salt
1 small shallot - roughly chopped
1 small carrot - roughly chopped
1 large celery stalk - roughly chopped
1/8 cup good red wine
3 Tbsp cashew milk

STRACCI:
1 1/2 – 2 lbs goldbar squash (about 4)
sea salt
flax seed oil (lends a rich, buttery flavor)

Directions:

SAUCE:
Toss the first 7 ingredients well in a large bowl and let
marinate 1 hour.

Transfer tomatoes to lined dehydrator trays and
dehydrate at 115 degrees for about 4 hours.

In a food processor, blend the grape tomatoes and the
sun-dried tomatoes together to a purée. Pour into
mixing bowl and set aside.

Next, add the criminis, walnuts, thyme, and
remaining 1 tsp sea salt to food processor and pulse
to a crumbly texture. Add to the tomato sauce
mixture.

Finally, pulse together the shallot, carrot, and celery
until finely diced and transfer to the sauce. Add wine
and cashew milk and stir together until well mixed.
Adjust seasonings if necessary.

STRACCI:
With a vegetable peeler, slice squash into thin sheets,
alternating on each side until seeds are visible. Set in a
large bowl, sprinkle and toss moderately with sea salt,
and allow to stand for about an hour.

Drain excess water, and drizzle with flax seed oil.
Transfer to dehydrator trays and dehydrate at 115
degrees for about 2 hours, or until "stracci" achieves a
chewy texture.

Top with pine nut parmesan (see page for recipe).

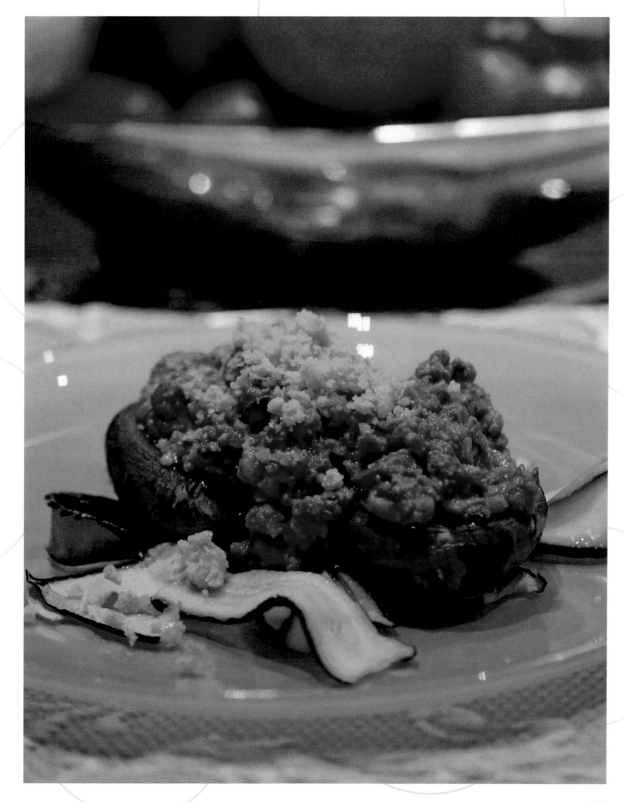

Quinoa Paella (X)($)

Serves 6:
Per serving: 376 Calories, 14g Fat, 52.5g Carbs, 9.9g Fiber, 14g Protein

Ingredients:

2 cups cooked quinoa (1 cup dry) – cooked until slightly underdone – a little crunchy
2 large roasted tomatoes – place them on a cookie sheet in the oven for 10 minutes each side on broil – then blend until smooth
1 Tbsp EVOO
1 small onion - thinly sliced
1/2 red bell pepper – chopped finely
1/2 cup hazelnuts - chopped
1/2 cup almonds - chopped
1 cup green peas
1/2 cup cooked artichoke hearts sliced
10 small tomatoes – halved
4 cloves garlic – crushed
1/4 tsp saffron threads soaked in 1/4 cup warm water
salt and pepper to taste
Parsley or cilantro chopped for the finish
(you can add subtract any of the vegetables that you like)

Directions:

Heat shallow paella or other shallow dish over low heat

Add EVOO, onion and bell pepper and cook slowly until soft and very slightly browned

Add cooked quinoa, peas hazelnuts, almonds and artichoke hearts

Stir gently and then add the blended tomatoes and crushed garlic, the saffron in warm water. If you do not have a rather soupy looking blend, you can add a little extra water or vegetable stock.

Cook on low for a couple of minutes – taste and adjust seasonings, then add the halved tomatoes just before serving sprinkle with parsley or cilantro if desired.

Serve with a green side dish

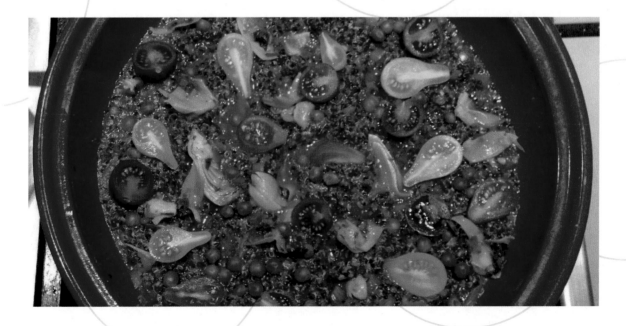

Vegetable Stroganoff ($)(E)

Serves: 4
Per serving: 203 Calories, 7.6g Fat, 1.1g Sat. Fat, 31g Carbs, 8.2g Fiber, 4.5g Protein

Ingredients:

1 large yellow onion – finely diced
2 cups well seasoned tomato sauce
2 cups chopped mushrooms
1 cup chopped baby artichokes (I use from a jar)
1 medium sweet potato – cut into 1" pieces
2 small carrots – diced
2 zucchini cut into ¾" circles
2 cups cooked beans – pinto, garbanzo, black, white etc.
2 Tbsp EVOO
1 bay leaf
2 cloves garlic – crushed
1 Tbsp chopped parsley – plus extra for finishing the recipe
1 tsp dried sage
1 tsp dried oregano
1 tsp smoked paprika
Cashew sour crème for topping (see page 238)

Directions:

In a medium sauté pan cook the onions over medium heat until soft and just staring to brown.

Add mushrooms and sauté a few minutes longer until mushrooms start to wilt.

Add tomato sauce and chopped sweet potato – cook ten minutes more.

Add the remaining ingredients.

Turn heat to low and simmer for about 20 minutes.

Taste, adjust seasoning to your likening and serve over rice, noodles, quinoa or any other GF grain such as millet, teff or buckwheat.

Spoon on 1-2 Tbsp of cashew sour crème and extra parsley.

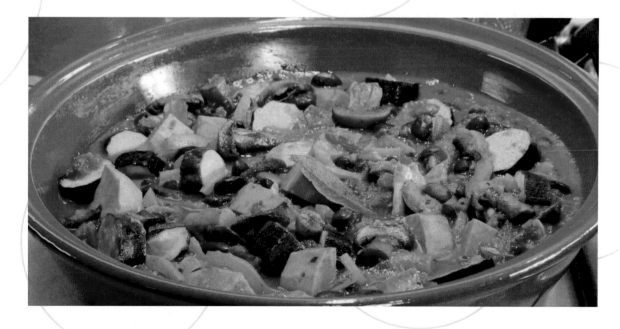

Tempeh Tikka (E)($)

Serves: 2

Per serving: 344 Calories, 17.8g Fat, 25.5g Carbs, 2.8g Fiber, 24g Protein

Ingredients:

1 8 oz package of tempeh
4 oz/100g plain coconut yogurt (if you cant find coconut yogurt just use coconut milk)
1 onion
1 Tbsp grated ginger
3 Tbsp lemon juice
1 tsp ground cumin
1 tsp ground turmeric
1 Tbsp garam masala (see page for recipe)
1 Tbsp chopped fresh mint
1 Tbsp chopped fresh cilantro
1/2 tsp mineral salt

Directions:

Chop tempeh into 1/14" squares and boil in a pan of water for 10 minutes.*

Drain and keep warm in single layers in bowl.

In your blender, add all of the remaining ingredients and blend till smooth.

Pour over the tempeh and marinate for 6 hours or overnight.

Either saute the tempeh without the marinade until a little crispy, heat the marinade and serve over the tempeh with some rice and a healthy salad.

Other Cooking Option: Thread the tempeh on skewers and BBQ - then add warmed sauce over the skewers.

* Tempeh can sometimes be a little bitter and this reduces that altogether.

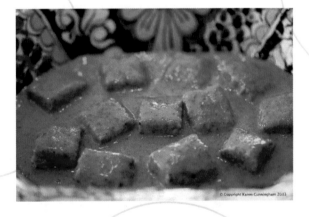

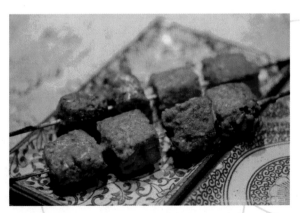

Ethiopian Lentils with Yams (E)($)

Serves: 4

Per serving: 110 Calories, 3.8g Fat, 0.6g Sat. Fat, 15.7g Carbs, 5.6g Fiber, 4.3g Protein

Ingredients:

1 small onion - diced
3 garlic clove - minced
1 tsp fresh ginger - minced
1 small sweet potato or yam - diced
1 Tbsp peanut oil
1/2 red sweet bell pepper - diced
2 tsp niter kibbeh (see page 368)
1/4 cup lentils (split red) - rinsed
2 tsp tomato paste
4 cups water - add one cup at a time and add more as your mixture gets dry. You want the final mix to be like a slightly juicy stew
1 tsp paprika
1 tsp ground coriander
1 tsp ground allspice
1/2 tsp ground cinnamon
1/2 tsp ground fenugreek
1/2 tsp ground ginger
salt and black pepper

Directions:

Sauté the onion, garlic, ginger and yam in oil at medium heat until the onions are almost translucent.

Add the red bell pepper and sauté for an additional minute.

Add the lentils, tomato paste and water. Add the paprika, coriander, allspice, fenugreek and ginger.

Lower heat slightly and allow the stew to simmer for 20 minutes or until the lentils are tender and all the water absorbed.

Add salt and black pepper as needed, and serve.

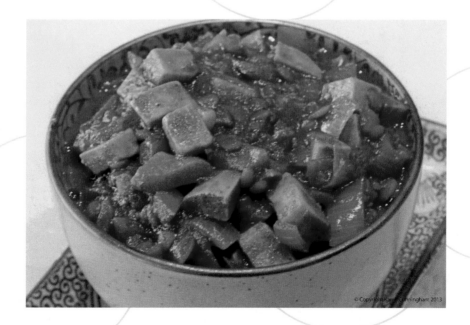

© Copyright Karen Cunningham 2013

Kathirikkai Gothsu ($)

Serves: 4
Per serving: 96 Calories, 2.3g Fat, 19g Carbs, 4.4g Fiber, 2.4g Protein

Ingredients:

2 ½ cups cubed eggplant (brinjal)
1 cup onion - roughly chopped
2 cups tomatoes - roughly chopped
2 green chilies - slit lengthwise
½ cup of tamarind extract, from fresh tamarind or
1/2 tsp of tamarind paste dissolved in 1/2 cup of water
½ tsp turmeric powder
¼ tsp asafoetida
½ tsp mustard seeds
3-4 curry leaves – crushed or 1 tsp mild curry powder
1 ½ tsp cracked pepper
1 ½ tsp ground coriander
2 tsp sesame seeds
1 tsp peanut oil
¼ tsp mineral salt

Directions:

Heat oil in a heavy bottomed pan on medium heat; add mustard seeds and allow it to crackle.

Stir in the asafoetida, curry leaves, onions and green chilies.

Sauté until the onions are tender.

Once the onions are tender, stir in the brinjal, tomatoes, turmeric powder, cracked pepper, coriander and salt.

Stir in 1/4 cup of water and simmer until the brinjal is tender.

Half way through the cooking process, stir in the tamarind water and cook until eggplant is soft.

Serve with Ven Pongal (see page 163) or plain lentils or rice and a green vegetable.

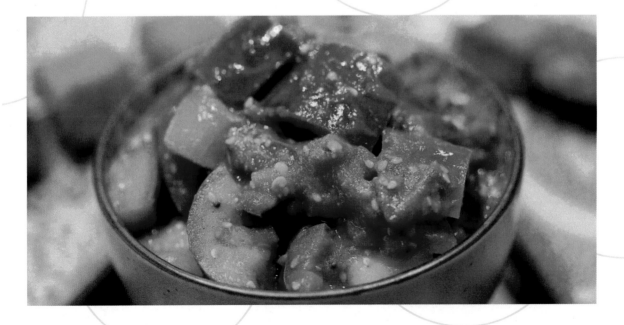

Mushroom Tacos ($)

Serves: 2-3
Per serving: 1.3g Fat, 18.2g Carbs, 6.4g Fiber, 4.7g Protein

Ingredients:

8 oz sliced mushrooms – sliced - any type will work
1 medium red onion – chopped small
¼ tsp mineral salt
1 Tbsp grapeseed oil
2 medium tomatoes – diced

Options: chopped avocado, peppers, cashew cheese (see page 243)

Directions:

Use small 6 inch besan as the taco shell.

Serve with a simple green salad – Seen here with Spinach salad with citrus vinaigrette and coconut chutney.

See page 296 for besan recipe.
See page 206 for citrus vinaigrette.
See page 186 for coconut chutney.

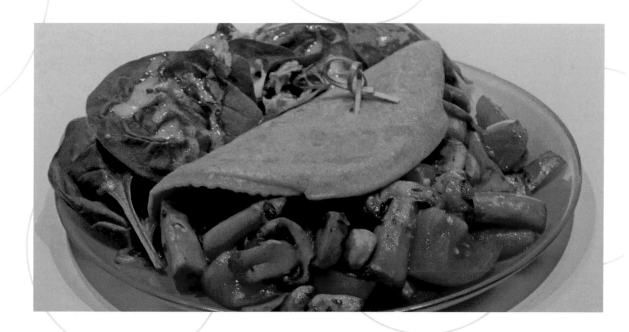

Nutmeat Loaf (R)(X)*

Serves: 12
Per serving: 280 Calories, 26g Fat, 2.4g Sat. Fat, 7.6 Carbs, 3.7g Fiber, 8g Protein

*Dehydrator required to keep this as a raw dish. You could use your regular oven on its lowest setting.

Ingredients:

1 1/3 cups walnuts (soaked for 3 hours then rinsed - do it, don't skip)
1 1/2 cups sunflower seeds (soaked for 3 hours then rinsed - do it, don't skip)
1 1/3 cups almonds (soaked for 3 hours then rinsed - do it, don't skip)
½ cup EVOO
2 medium garlic cloves
1/2 Tbsp ginger
1 1/2 tsp Celtic sea salt
1 Tbsp dried basil
½ Tbsp dried rosemary
2 Tbsp ground flax seed meal

Chop (by hand or in food processor):
2 ½ cups fresh white button mushrooms
1/2 cup fresh parsley
1/2 cup white onion – roughly chopped
1 cup red bell pepper

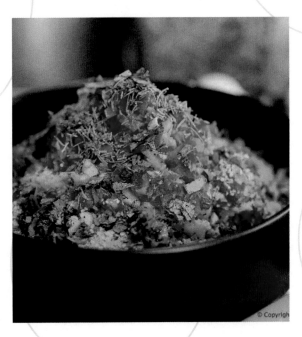

Directions:

Soak the walnuts, sunflower seeds and almonds for three hours. Drain. Rinse with clean water. Drain again.

Process walnuts, sunflowers, almonds, oil, garlic, ginger and sea salt in your food processor. You might need to add a little bit of liquid to help facilitate movement in the food processor. Add water carefully, 1 Tbsp at a time. Process until doughy. Small chunks of nuts are okay. Transfer nut mixture into a big mixing bowl.

Process the mushrooms, parsley and bell pepper separately, placing each ingredient in the bowl with the nut mixture. Be careful not to over process – you want small chunks not a purée. Maybe pulsing the food processor is a good idea if using it so you can really control your mixture.

Then add the rosemary, basil and flax seed to nut mixture. Mix all ingredients together using gloved hands. On a Paraflexx (you could use parchment paper as well) sheet covered Dehydrator tray form into small, single-serving slices, approximately ¾" thick by 2 1/2" wide. This will not work as a whole loaf (Outside too dry, inside sloppy)

Dehydrate on high for 2 hours. Reduce temperature to 105 degrees and continue dehydrating until to your desired result. The outside will look dark brown like it has been roasted. The inside should also be brown when completely done.

* I like to serve this with raw nutmeat loaf recipe with raw ketchup and some greens.

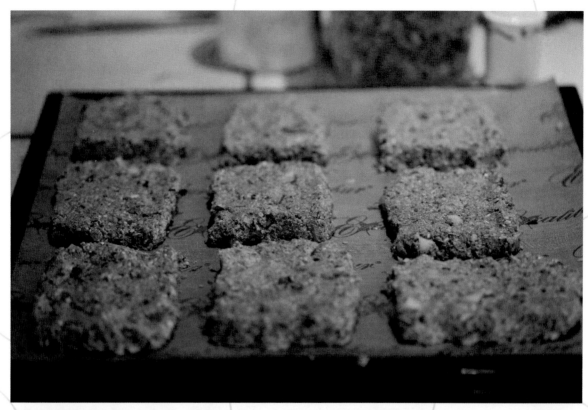

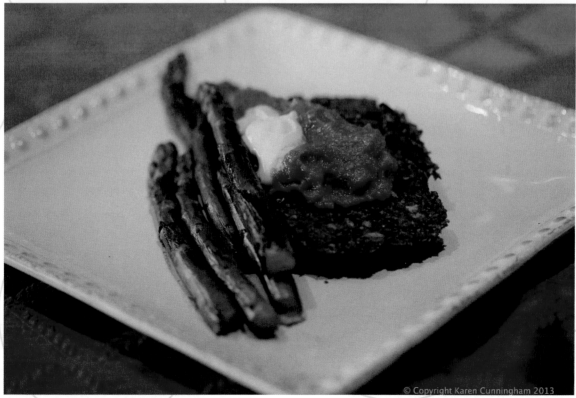

Spicy Vegetable Curry (E)($)

Serves: 4
Per serving: 662 Calories, 19.8g Fat, 102.3g Carbs, 7.3g Fiber, 20.7g Protein

Ingredients:

1 Tbsp EVOO
2 cups onion - finely chopped
1 tsp salt - divided
2 tsp tamarind pulp
1 Tbsp fresh ginger - finely chopped peeled
1 Tbsp fresh garlic - finely chopped
1 1/2 tsp ground coriander
1/2 tsp ground turmeric
1/2 tsp crushed red pepper
1 (3-inch) cinnamon stick
3 cups sweet potato - chopped, peeled
1 cup water
1 (13.5-oz) can light coconut milk
8 oz organic tempeh, cut into 3/4-inch cubes
1 Tbsp fresh lime juice
2 tsp tamari sauce

Rice:
1 1/2 cups uncooked basmati rice
1/3 cup chopped fresh cilantro
1/4 tsp salt

Directions:

To prepare curry, heat oil in a large nonstick skillet over medium-high heat.

Add onion and 1/2 tsp salt. Cook 2 minutes or until onion is tender, stirring occasionally. Stir in tamarind; cook 2 minutes, stirring to break up tamarind.

Add ginger and next 5 ingredients (through cinnamon); cook 2 minutes, stirring frequently. Add remaining 1/2 tsp salt, potato, water, milk, and tempeh; bring to a boil. Cover, reduce heat, and simmer 15 minutes or until potatoes are tender.

Uncover; stir in juice and soy sauce. Simmer 3 minutes or until slightly thickened.

Discard cinnamon stick.

To prepare rice, cook rice according to package instructions, omitting salt and fat. Stir in cilantro and 1/4 tsp salt. Serve with curry.

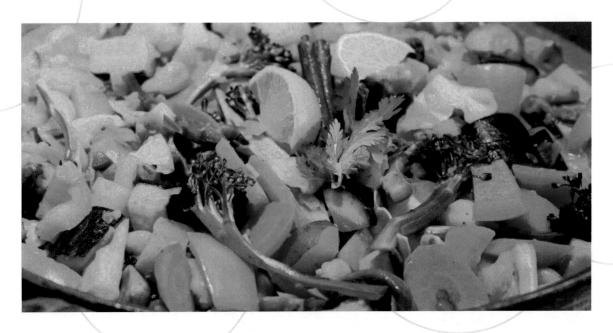

Vegetable Tagine ($)

Per serving: 405 Calories, 18g Fat, 49g Carbs, 15.2g Fiber, 17g Protein

Ingredients:

6 Tbsp EVOO
1 large yellow onion - thinly sliced
2 tsp ground cumin seed
1 cinnamon stick – 3 inches or 1 tsp ground cinnamon
1 tsp grated fresh ginger
3 medium cloves garlic - thinly sliced
3 medium carrots - peeled, medium dice
1 cup diced tomatoes with juice
1 quart (4 cups) vegetable broth
Pinch saffron threads
1 medium head cauliflower - large dice
1 1/4 cup green olives - pitted and halved
2 cups cooked chickpeas
1 Tbsp preserved lemon - finely chopped
1/2 cup dried currants
1 cup toasted almonds
½ cup cashew sour crème (see page 238)

Directions:

Heat EVOO in a large Tagine, Dutch oven or heavy-bottomed pot with a tightfitting lid over low heat.

When oil shimmers, add onion, season with salt and freshly ground black pepper, and cook, stirring occasionally, until soft and translucent, about 5 minutes.

Stir in cumin and cinnamon stick, and toast until aromatic, about 1 minute; add ginger and garlic, and cook until just softened, about 1 minute more.

Add carrots, season with salt and freshly ground black pepper, and cook until slightly tender, about 3 minutes.

Add tomatoes and their juice, vegetable broth, and saffron and stir to combine.

Bring mixture to a simmer and cook, covered, until vegetables are almost completely cooked but still raw in the center, about 7 minutes.

Add cauliflower, olives, chickpeas, preserved lemon, and currants and simmer, stirring occasionally, until cauliflower is just tender, about 10 minutes more.

Taste tagine and adjust seasoning if necessary.

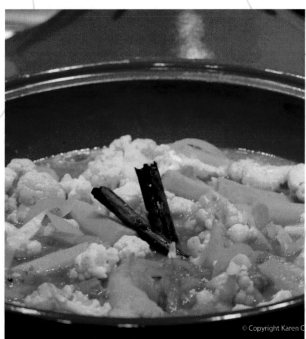
© Copyright Karen C

Zucchini Fettuccine with Cashew and Basil Alfredo (R)(Q)($)
Serves: 1
Per serving: 387 Calories, 28g Fat, 27.6g Carbs, 6.7g Fiber, 14.2g Protein

Ingredients:

1-2 tsp lemon juice
1/4 cup raw cashews*
1 stalk celery
1 clove garlic
1 tsp nutritional yeast
1 Tbsp onion – finely chopped
1 tsp fresh thyme
3 basil leaves
1/4 cup dater
1 medium zucchini
¼ cup salt cured olives
2 Tbsp raw pumpkin seeds

*soak cashews in advance if possible for 20 minutes

Directions:

Put cashews, celery, garlic, onion, thyme, nutritional yeast and basil in the blender.

Add just enough water to blend into a smooth thick sauce.

Peel zucchini into long strips resembling fettuccine noodles.

Pour sauce over the zucchini and top with black pepper.

Put in serving dish and sprinkle olives and pumpkin seeds over top

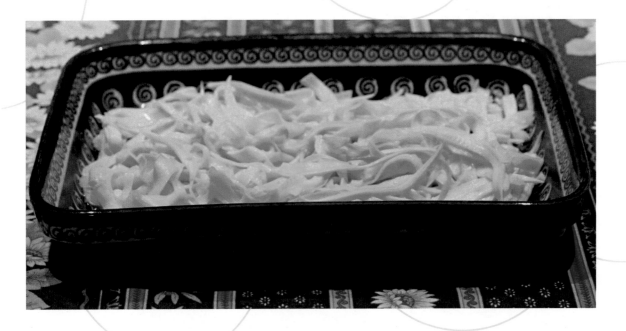

Mixed Vegetable Tagine ($)(E)

Serves: 4
Per serving*: 185 Calories, 5.4g Fat, 30.5g Carbs, 6g Fiber, 6.2g Protein
*Analyzed using a variety of squash, carrot, parsnips.

Ingredients:

1 Tbsp EVOO
1 large onion - thickly sliced
3 large garlic cloves - finely chopped
½ tsp each ground cumin, turmeric and cinnamon
1 tsp ground ginger
1½ tsp harissa paste or
1 tsp cayenne
2 Tbsp date purée (see page 304)
2 lbs seasonal vegetables (such as)
half a small butternut squash
2 large carrots
3 medium parsnips and
1 large sweet potato - all peeled and cut into chunks
2 ½ cups hot vegetable stock
2 Tbsp chopped fresh coriander

Directions:

Heat the oil in a large non-stick saucepan and gently cook the onion and garlic for 5-7 minutes.

Tip in the ground cumin, turmeric, cinnamon and ginger, harissa paste and honey and cook for another minute before stirring in the vegetables, stock and 1 tsp salt.

Bring to the boil, cover and simmer for 25 minutes.

Stir in the Quorn or tofu and continue simmering for a further 5 minutes, then taste and add more salt and harissa paste if you like. Scatter with the chopped coriander and serve

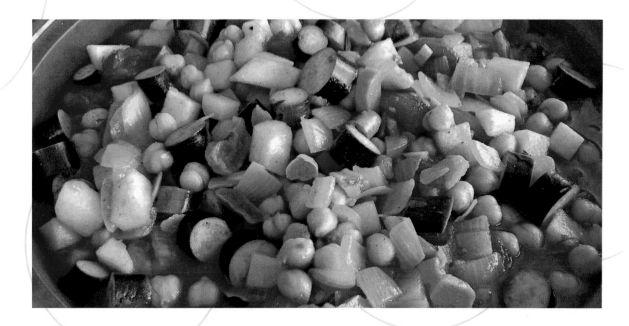

Lentil Bolognese (E)($)
Serves 10-12
Per serving: 198 Calories, 6.6g Fat, 26g Carbs, 9.8g Fiber, 10.6g Protein

Ingredients:

1/4 cup EVOO
2 yellow onions - minced
5 carrots - minced
3 celery stalks - minced
1 bulb garlic - minced
1 cup dried red lentils
4 lbs diced tomatoes
3 Tbsp dried basil
1 tsp dried oregano
1 Tbsp garlic powder
1 Tbsp miso paste
6 cups vegetable stock (or more – as needed)
2 Tbsp tomato paste
mineral salt and pepper to taste

Directions:

Heat oil on medium in a large, deep pan. Add onions, and cook until translucent.

Add carrots, celery and garlic and cook for about 5 more minutes

Put everything in the crock-pot on high for 6 hours, adding vegetable stock or water as needed.

I like my dishes to have more sauce, rather than be in the dry side

Reduce heat to low and cook for another 6 hours, adding water or vegetable stock as needed.

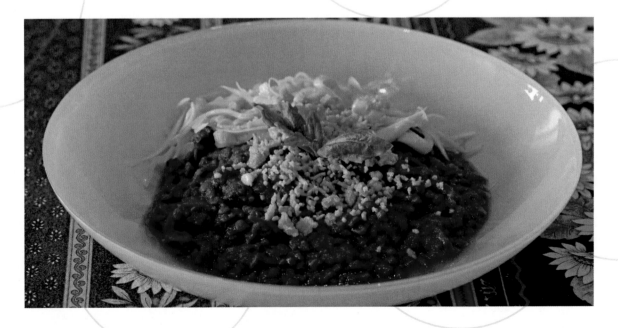

Coconut Lentils (E)($)

Per serving: 292 Calories, 15.8g Fat, 28.6g Carbs, 13.5g Fiber, 11.5g Protein

Ingredients:

1 medium onion - finely chopped
2 Tbsp coconut oil
1 Tbsp fresh peeled ginger – finely diced
2 garlic cloves - finely chopped
1 tsp ground cumin
1/2 tsp ground coriander
1 tsp turmeric
2 cups vegetable stock
1 1/2 cups dried red lentils (other lentils can be used, but they will take longer to cook)
14 oz unsweetened coconut milk (or more)
1 lb zucchini (2 medium) - small dice ¼"

Options :1 cup loosely packed fresh cilantro sprigs, and or 1 cup diced avocado

Directions:

Cook onion in oil in a 3 1/2- to 4-quart heavy pot over moderate heat, stirring occasionally, until edges are golden, about 6 minutes.

Add ginger, cumin, coriander, turmeric, salt, and chili and garlic and cook, stirring, 1 minute.

Stir in vegetable stock, lentils, and coconut milk, then simmer, covered, stirring occasionally, 5 minutes.

Stir in zucchini and simmer, covered, until lentils and zucchini are tender, about 15 minutes.

Season with mineral salt and serve with cilantro sprigs or avocado scattered on top.

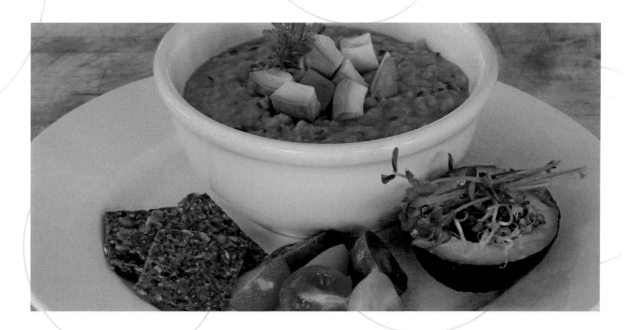

Chipotle Beans ($)(E)(Q)

Per serving: 414 Calories, 8.5g Fat, 67g Carbs, 19g Fiber, 20g Protein

Ingredients:

6 cups cooked mixed beans – garbanzo – black – giant white –kidney – pinto
2 onions – chopped
1 Tbsp EVOO
2 dried chipotle peppers – soaked in water for 1 hour
2 cups puréed tomatoes
½ tsp ground coriander
½ tsp mineral salt
½ tsp smoked or sweet paprika

Directions:

After soaking the chipotle peppers, remove from the soaking liquid and reserve liquid.

Slit the peppers lengthwise and remove the seeds.

Add tomato purée, peppers and spices to a blender and process until smooth.

Meanwhile heat the EVOO on medium-low heat and gently sauté the onion until translucent.

Add the tomato/pepper mixture to the pan and cook another couple of minutes, stirring in the onions.

Add the beans and cook for about ten minutes more.

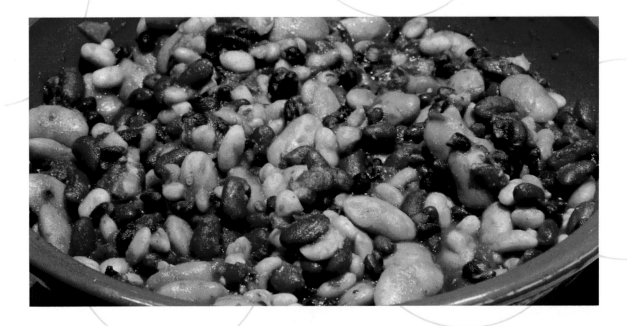

Pasta Primavera (Q)($)(E)

Serves: 6
Per serving: 610 Calories, 16.1g Fat, 103g Carbs, 9.4g Fiber, 14.3g Protein

Ingredients:

3 carrots - julienned
2 medium zucchini or 1 large zucchini - julienned
1 onion - julienned
2 cloves crushed garlic
1 yellow or orange bell pepper - julienned
1 red bell pepper - julienned
1/2 small cauliflower broken into florets (we love this
purple cauliflower for it's exceptional flavor.
1/4 cup olive oil
mineral salt
freshly ground black pepper
1 Tbsp dried Italian herbs or herbes de Provence
1/4 tsp sweet paprika
pinch of ground nutmeg
1 pound of your favorite short pasta
1/2 cup grated pine nut parmesan (see page 234)

Directions:

Preheat the oven to 450 degrees.

In a large baking pan, mix all of the vegetables, except
the cauliflower with the oil, salt, pepper, paprika,
nutmeg and dried herbs to coat.

If your pan looks too crowded, divide the vegetables
into two pans.

Bake until the carrots are tender and the vegetables
begin to brown, stir only once or twice.

This should take about 20 minutes total.

Meanwhile, cook the gluten free pasta in a large pot of
boiling salted water until al dente, tender but still firm
to the bite, according to the directions of your chosen
pasta.

Drain, reserving 1 cup of the cooking liquid.

At the same time that you cook the pasta, gently steam
or boil the cauliflower in a small amount of water until
it is to your taste.

We like it crunchy, so I steam it for about two minutes
only.

Set aside and keep warm

Toss the pasta with the vegetable mixtures in a large
bowl to combine.

Add enough vegetable stock to moisten.

Season the pasta with salt and pepper, to taste.

Sprinkle with the Vegan Parmesan and serve
immediately.

NOTE:
This reheats well and keeps for a few days in the
refrigerator

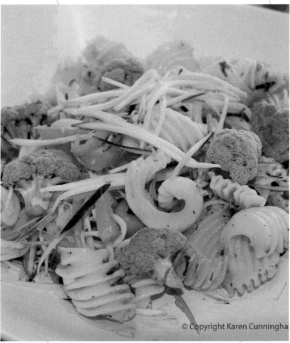
© Copyright Karen Cunningha

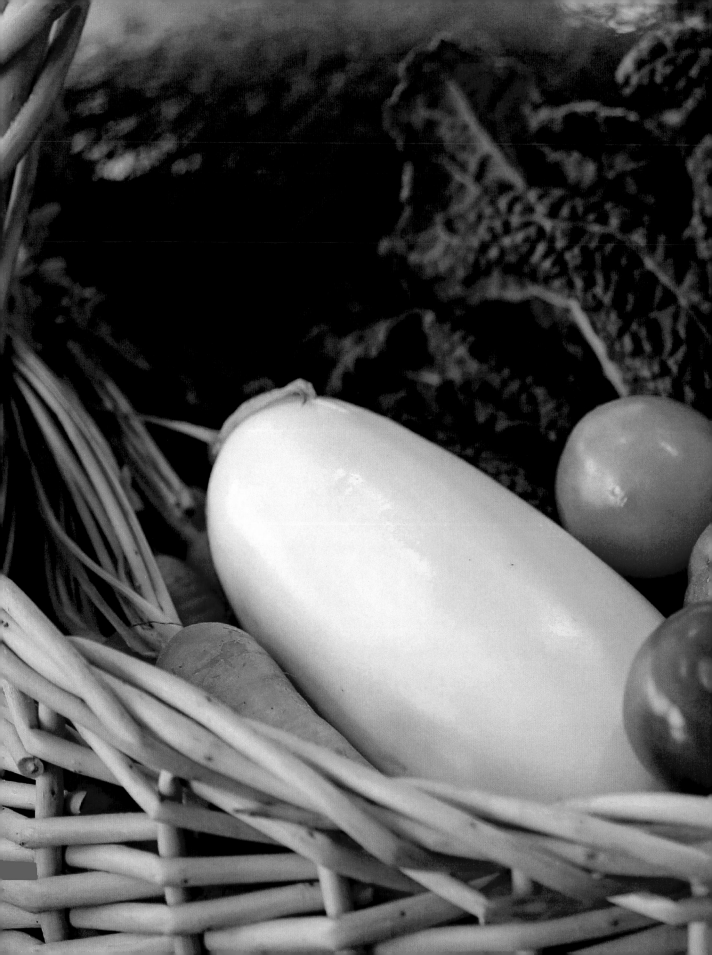

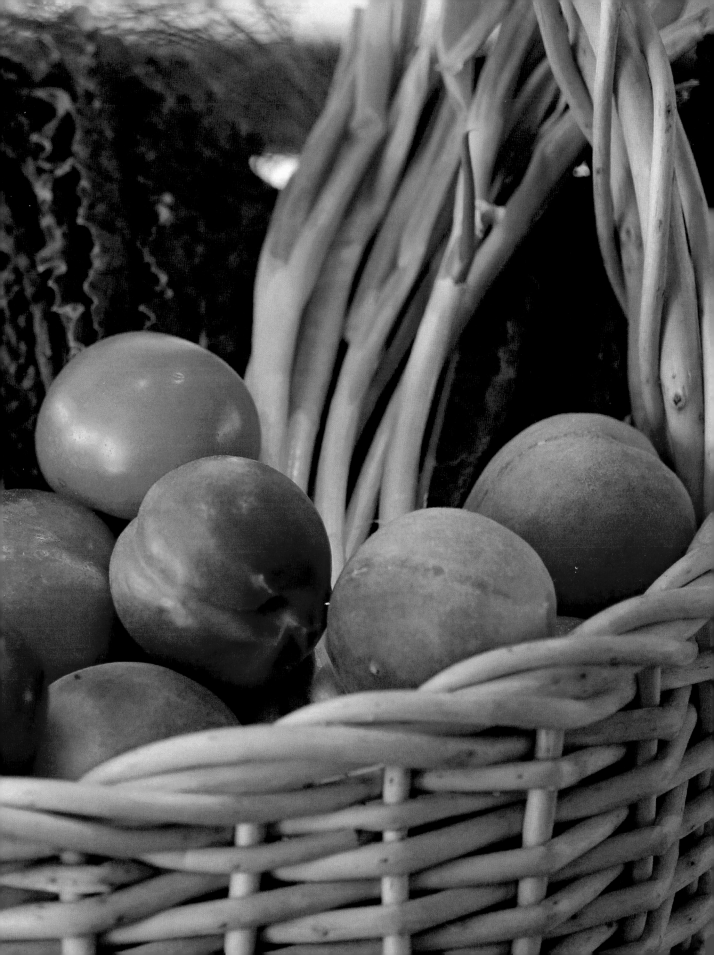

Mixed Vegetable Curry ($)

Serves: 6

Per serving: 559 Calories, 42g Fat, 43g Carbs, 20g Fiber, 14 Protein

Ingredients:

2 Tbsp EVOO
1 tsp cumin
1 tsp chili powder - beware of heat level
3 tsp turmeric
1 tsp ground coriander
1 tsp fennel seeds
1 tsp dried ginger
1 tsp ground cinnamon
1 tsp cayenne - beware of heat level
1 cup vegetable stock
1 cup coconut milk
1 cup almond milk
1 large yellow onion, chopped
2 small eggplants – cut into 1 inch squares
2 1/2 cups diced root vegetables
2 cups cauliflower – cut into 2-3 inch pieces
1 cup red bell peppers - cut into thin matchstick strips
1 cup cilantro – torn into small pieces with no stalks
1 cup chopped toasted almonds (or peanuts if you are not detoxing)

Directions:

Sauté onion and eggplant in oil on medium to low heat - 8 - 10 minutes until soft.

Add root vegetables

Add stock, coconut and almond milk.

Stir to combine ingredients

Cover and cook for about 5 minutes – then

Add cauliflower and peppers and cook another 5 minutes or so

Test your vegetables to see if they are cooked to your taste.

Optional 1 cup cooked beans – garbanzo, black beans, kidney beans, etc.

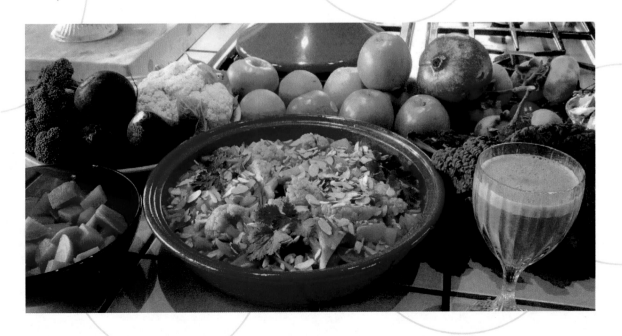

Cashew Coconut Curry ($)

Serves: 6

Per serving;:589 Calories, 47g Fat, 38.5g Carbs, 7.3g Fiber, 11.5g Protein

Ingredients:

1 lb pumpkin or butternut squash – peeled and cut into 1 ½ inch pieces
1 potato – peeled and chopped
1 carrot – peeled and chopped
4 oz button mushrooms
1 tsp mineral salt salt
3 Tbsp grapeseed or hemp oil
1 onion - halved and cut into half-moons
1 or 2 red or green serrano chiles - minced
1 cinnamon stick (2 1/2 in. long)
2 Tbsp curry powder
1 tsp turmeric
1 tsp cumin seeds
16oz coconut milk
2 cups dry roasted cashews
1 Tbsp lemon juice
3 Tbsp unsweetened desiccated coconut
pinch saffron
3 Tbsp cilantro leaves to garnish (optional)

Directions:

Mix the coconut and saffron together with a couple of drops of water and set aside – this makes a very pretty duo toned topping.

Sprinkle vegetables with 1/2 tsp salt.

Heat 1 Tbsp oil in a large nonstick frying pan over medium-high heat.

Brown the vegetables in oil, turning once, 6 to 8 minutes; reduce heat if vegetables brown too fast or stick.

Add chilies, spices and coconut milk and simmer until vegetables are just soft.

Then add the lemon juice and stir gently.

Then add the cashews just before serving.

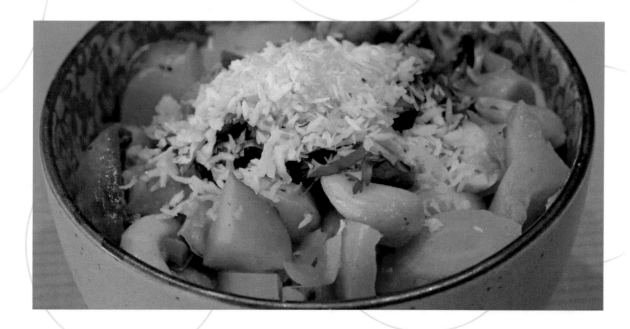

Socca Lunch ($)

Serves: 1-2
Per pancake with topping: 270 Calories, 23g Fat, 12.3g Carbs, 4.8g Fiber, 5.2g Protein

Ingredients:

2 socca pancakes (see page 297)
2 Tbsp hummus
2 slices tomato
2 slices avocado
1 tsp cashew sour crème (see page 238)
1 Tbsp roasted bell pepper pesto
1 Tbsp sprouts
fresh cracked black pepper

Directions:

See picture and spread over your socca pancakes and enjoy.

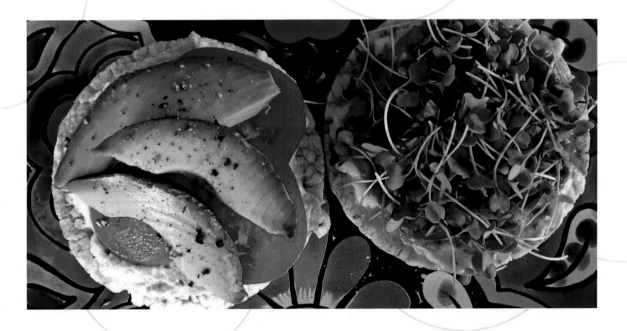

Masala Dosa ($)

Serves: 4
Per ¼ filling: 128 Calories, 3.7g Fat, 22g Carbs, 3.8g Fiber, 2.5g Protein

Ingredients:

2 medium potatoes – peeled, steamed and partially mashed
1 carrot – peeled and grated
1 large onion - thinly sliced
2 tsp fresh ginger - chopped
2 tsp chopped garlic
5 small green chilis – chopped (less if you don't like the heat)
¼ tsp cayenne pepper (optional for extra heat)
¼ tsp turmeric
½ tsp garam masala (see page 371)
½ tsp mustard seeds
½ tsp cumin seeds
3 curry Leaves
2 Tbsp cilantro leaves – chopped
1 tsp lime juice
1 Tbsp grape seed oil
pinch mineral salt

Directions:

Heat oil in a mid sized pan to medium heat, add mustard seeds.

When they splutter, add cumin seeds and fry for a minute.
Add chopped ginger, garlic, sliced onion, green chilies and curry leaves. Sauté till the onions turn light golden brown.
Add turmeric, cayenne and garam masala powder and mix well.
Add the mashed potatoes, salt and 1/4 a cup of water. When the mixture boils, lower the heat and cook for about 10 minutes, stirring often.
Finally add lime juice and coriander leaves, mix well and turn off the heat. Masala Filling is ready.

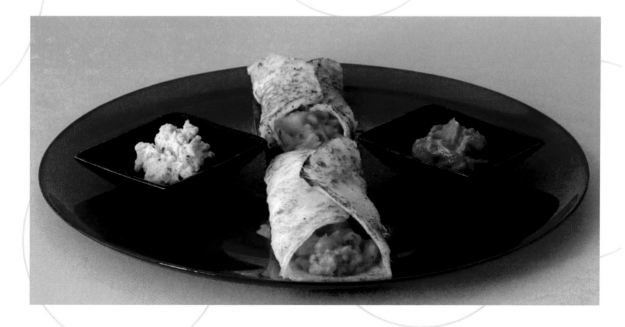

Beet Burgers ($)
Makes 12 patties
Per burger: 200 Calories, 9.2g Fat, 0.7g Sat. Fat, 22.3g Carbs, 7.6g Fiber, 9.2g protein

Ingredients:

1 1/4 cups cooked, cooled brown rice
1 cup cooked brown or green lentils - cooled, drained well
1 cup shredded beets
1/2 tsp salt
Fresh black pepper
1 tsp thyme - rubbed between your fingers
1/2 tsp ground fennel (or finely crushed fennel seed)
1 tsp dry mustard
3 Tbsp very finely chopped onion
2 cloves garlic, minced
2 Tbsp smooth almond butter
1/2 cup ground flax
EVOO for the pan

Directions:

Peel beets and shred with the shredder attachment of your food processor, then set aside. Change the attachment to a metal blade.

Pulse the brown rice, shredded beets and lentils about 15 to 20 times, until the mixture comes together, but still has texture. It should look a lot like ground meat.

Now transfer to a mixing bowl and add all the remaining ingredients. Use your hands to mix very well.

Everything should be well incorporated, so get in there and take your time, it could take a minute or two.

Place the mixture in the fridge for a half hour to chill.

Preheat a cast iron pan over medium-high. Now form the patties. Each patty will be a heaping 1/2 cup of mixture.

To get perfectly shaped patties, use a 3 1/2 inch cookie cutter or ring mold (I have pics of how to do it here.) Otherwise, just shape them into burgers with your hands.

Pour a very thin layer of oil into the pan and cook patties for about 12 minutes, flipping occasionally. Do two at a time if your pan isn't big enough.

Drizzle in a little more oil or use a bottle of organic cooking spray as needed.

Burgers should be charred at the edges and heated through.

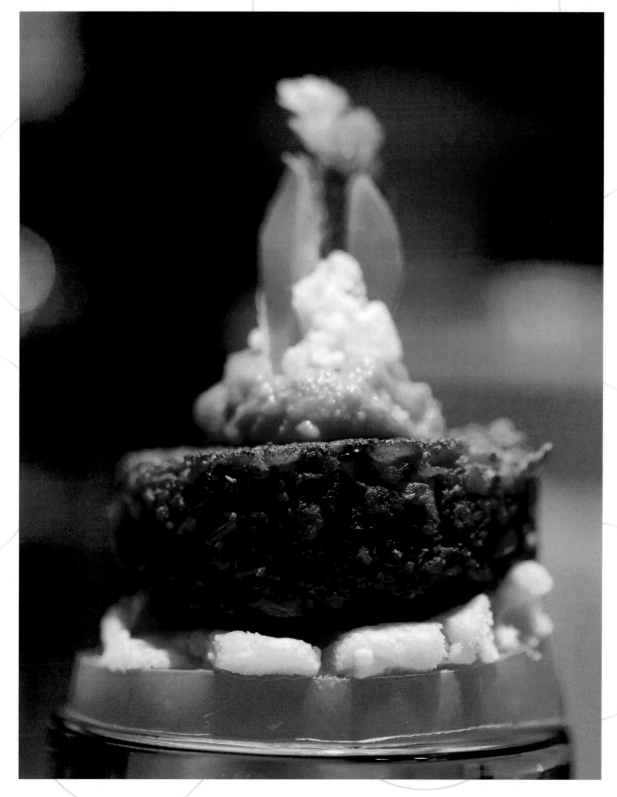

Beet Sliders ($)
Per serving: 191 Calories, 4.4g Fat, 28.4g Carbs, 9g Fiber, 8.7g Protein

Ingredients:

1 1/4 cups cooked, cooled brown rice
1 cup cooked brown or green lentils, cooled, drained well
1 cup shredded beets
1 Tbsp miso paste
1 Tbsp hemp or chia seeds
¼ tsp ground black pepper
1 tsp dried thyme
1 tsp dried rosemary
1/2 tsp ground fennel (or finely crushed fennel seed)
1 tsp dry mustard
1 red onion - finely chopped
2 cloves garlic - minced
2 Tbsp smooth sunflower butter (could use almond, cashew or peanut butter)
1/2 ground flax seed
grapeseed or peanut oil for the pan

Directions:

In a small pan sauté the onion on medium heat in a little oil until it just starts to lightly brown – remove from the heat and place into a large mixing

Peel beets and shred with the shredder attachment of your food processor, then set aside. Change the attachment to a metal blade. Pulse the brown rice, shredded beets and lentils about 15 to 20 times, until the mixture comes together, but it still has lots of texture.

Now transfer to a mixing bowl and add all the remaining ingredients. Use your hands to mix very well. Everything should be well incorporated, so get in there and take your time, it could take a minute or two.

Place the mixture in the fridge for a half hour to chill.

Preheat a cast iron pan over medium-high. Now form the patties. Each patty will be a heaping 1/2 cup of mixture. To get perfectly shaped patties, use a 3 1/2 inch cookie cutter or ring mold (I have pics of how to do it here.) Otherwise, just shape them into burgers with your hands.

Pour a very thin layer of oil into the pan and cook patties for about 12 minutes, flipping occasionally. Do two at a time if your pan isn't big enough. Drizzle in a little more oil or use a bottle of organic cooking spray as needed. Burgers should be charred at the edges and heated through.

Serve immediately.

NOTE:
They taste pretty great heated up as well. You can cook them in advance, refrigerate, then gently heat in the pan later on.

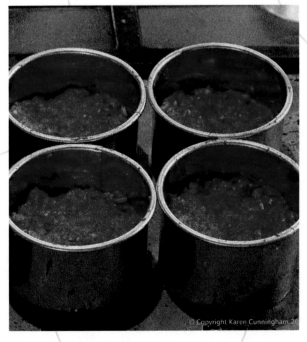

© Copyright Karen Cunningham 20

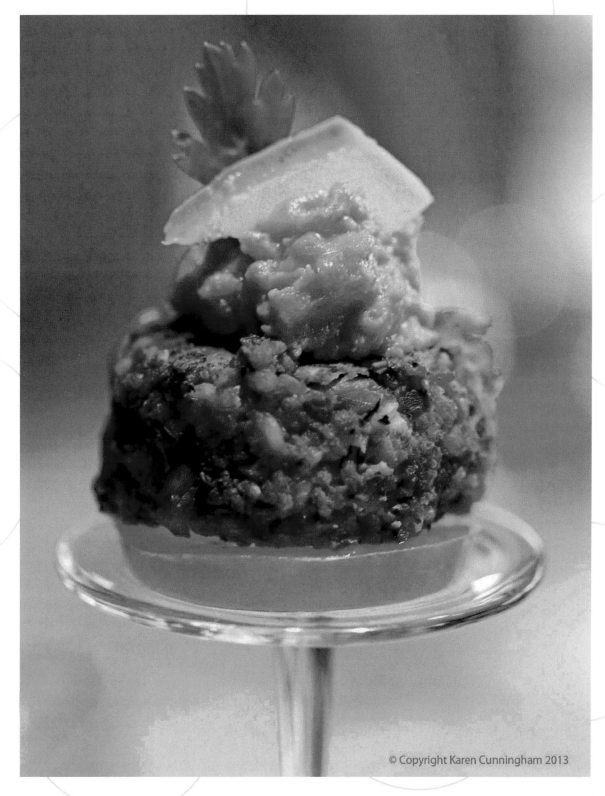

Beet Ravioli with Pine Nut Sauce and Rosemary Sauce (X)
Serves: 6
Per serving: 561 Calories, 57g Fat, 5g Sat. Fat, 12.6g Carbs, 3.6g Fiber, 9.6g Protein

Ingredients:

2 Medium Beets – peeled and sliced thinly on a
mandolin
2 Tbsp EVOO
1 Tbsp Lemon Juice
¼ tsp mineral salt
Fresh ground black pepper

Directions:

In a glass bowl marinate the beet slices with the other
ingredients for at least 30 minutes

Assembly
Lay half the beet slices on a working surface. Add a
dollop of the pine nut sauce* on each one and then
layer the remaining slices on top and gently press
together.

Spoon the pine nut sauce over each serving plate and
layer the beet slices over the sauce. Top each plate
with a drizzle of the **rosemary sauce and serve with
a salad

*For pine nut sauce see page 223
**For rosemary sauce see page 223

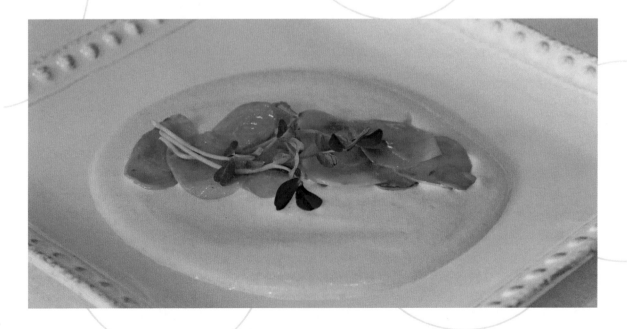

Cashew Vegetable Curry (E)(Q)($)

Serves: 6

Per serving: 392 Calories, 28.7g Fat, 28.2g Carbs, 4.2g Fiber, 10.3g Protein

Ingredients:

1 butternut squash – peeled and cut into 1 ½ inch pieces
1 sweet potato – peeled and chopped
1 carrot – peeled and chopped
4 oz button mushrooms - halved
1 tsp mineral salt
3 Tbsp grapeseed or hemp oil
1 onion - halved and cut into half-moons
1 or 2 red or green serrano chiles - minced
1 cinnamon stick (2 1/2 in. long)
2 Tbsp curry powder
1 tsp turmeric
1 tsp cumin seeds
16oz vegetable stock
2 cups dry roasted cashews

Directions:

Heat oil in medium sized pan and gently sauté the onion for a few minutes.

Add all of the remaining ingredients, cover and simmer for about 30 minutes – stirring occasionally.

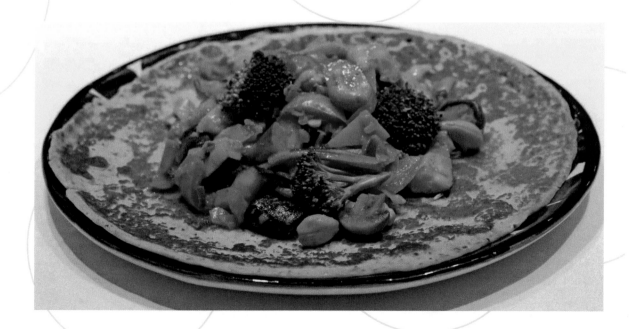

Mexican Style Peppers (E)(Q)($)

Serves: 4
Per serving: 210 Calories, 3.2g Fat, 36.5g Carbs, 7.1g Fiber, 9.8g Protein

Ingredients:

2 whole red, yellow or orange bell pepper – tops removed and seeded
1/4 cup corn kernels
1/2 cup cooked black beans
½ cup diced tomato
2 tsp cilantro – chopped
2 tsp lime juice
½ cup cooked quinoa
½ tsp chili powder
1 tsp onion flakes
½ tsp cumin
½ cup water
2 Tbsp cashew cheese (see page 243)

Directions:

Preheat oven to 375F. Cut tops of peppers and reserve them. Remove all pepper seeds (they can be very bitter).

Heat all other ingredients plus 1/2 cup water over med heat until it simmers.

Place peppers in an oven proof glass dish and spoon mixture into peppers.

Spoon cashew cheese over each pepper and place tops on peppers.

Cover with foil and bake 20 minutes or until peppers are tender.

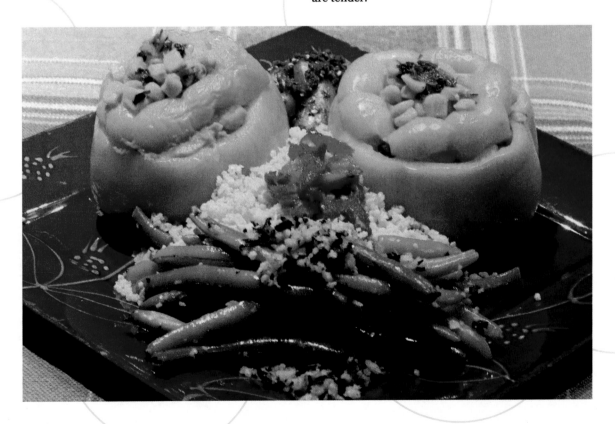

Avocado Green Herb Pesto Pasta (Q)(E)($)(R)*

Serves: 2

Per serving: 223 Calories, 10g Fat, 29g Carbs, 10g Fiber, 8g Protein

*For avocado basil pesto recipe see page 207

Ingredients:

3 cups raw spiral zucchini pasta
1 cup cooked peas
2 cups baby heirloom tomatoes
1/4 cup macadamia nut parmesan
mineral salt and cracked pepper

Directions:

Blend the pesto ingredients.

Mix with the pasta and vegetables.

Serve with macadamia parmesan and extra chopped parsley if you like.

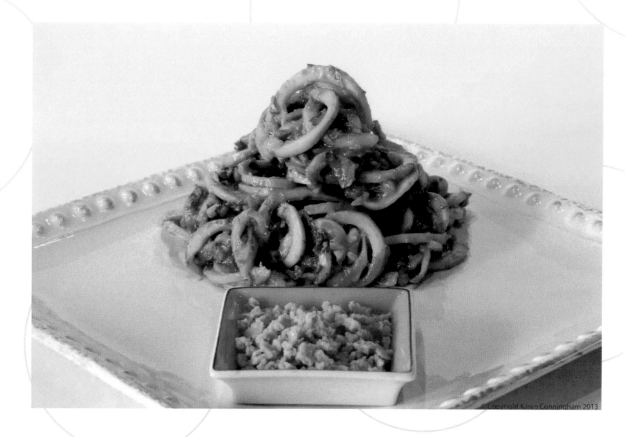

Kung Pao Vegetables (E)(Q)($)
Serves: 2
Per serving*: 326 Calories, 20g Fat, 26.2g Carbs, 7.6g Fiber, 15.9g Protein
*analyzed with sauce

Ingredients:

2 cups of your favorite vegetables (try to use as many colors as you can) - cut into bite sized pieces
½ red onion - sliced
1 Tbsp grapeseed oil
2 -3 Tbsp kung pao sauce
¼ cup peanuts or almonds – chopped (use almonds if you are cleansing)

Directions:

Heat oil in a wok on medium to high and sauté vegetables for a few minutes

Add the kung pao sauce and stir for another minute

Remove from heat and serve with the nuts sprinkled over the top

Kung Pao Sauce (E)(Q)($)
Per serving: 105 Calories, 3.7g Fat, 10g Carbs, 1.3g Fiber, 8.3g Protein

Directions:

3 Tbsp minced garlic
2 Tbsp minced ginger
2 Tbsp sambal oelek
1 cup tamari sauce
1 Tbsp date purée (see page 304)
1/2 cup apple cider vinegar
1 Tbsp grapeseed oil for cooking

Directions:

Mix.

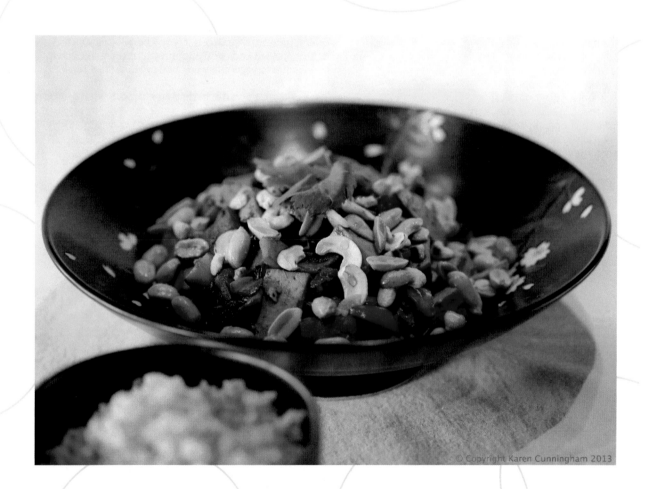

© Copyright Karen Cunningham 2013

Vegetable Pot Pie ($)

Per servings: 229 Calories, 13g Fat, 22g Carbs, 5.2g Fiber, 7g Protein

Ingredients:

1 Tbsp EVOO and sauté
1 onion - chopped
2 carrots - chopped
1 stick of celery - chopped
4 tomatoes - chopped
1 tsp not-poultry seasoning
1 cup frozen organic corn kernels
1/2 cup chopped parsley
1 cup chestnut purée (see page 189)
2 cups vegetable stock

*See page 294 for garbanzo pie crust recipe

Directions:

In a large pan add EVOO and sauté onion, carrots, celery, tomatoes, seasoning, corn and parsley. Once lightly sautéed add chestnut purée and vegetable stock and whatever vegetables you like to make stew thick.

Then add your favorite herbs and spices.

Then ladle into individual oven proof bowls.

This recipe can sit for a day or two if you before proceeding

Heat oven to 350 and put crustless pies into the oven for 30 minutes to warm. Then add the crust*.

Cut into sizes that will cover your pies.

Bake at 375 alone for a more crunchy crust = 10-15 minutes, or if you cover the pies at this time the crust will end up a little softer = 15-20 minutes
Directions:

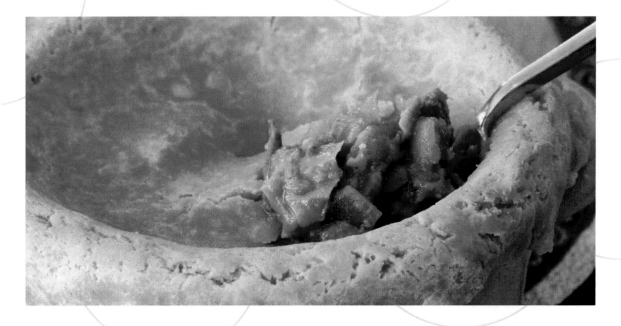

Omlette (E)($)

Serves: 2
Per serving: 214 Calories, 10.7g Fat, 38.3g Carbs, 4.9g Fiber, 21.3g Protein

Ingredients:

1 (14 oz) package tofu
1 Tbsp almond milk
2 Tbsp nutritional yeast
1 Tbsp potato or tapioca starch
1/2 tsp onion powder
1/4 tsp cumin
1/4 tsp miso paste
1/4 tsp turmeric
1/2 tsp Bragg's liquid amino acids
1/4 tsp paprika
mineral salt & pepper to taste

Directions:

Blend all ingredients and then cook on a griddle adding whatever ingredients you like in an omelet.

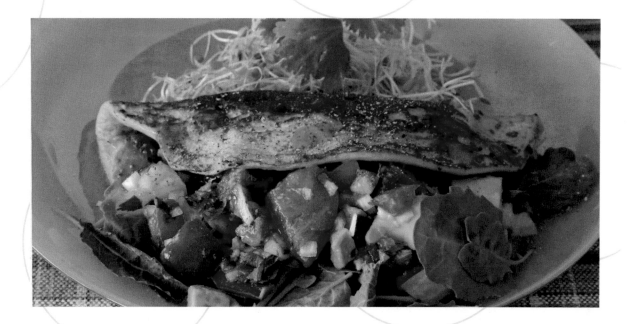

Buckwheat Meatballs ($)

Serves: 2
Per serving: 191 Calories, 5.3g Fat, 26.5g Carbs, 6.6g Fiber, 10g Protein

Ingredients:

1/2 cup toasted buckwheat, aka kasha (dry measure)
1 cup water (or more)
pinch sea salt
2 Tbsp ground flax seeds
1/4 cup water
3 Tbsp tomato paste
1 Tbsp dry mustard
2 Tbsp tamari
1 tsp dried oregano
1 tsp dried sage
1/2 tsp dried thyme
1 tsp onion powder
1 tsp garlic powder
1/2 tsp ground cumin
1 tsp smoked paprika

Directions:

Preheat the oven to 350 degrees. Mix the ground flax with the 1/4 cup water and leave to sit.

Toast buckwheat in a large frying pan, stirring constantly until it browns and smells fabulous. Remove from heat and put it in a small pot with the water and pinch of salt, and bring to a boil. Turn down to simmer, covered, for about 5 – 10 minutes until soft.

Mix together the seasonings in a large bowl, then add the cooked buckwheat and soaked flax and stir to combine.

Shape spoonfuls of the mix into small balls onto cookie sheet. Bake 30 minutes or until nice and crunchy. Once the meatballs are done, take them out of the oven, and let them cool for a few minutes before handling them. Serve with your favorite spaghetti sauce.

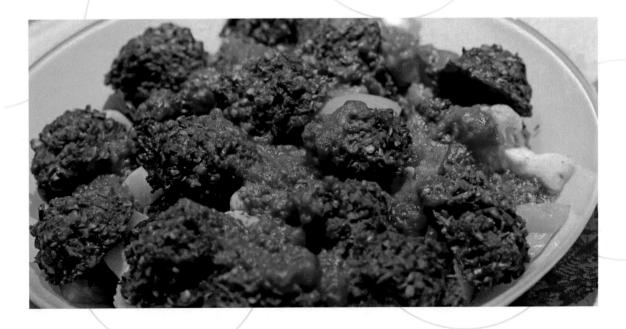

Zucchini Pomodoro (E)($)

Serves: 4
Per serving: 177 Calories, 10g Fat, 21g Carbs, 5.3g Fiber, 5.3g Protein

Ingredients:

3 zucchini – spiral cut
2 Tbsp grapeseed oil
2 cloves garlic, peeled and minced
1 small onion, finely chopped
2 tsp olive oil
1 can (28 oz) diced plum tomatoes
3 Tbsp tomato paste
1 tsp apple cider vinegar
1 tsp dried oregano
1 tsp dried basil
1/2 tsp red pepper flakes
½ cup chopped parsley leaves
fresh basil – as much as you love

Directions:

Sauté garlic and onion in grapeseed oil in medium saucepan over medium heat 5 minutes.

Add remaining ingredients except fresh basil and cook, stirring occasionally, for 30 minutes.

Serve over spiraled zucchini.

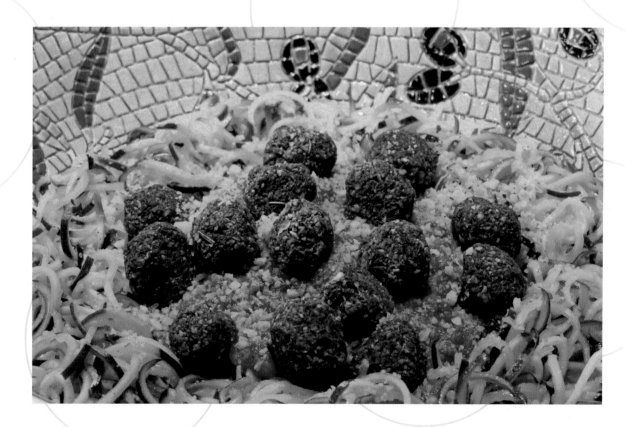

Orange Vegetable Tagine ($)

Serves: 6
Per serving: 334 Calories, 14.3g Fat, 41g Carbs, 10g Fiber, 11.3g Protein

Ingredients:

1/2 cup of sliced green cabbage
1 sliced onion – large chunks
all other vegetables cut into 1 inch pieces
1/2 cup of butternut squash
1/2 cup of yellow zucchini
1/2 cup carrots
1/2 cup sweet potatoes
1/2 cup turnips
1/2 cup parsnips
1/2 cup chopped parsley
1/2 cup chopped coriander
1/2 cup toasted slivered almonds
2 cups cooked garbanzo beans
2 Tbsp olive oil

CARAMELIZED ONION TOPPING
1/2 onion, sliced
1 Tbsp dried currants
1/4 tsp cinnamon
1/4 cup orange juice
1 Tbsp orange blossom water

SPICE MIX
1 tsp of cumin
1/2 tsp ginger
1/2 tsp of turmeric
1/4 tsp of saffron
1/2 tsp of harrissa (spicy sauce)
1/2 tsp of ras el haonut (see page 371)
1/2 cup of water

Directions:

Beginning the Vegetable Tagine:
Pour 1 Tbsp olive oil in the tagine first, spread evenly.

Layer the vegetables in the following order: Onions, then all of the hard vegetables, then the squash garbanzo beans and then the cabbage.

Prepare Spices :
Mix all the spices together and add 1/2 water to make a little sauce and pour over the vegetables.

Cover and cook over low heat for about 15 minutes or until the vegetables are cooked to your taste

Make Caramelized Onion Topping:
While the tagine is cooking, make the caramelized onions. Preheat a saute pan on medium heat. Heat 1 Tbsp EVOO in the pan.

Add the onions and cook for 5 minutes, stirring to avoid burning the onions. Once the onions are golden brown add the dried currants.

After a few minutes the currents will puff up a little, then add in the cinnamon and the orange juice. Stir for a few moments then add the orange blossom water, keep stirring and remove from the heat.

Finish the Vegetable Tagine:
Add the caramelized onions to your tagine by sprinkling them on top, cook for another 5 minutes, then turn off the heat and let sit for 10 minutes.

Before serving add the parsley, cilantro and almonds.

NOTE:
You can substitute any of your favorite vegetables for this dish.

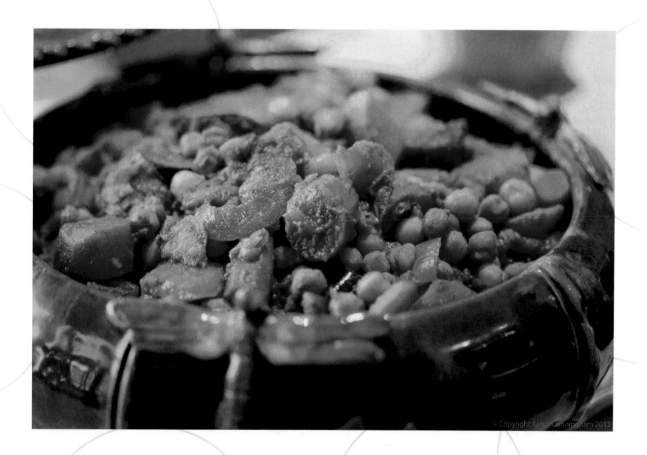

Vegetable Kebabs (E)($)

Serves: 4
Per serving: 161 Calories, 7.5g Fat, 21.4g Carbs, 7.7g Fiber, 6.2g Protein

Ingredients:

1 bunch asparagus – ends snapped
½ white cabbage (purple would be good too) – cut into 8 pieces
2 zucchini – cut into 1/12 inch pieces
8 medium sized whole mushrooms
4 tomatoes – quartered
1 large red onion - cut into 8 pieces
1 large yellow bell pepper – cut into 8 pieces
2 Tbsp grapeseed oil
mineral salt and pepper if desired

Directions:

Thread the vegetables onto skewers and BBQ until just staring to turn brown – undercooked is better.

Serve with mango habañero sauce or mango yoghurt sauce.

See page 193 for mango habañero sauce.
See page 214 for mango yoghurt sauce.

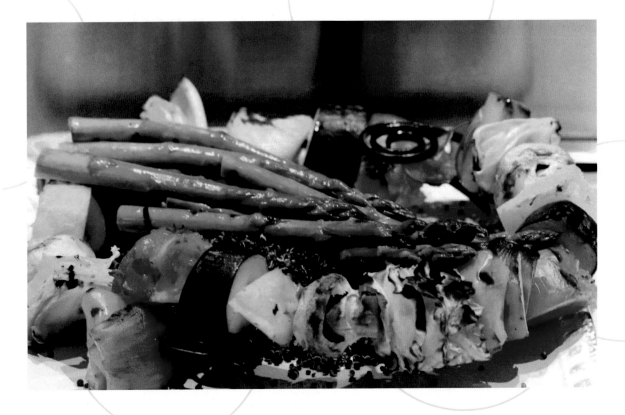

Cauliflower with Cheese ($)

Serves: 6
Per serving: 176 Calories, 11.8g Fat, 13.9g Carbs, 4.4g Fiber, 7.7g Protein

Ingredients:

1 medium sized cauliflower – center stem and leaves removed
1 cup cashew cheese (see page 243)
½ cup dry roasted pumpkin seeds

Directions:

In a steamer basket over a large pot – steam the head of cauliflower until it is just soft – a skewer should only just be able to go through it. This will be 10-20 minutes depending on the size of your cauliflower

Remove from the heat and platter.
Pour the cashew cheese and pumpkin seeds over the top

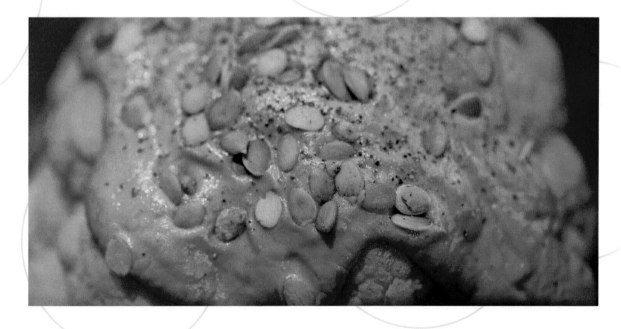

Orange Ginger Stir Fry (Q)(E)($)

Serving:
Per serving*: 128 Calories, 2.8g Fat, 24g Carbs, 5.7g Fiber, 4.2g Protein
*Analyzed using½ cup sauce, no rice, and mixture of carrots, green vegetables, and bell peppers

Ingredients:

Approximately 3 cups of your favorite vegetables. This recipe used:

carrot
onion
red and yellow bell peppers
baby kale
asparagus
zucchini
green beans

Other Ingredients:
1 tsp grapeseed oil
1/2 cup of orange ginger stir fry sauce (see page for recipe)
1/2 cup water

Directions:

In a wok add grapeseed oil over medium high heat
If using onions in your stir fry, add them first and stir fry for about 2 minutes.

Add the remaining vegetables, sauce and water.

Stir fry for about 4-5 minutes.

NOTE
You can add a little more sauce if you like your stir fry with more sauce

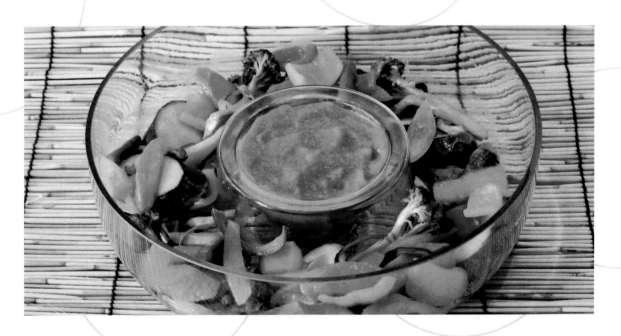

Grilled Tempeh Pineapple Skewers (E)($)

Serves: 2 as a main, 4 as a starter
Per serving (as a main): 340 Calories, 12.6g Fat, 39.5g Carbs, 2.2g Fiber, 23.3g Protein
Per serving (as a starter): 170 Calories, 6.3g Fat, 19.8g Carbs, 1.1g Fiber, 11.7g Protein

Ingredients:

8oz package of tempeh
2x1 inch thick slices fresh pineapple

MARINADE:
8oz unsweetened pineapple juice
1 Tbsp tamari sauce
2 cloves garlic – minced
1 inch pieces of fresh ginger – grated
½ yellow bell pepper – chopped fine
4x6 inch bamboo or stainless steel skewers

Directions:

Mix the marinade ingredients and place into a shallow dish.

Cut the tempeh into 1 inch square and marinate in the mixture overnight or for at least 6 hours.

When ready to proceed cut the pineapple into 1 inch squares and thread the pineapple and tempeh onto the skewers.

Turn griddle to high and brown the skewers.

Meanwhile heat the remaining marinade and allow to simmer gently while you are cooking the skewers.

Serve the marinade over the skewers.

This is best served over a little rice, and the Kitchen Sink* salad makes a perfect accompaniment.

*see page for recipe

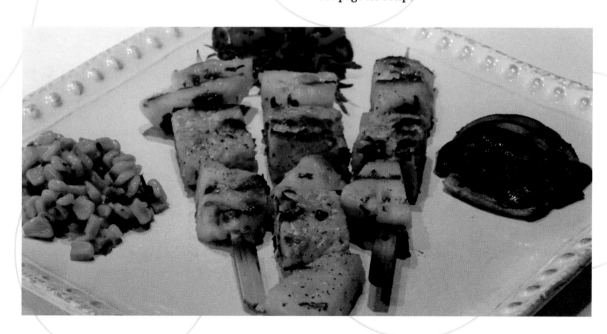

Spinach and Mushroom Shepherd's Pie (NCF)($)
Serves: 4 -6
Per serving: 454 Calories, 17g Fat, 65g Carbs, 12.3g Fiber, 15g Protein

Ingredients:

4-6 mixed sweet potatoes (we found some purple –
white and orange ones for this recipe)
2 Tbsp EVOO
1/2 cup unsweetened almond or hemp milk
mineral salt to taste
1 large onion - finely chopped
3 cloves garlic - minced
16 oz cremini or baby bella mushrooms – sliced
1 cup plain cashew crème (see page 239)
2 Tbsp apple cider vinegar
1 to 2 Tbsp Bragg's liquid aminos or tamari sauce
1 tsp dried thyme
1 Tbsp miso paste
1 tsp smoked paprika
1 tsp sage
freshly ground pepper to taste
8 to 10 oz baby spinach
1 cup pine nut parmesan

Directions:

Peel and slice the potatoes.

Place in a large saucepan with enough water to cover.

Bring to a simmer, then cover and simmer until
tender, about 10 minutes.

Drain and transfer to a small mixing bowl.

Preheat the oven to 350 degrees.

While the potatoes are cooking, heat the oil in a
medium skillet.

Add the onion and sauté over medium heat until
translucent.

Add the garlic and mushrooms and continue to sauté
until the onion is golden.

Stir in the brags liquid aminos and seasonings and
cook over low heat for 5 minutes.

Add the spinach, a little at a time, cooking just until it'
s all wilted down.

Remove from the heat; taste to adjust seasonings to
your liking.

Lightly oil a 9x9 pyrex dish layer some of the potatoes
on the bottom, keep the same amount aside for the
top.

Mix the spinach and mushroom mix with the
remaining potatoes and put into dish – pressing
slightly

Lay the remaining potatoes over the top and finish
with the pine nut parmesan.

Bake for 30 to 35 minutes.

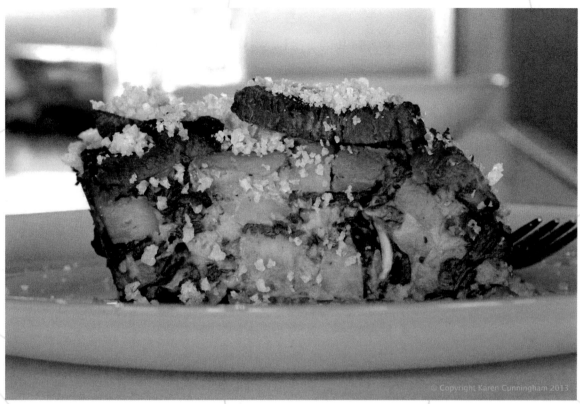

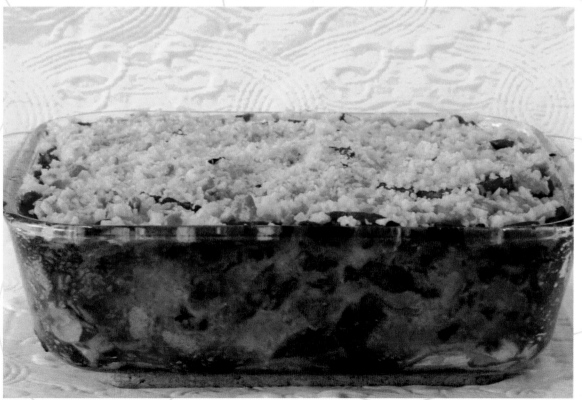

Kitchen Sink Salad (E)(R)(Q)($)

Serves 3-4
Per serving (1/4th recipe): 274 Calories, 20.3g Fat, 23.5g Carbs, 8.3g Fiber, 3.9g Protein

Ingredients:

1 tomato per person - quartered
1 Large cucumber – peeled and chopped
1 yellow bell pepper – peeled and chopped
1 red bell pepper – peeled and chopped
1 orange bell pepper – peeled and chopped
1 medium red onion – peeled and chopped
¼ red cabbage – chopped
1 cup Napa cabbage - chopped
4 Tbsp parsley – chopped
2 carrots - peeled and chopped
1 avocado – peeled – deseeded and chopped
½ cup pitted olives – cut in halves
citrus vinaigrette – 3 Tbsp per person (see page 206)

Directions:

Put all vegetables in a large mixing bowl except for the tomatoes and toss with the vinaigrette.

Arrange onto serving plates and add the tomato.

Finish with mineral salt and pepper to taste or add a few sprinkles of your favorite topping.

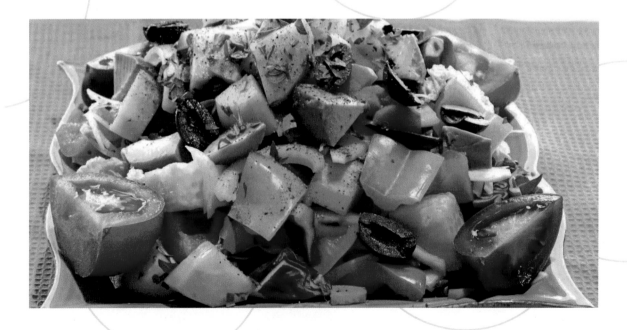

Braised Cabbage with Carrots and Onions(E)(Q)($)

Serves: 4

Per serving: 123 Calories, 10.6g Fat, 7.5g Carbs, 2.1g Fiber, 0.8g Protein

Ingredients:

1/2 green cabbage – coarsely chopped
1 sweet onion sliced
3 carrots
3 Tbsp EVOO
salt and pepper
apple cider vinegar to drizzle
sprinkling of red pepper flakes – per your taste

Directions:

Add chopped vegetables to a wok or large based saucepan and gently sauté for about 30 minutes

Then place the pan under a broiler for a few minutes to brown the dish. The slow cooking makes for a very sweet dish indeed.

A sprinkle of apple cider after the dish has browned makes for even more delicious flavor.

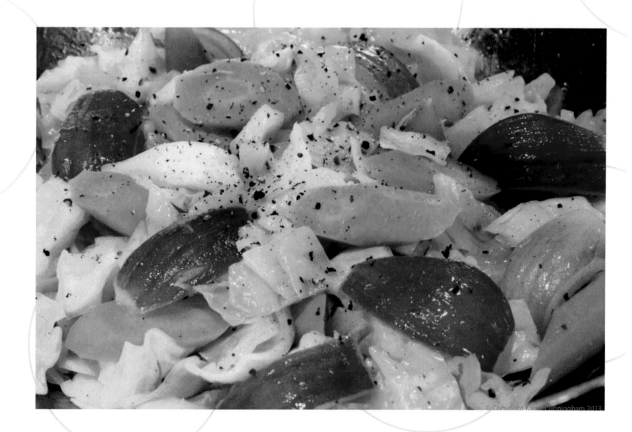

Quinoa Paella with Spring Vegetables ($)

Serves: 6
Per serving: 294 Calories, 11.2g Fat, 39g Carbs, 8.8g Fiber, 11.6g Protein

Ingredients:

2 small carrots – peeled and chopped into ½ inch pieces
2 small turnips - peeled and chopped into ½ inch pieces
10 asparagus spears – ends snapped off
1/3 cup cooked fava beans
4 baby artichokes in water (from jar) – or fresh from deli – cut into quarters
1 lemon
2 cups vegetable stock
1/4 cup EVOO
2 cups scallions – sliced into thin strips
2 cloves garlic - finely chopped
1 1/4 cups quinoa
1 cup puréed tomatoes
1/2 tsp spanish sweet smoked paprika
1/4 tsp saffron - steeped in 1Tbsp warm water

Directions:

Preheat oven to 300 degrees.
Use a (13½ -inch) paella pan suitable for use on the stove and in the oven or a frypan that can also go into the oven

Cut the tips off the asparagus – you want 2 inch lengths and set aside
Cut the remaining asparagus into ½ inch pieces

Heat the EVOO in a paella pan over medium heat, and sauté the carrots, turnips, broad (fava) beans, asparagus (except the chopped tips), artichokes and spring onions for 2 minutes.

Add the garlic to the center of the pan and continue cooking until the vegetables are softened and lightly browned.

Add the quinoa and sauté until translucent, without allowing it to burn, just as if it were rice for a paella. Add the (sofrito) – tomatoes, paprika and saffron mixture, and stir with a wooden spatula, scraping the bottom of the paella pan thoroughly. Allow to thicken, cook for a few seconds more, taking care that it does not burn.

Pour in the hot vegetable stock, stir and bring to a boil. Continue to cook over high heat stirring often. After 5 minutes, the quinoa rises to the surface.

Carefully transfer the paella pan to the oven for 12 minutes. Remove the paella pan from the oven and allow to rest for 3 minutes.

Meanwhile, place the asparagus tips in a bowl of boiling water and let sit for ten minutes, then drain the chopped asparagus tips and sprinkle all over the paella.

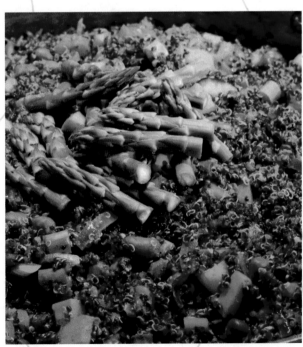

Vegetarian Gumbo ($)
Per serving: 324 Calories, 8.8g Fat, 44.6g Carbs, 11.3g Fiber, 18.6g Protein

Ingredients:

2 cups water
1/4 cup grapeseed oil + 2 Tbsp
1/4 cup garbanzo flour
2 onions - diced
1 red bell pepper - diced
4 stalks celery - chopped
4 tomatoes – chopped
2 zucchini – diced
2 oz brown mushrooms - chopped
1/4 cup hot sauce
1/4 tsp cayenne pepper (or to taste)
1/2 tsp thyme
1/2 tsp oregano
1 tsp File (sassafras)
1/4 cup fresh parsley - chopped
3 cloves garlic - minced
6 cups vegetable broth
2 bay leaves
16 oz cooked kidney beans
mineral salt and pepper to taste

Directions:

In a small pot, whisk together the 1/4 cup oil and flour over low heat to form a roux, stirring continuously for about 10 to 15 minutes. Once it turns a dark reddish brown, remove from the heat and set aside.

In a large soup or stock pot, sauté the onions, bell pepper, celery, zucchini, mushrooms and tomatoes for a few minutes in the 2 tablespoons of oil, until just soft. Reduce the heat and add the hot sauce, file powder, cayenne, thyme, oregano, parsley and garlic and cook, stirring for one or two more minutes.

Add the four and oil roux and the vegetable broth and stir well to combine. Add the bay leaves. Bring to a simmer, and allow to cook for 15 minutes.

Add the, kidney beans, and cook for 5 more minutes. Remove bay leaves before serving.

Serve with steamed collard greens or kale and cooked buckwheat.

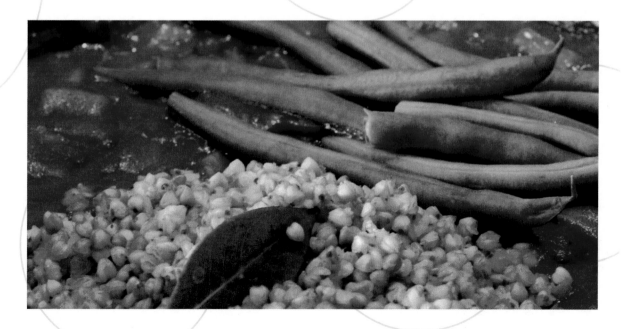

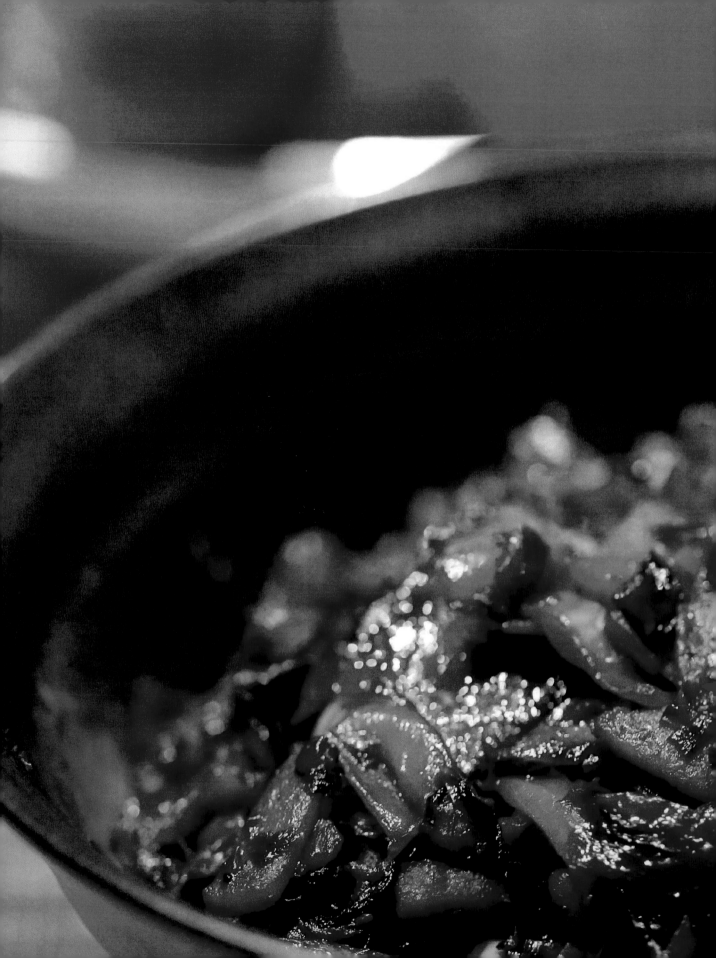

Sides

Buckwheat Pilaf ($)
Serves 6 (134g)
Per serving: 114 Calories, 3.6g Fat, 17g Carbs 2.5g Fiber, 4.6g Protein

Ingredients:

1 Tbsp EVOO
1 yellow onion - chopped
1 cup buckwheat groats (toasted buckwheat)
3 garlic cloves - minced
1/2 tsp cumin seed
1/2 tsp mustard seed
1/4 tsp ground cardamom
2 cups vegetable stock or broth
1 tomato, peeled and seeded, then diced
1/2 tsp salt
2 Tbsp fresh cilantro (fresh coriander) - chopped

Directions:
In a saucepan, heat the EVOO over medium heat.

Add the onion and saute until soft and translucent, about 4 minutes. Add the buckwheat groats, garlic, cumin seed, mustard seed and cardamom.

Saute, stirring constantly, until the spices and garlic are fragrant and the buckwheat is lightly toasted, about 3 minutes.

Carefully pour in the stock. Bring to a boil, then reduce the heat to medium low, cover and simmer until the liquid is absorbed, about 10 minutes.

Remove from the heat and let stand, covered, for 2 minutes.

Stir in the tomato and salt. Transfer to a serving bowl and sprinkle with the cilantro. Serve immediately.

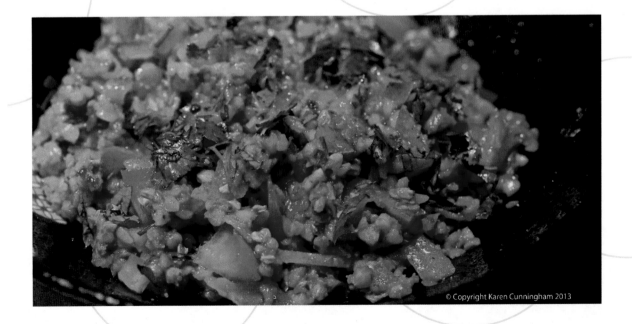

Blaukraut ($)

Serves 4 (414g)
Per serving: 177 Calories, 6.7g Fat, 29g Carbs, 9.8g Fiber, 4.5g Protein

Ingredients:

1 red cabbage, approximately 2 lbs
2 Tbsp EVOO
1 tsp ground cumin
1/2 tsp ground cinnamon
1 bay leaf
2 Tbsp Bragg's Organic Apple Cider Vinegar
1 large green apple - peeled, cored and chopped into smallish pieces
1 sweet onion - roughly chopped
1/2 onion - finely chopped
Salt to taste if necessary

Variations:
Add 1 diced carrot along with the onions.
Add 2 tsp caraway seeds with the onions for a variation in flavor.
Add 1/4 cup red or white wine with the water or stock

Directions:

Heat the EVOO in a large pot or skillet on low heat.

Add onions and sauté till translucent.

Turn up the heat to medium and add sliced apple and sauté until soft.

Add the cabbage in batches and sauté until wilted.

Immediately stir in the vinegar.

Add the rest of the ingredients and season to taste with salt and pepper.

Simmer covered over low heat for 30-45 minutes, adding water if necessary

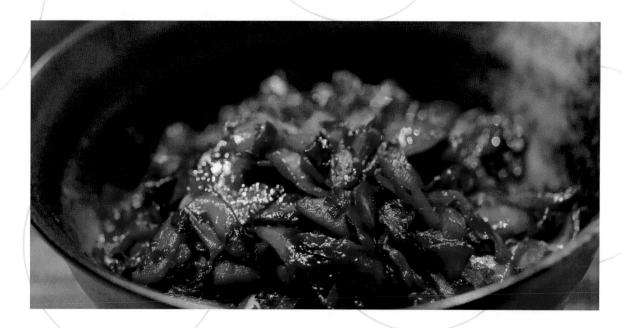

String Bean Mint Salad (E)($)(Q)

Serves: 2
Per serving: 64 Calories, 0.2g Fat, 13.9g Carbs, 6.2g Fiber, 3.3g Protein

Ingredients:

1/2 lb green beans
1/2 lb wax beans
garlic – as much as you like – minced or chopped
1 bunch mint chopped finely
lemon juice from half a lemon
salt and pepper to taste

Directions:

Cook for just a couple of minutes until color just changes.

Drain rinse in cold water and set aside.

Meanwhile, in a separate bowl mix garlic, lemon juice, 1/2 of the mint.

Combine beans and lemon juice mix.

Season with salt and pepper.

Set aside for one hour before serving.

Then sprinkle remaining mint over the top just before serving.

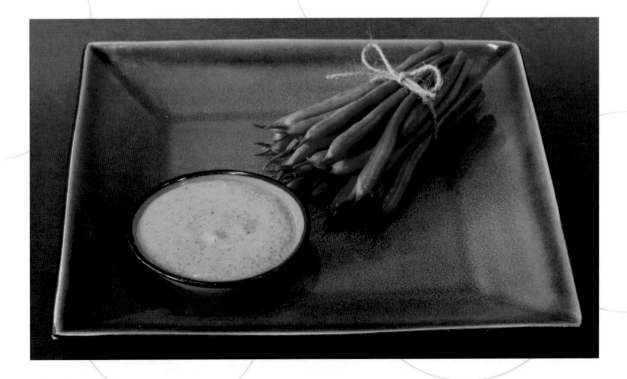

Cannellini Bean Mash (E)(Q)($)

Serves: 4

Per serving: 200 Calories, 4g Fat, 30g Carbs, 12.5g Fiber, 11.9g Protein

Ingredients:

1 13 oz can cannellini beans
2 cloves garlic
EVOO
1/4 cup chopped parsley
pepper to taste
drizzle of garlic infused EVOO if wished

Directions:

Chop the garlic cloves finely.

Open the tin of cannellini beans and drain. In a frying pan, drizzle in about one Tbsp of the EVOO and fry the garlic gently on low heat without coloring.

Once it begins to soften, pour in the drained cannellini beans and heat gently.

The beans will start to break down on cooking. As they do so, squash them down into the pan with the back of the spoon or fork you are using. Mash them gently but so that they retain some texture.

If extra garlic pungency is desired, drizzle over a tiny dash of the garlic infused EVOO.

Taste and season carefully with salt and pepper - canned beans and pulses can be salty and may not need much seasoning.

For an extra smooth result, blitz in a food processor or hand-held blender.

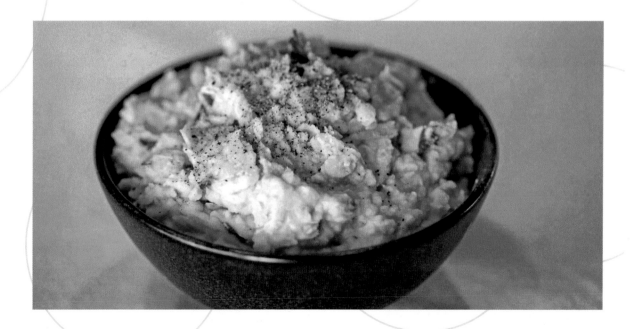

Green Rice with Smoked Paprika (E)($)

Serves: 6
Per serving: 262 Calories, 14.6g Fat, 29.3g Carbs, 3.7g Fiber, 5.4g Protein

Ingredients:

2 cups cooked brown rice
3 cups water
1/2 tsp mineral salt
1 big handful peas (fresh or frozen)
3 Tbsp arugula-shallot butter (see recipe at bottom) -
I always use EVOO
1 big handful chopped arugula
12 mint leaves - torn
a generous dusting of smoked paprika
1/2 cup toasted pine nuts (or almonds)
lemon wedges

Arugula Shallot Butter: purée 4 Tbsp EVOO, a big
handful of arugula, 1 medium shallot (peeled), and a
couple pinches of salt in a processor for at least 30
seconds - until it is no longer chunky. Add 1/2 tsp of
maple syrup if you need to balance out the flavor a bit.

Directions:

Cook brown rice in salted water until just cooked –
should be just a little chewy. (*The consistency of the
rice is important here - you don't want it too wet. Too
dry is no good either. If you need to work in a bit
more water, go for it.*)

Then stir in a big dollop of arugula butter, I start with
about 3 Tbsp, and add from there.

Stir in the arugula and mint. Season with more salt if
needed.

Serve topped with a generous dusting of smoked
paprika, plenty of nuts, and a squeeze of lemon juice if
you like.

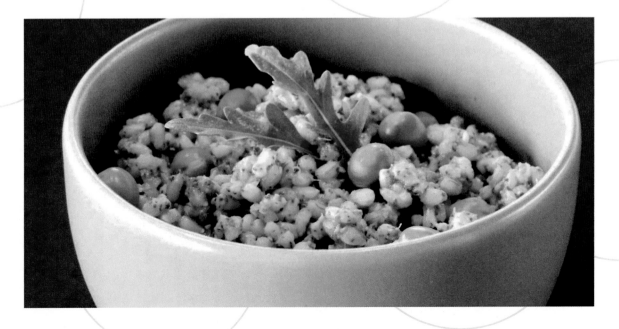

Ethiopian Cabbage with Carrots (E)($)

Per serving: 230 Calories, 13g Fat, 30g Carbs, 5.5g Fiber, 3.3 Protein

Ingredients:

1/2 cup EVOO
4 carrots - thinly sliced
1 onion - thinly sliced
1 tsp sea salt
1/2 tsp ground black pepper
1/2 tsp ground cumin
1/4 tsp ground turmeric
1/2 head cabbage - shredded
5 potatoes - peeled and cut into 1-inch cubes

Directions:

Heat the EVOO in a skillet over medium heat.

Cook the carrots and onion in the hot oil about 5 minutes.

Stir in the salt, pepper, cumin, turmeric, and potatoes and cook another 15 to 20 minutes.

Add the cabbage cover and reduce heat to medium-low and cook until potatoes are soft.

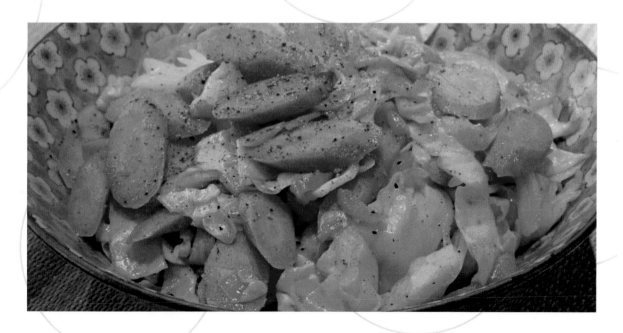

Refried Pinto Beans (Q)(E)($)

Per serving: 370 Calories, 4.7g Fat, 61.4g Carbs, 15.1g Fiber, 20.9g Protein

Ingredients:

2 cups cooked pinto beans
1 Tbsp EVOO
2 Tbsp vegetable stock
¼ cup onion – finely chopped
2 tsp garlic – chopped
¼ tsp mineral salt
¼ tsp green pepper (optional) – finely chopped

Directions:

Heat oil in pan at low-medium heat

Add onion and cook until onion Is translucent

Add remaining ingredients and cook for about 5 minutes slightly mashing as you go.

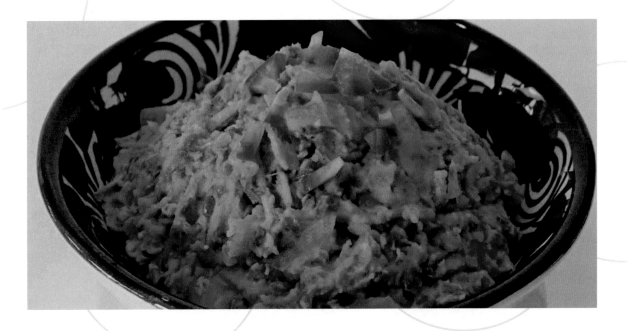

Ven Pongal (E)($)

Serves 4

Per serving: 324 Calories, 10.5g Fat, 48.5g Carbs, 4.4g Fiber, 9.3g Protein

Ingredients:

1 cup brown rice
½ cup yellow moong dal/mung dal (split moong dal)
1 tsp finely chopped ginger
¼ tsp asafoetida
1 tsp whole peppercorns
1 tsp cumin seeds
1 tsp black pepper powder
4-5 chopped curry leaves or 1 tsp mild curry powder
2 Tbsp halved cashew nuts – lightly dry toasted
2 Tbsp coconut or peanut oil
¼ tsp mineral salt

Directions:

Heat a pan on medium heat and roast the yellow moong dal until a lightly roasted aroma is released. Don't let it turn brown.

Move dal to a bowl.

Place rice in the same pan as the dal was roasted and add 4 cups of water and salt.

Cook rice for about ten minutes and then add the dal to the same pot.

Cook until both grains are just soft, you may need to add more water.

If mix is still watery, drain off excess water.

Place a small pan on medium heat; add 1 Tbsp of the oil and roast the peppercorns for a few seconds.

Add cumin seeds, ginger, curry leaves, pepper powder, asafoetida and saute for a few more seconds.

Turn off heat and set aside.

Once the rice-dal mixture is cooked; add the roasted spices to the rice-dal mixture.

Add the remaining oil and mix gently till the spices have blended well into the rice.

Sprinkle the cashews over the top and serve

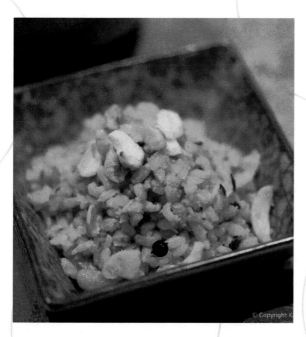

Mexican Inspired Millet (E)($)

Serves: 8

Per serving (1/8th recipe): 309 Calories, 14.3g Fat, 40.7g Carbs, 2.7g Fiber, 5.6g Protein

Ingredients:

12 ounces ripe tomatoes - chopped
1 medium white onion - chopped
3 medium jalapenos – chopped with seeds removed
2 cups brown rice
1/4 cup EVOO
4 garlic cloves - minced
2 cups vegetable broth
1 Tbsp tomato paste
¼ tsp mineral salt
1/2 cup fresh cilantro, minced
1 Tbsp lime juice

Directions:

Saute the onion in 1 Tbsp EVOO until translucent.

Blend tomatoes until smooth.

Add remaining ingredients, except for lime juice and cilantro to the pan and gently cook until millet is cooked (20 minutes or so).

Remove from pan, adjust seasonings and then add the lime and cilantro.

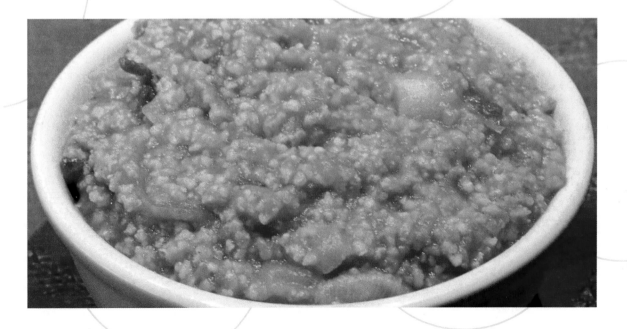

Nutty Black Rice (E)($)

Serves 4

Per serving (includes dressing and all optional nuts): 411 Calories, 22.6g Fat, 4.6g Sat. Fat, 45g Carbs, 7.6g Fiber, 12.1g Protein

Ingredients:

RICE:
2 cups cooked black rice
*All following items are optional:
½ cup unsweetened desiccated saffron coconut (Mix 1 pinch of saffron threads with 2 Tbsp warm water and mix into the coconut till you have some orange and white coconut)
¼ cup toasted almonds
¼ cup toasted cashews
¼ cup toasted pumpkin seeds
2 Tbsp sesame seeds
2 Tbsp chia seeds
2 Tbsp hemp seeds
1 Tbsp grated orange zest

DRESSING
2 Tbsp EVOO
1 tsp sesame oil
1/3 cup orange juice
1 Tbsp Orange flower water
½ tsp dry mustard
1 tsp poppy seeds

Directions:

RICE

Mix all ingredients together, except for the coconut and reserving a few nuts and some orange zest for the topping

DRESSING:

Whisk together.

Mix dressing with the rice mix

Finish by sprinkling the coconut over the top and sprinkling the remaining nuts and orange zest on top.

Great with a big mixed vegetable salad.

Can be served warm or cold

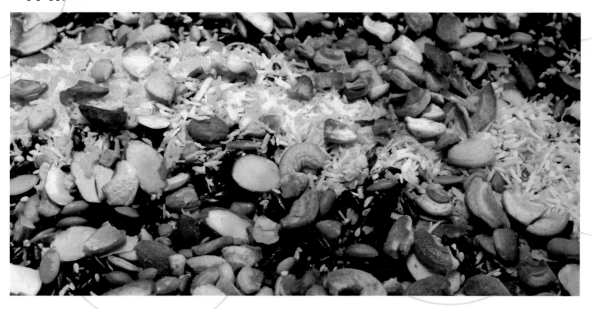

Brown Rice Peas and Saffron (E)($)
Serves: 2
Per serving: 409 Calories, 2.8g Fat, 84.2g Carbs, 7.2g Fiber

Ingredients:

2 cups cooked brown rice
1 cup fresh green peas
1 pinch of saffron threads – steeped in ¼ cup warm
water
¼ cup finely chopped white onion
¼ tsp mineral salt

Directions:

Steam the green peas for a couple of minutes until just bright green.

Mix all ingredients together leave for the flavors to combine for about an hour and serve warm.

Reheat by gently sautéing in a pan – you can add a little extra water if necessary.

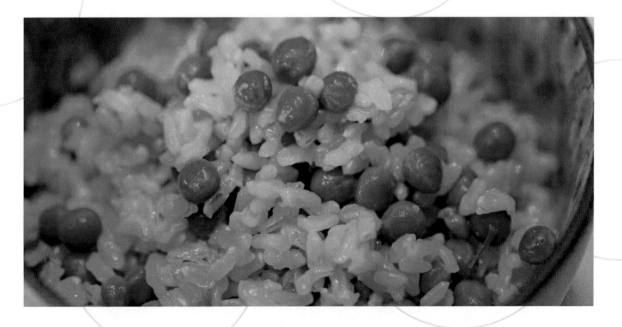

Peas Be With You (E)($)

Serves: 8

Per serving: 327 Calories, 4.8g Fat, 62.9g Carbs, 6.1g Fiber, 10.2g Protein

Ingredients:

2 cups cooked brown Rice
1 cup frozen green peas - thawed
1 cup fresh sugar snap peas or snow peas
1 cup pea sprouts
2 cups spearmint leaves
1/2 tsp mineral salt - chop together until they are a fine paste
1 brown onion - finely chopped
1 Tbsp EVOO
2 cloves garlic - chopped
1 cup vegetable stock
1 cup raw lemon cashew cheese - optional

Directions:

Saute onion in EVOO in medium saute pan on medium-low for a few minutes until translucent.

Add garlic and cook another 2 minutes

Add in the cooked rice and mint mixture - stir well.

Add the rest of the ingredients and stir until warmed.

Serve with cashew cheese if desired.

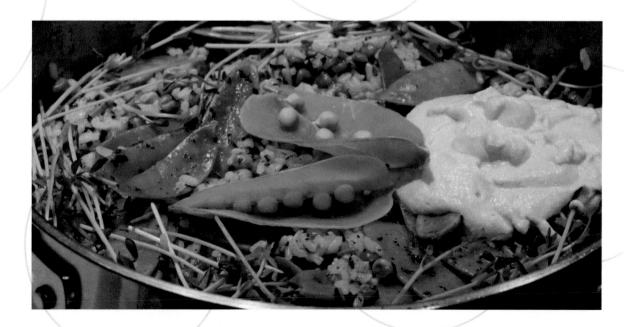

Peas Rice and Roasted Tomatoes (E)
Serves: 2
Per serving: 428 Calories, 3.1g Fat, 88.3g Carbs, 8.3g Fiber, 12.2g Protein

Ingredients:

2 cups cooked brown rice
1 cup fresh green peas
1 pinch of saffron threads – steeped in ¼ cup warm water
¼ cup finely chopped white onion
¼ tsp Mineral salt
1 tsp dried rosemary
¼ cup sundried tomatoes

Directions:

Steam the green peas for a couple of minutes until just bright green.

Mix all ingredients, except for the sundried together leave for the flavors to combine for about an hour and serve warm.

Reheat by gently sautéing in a pan – you can add a little extra water if necessary.

Top with the sundried tomatoes.

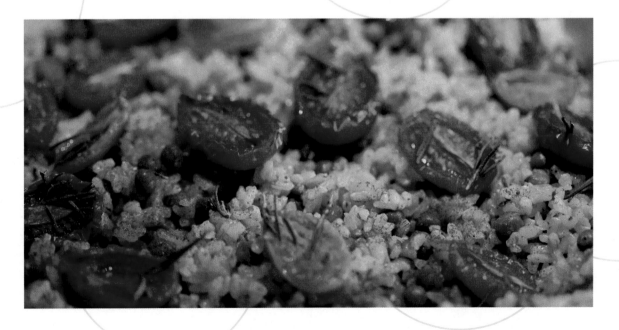

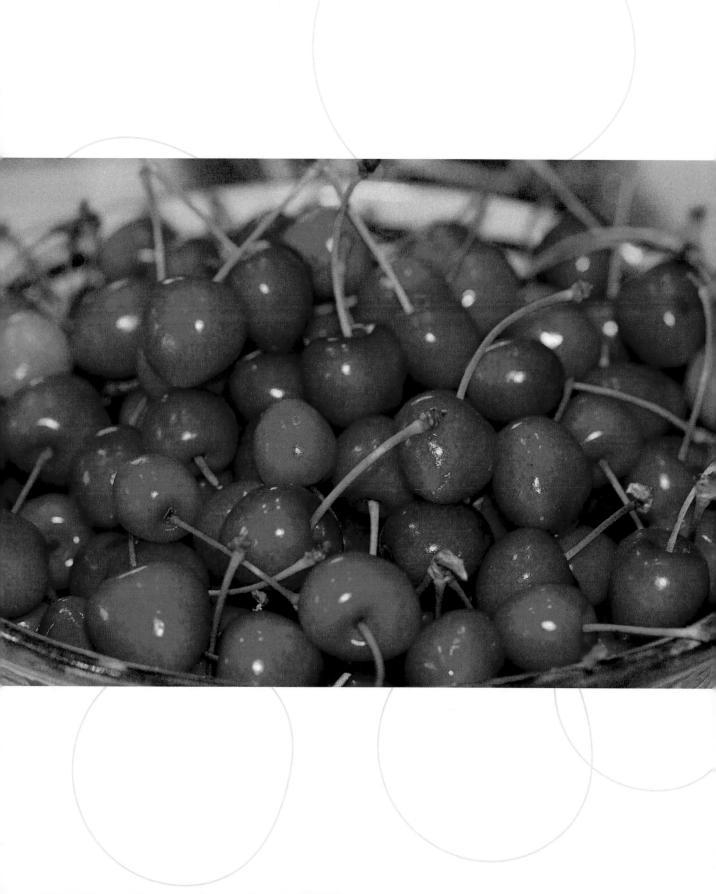

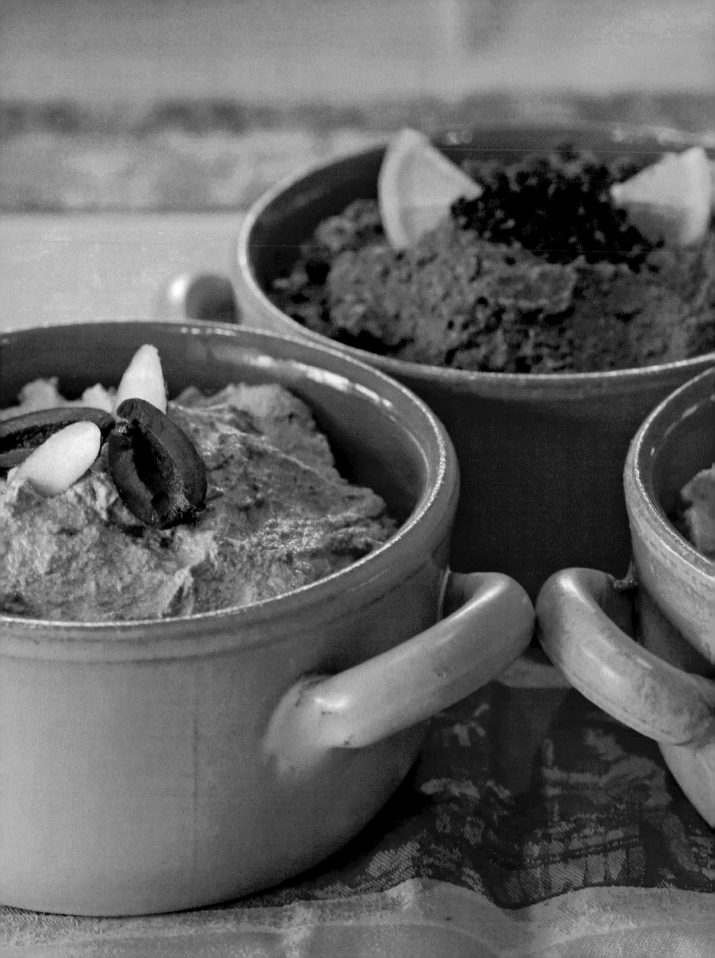

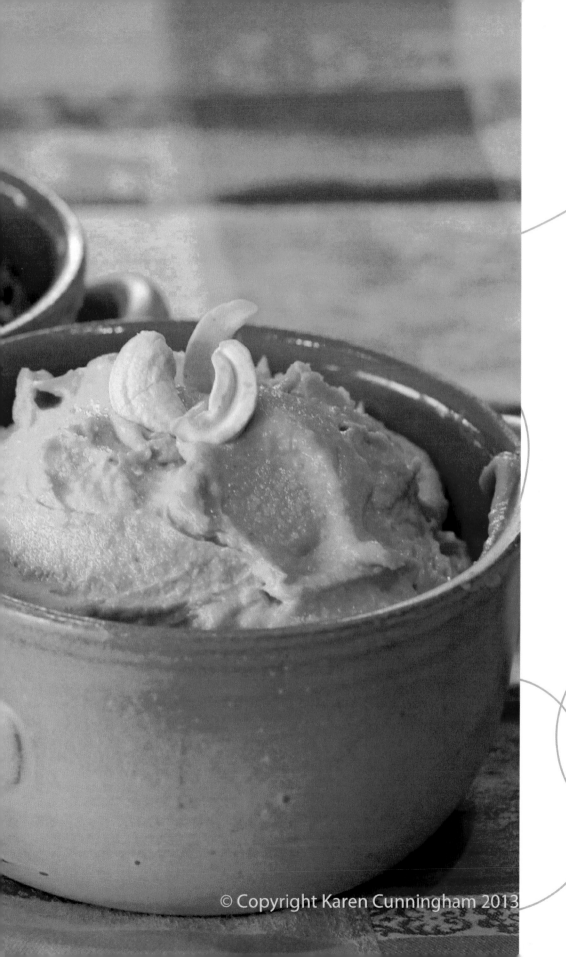

Dips, Dressings and Sauces

Midnight Hummus (E)($)

Per serving (~3 Tbsp): 90 Calories, 4.5g Fat, 0.6g Sat. Fat, 10g Carbs, 3g Fiber, 4g Protein

Ingredients:

3 medium cloves garlic, peeled
2 cups beluga lentils (or black beans), cooked
1/4 cup black sesame tahini
or 1 cup whole black sesame seeds – you will need
more water
1/3 cup EVOO
juice of ½ lemon or more to taste
2 tsp ground cumin
1/4 tsp salt or more to taste
fresh ground black pepper to taste
Chopped fresh tomatoes or peppers for decoration
and delight

Note:
Having trouble finding beluga lentils? Black beans
make a great substitute.

Directions:

Place garlic into your food processor and pulse until
finely minced.

Add the remaining ingredients and process for 1
minute.

Scrape down the sides of the food processor. Taste
and adjust for lemon juice, salt, and pepper. Process
until well combined and smooth.

Serve this versatile hummus on whole grain crackers,
as a dip for crisp vegetable crudités scattered with
white sesame seeds, or spread inside of a warm pita
with a slice of tomato, sprinkle of feta cheese – and
maybe a few mint leaves.

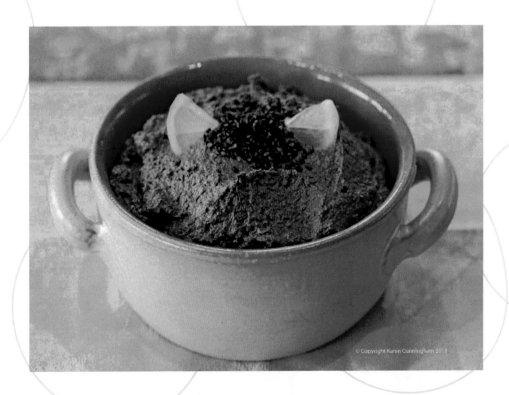

Mediterranean Olive Dip ($)(E)

Per serving (2 Tbsp): 87 Calories, 8.4g Fat, 0.9g Sat Fat, 2.6g Carbs, 1.3g Fiber, 2g Protein

Ingredients:

1 1/2 cups raw almonds – soaked in water for two hours
1/2 cup salt cured pitted olives or kalamata olives
2 cloves garlic
2 Tbsp Lime Juice
1/4 cup EVOO
3/4 cup water
1 Tsp dried oregano
1/4 Tsp ground coriander
1/4 Tsp white pepper (black will do)

Directions:

Blend in high speed blender and enjoy

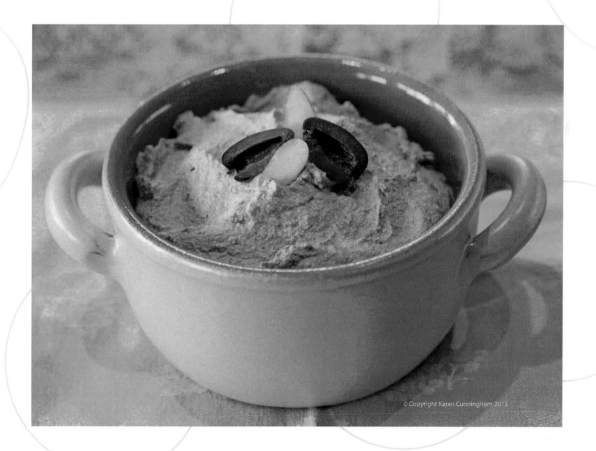

© Copyright Karen Cunningham 2013

Beet Hummus (E)($)

Per Serving (~2 Tbsp): 90 Calories, 4.5g Fat, 0.6g Sat. Fat, 10g Carbs, 3g Fiber, 4g Protein

Ingredients:

3 medium sized beets about the size of tennis balls
1/2 cup tahini
4 cloves of garlic
1-2 Tbsp lemon juice
sea salt to taste (I usually leave this out)
4 Tbsp EVOO
pinch of ground cumin
chopped flat leaf parsley to garnish

Directions:

Steam uncut beets for about 50 minutes or until a skewer penetrates the beet without too much resistance.

Let beets cool to handle, then peel with your fingers (I use gloves) . The skins should slip off very easily

purée all ingredients.

Check for seasoning then pour into a serving bowl and garnish with the chopped parsley and a light drizzle of EVOO.

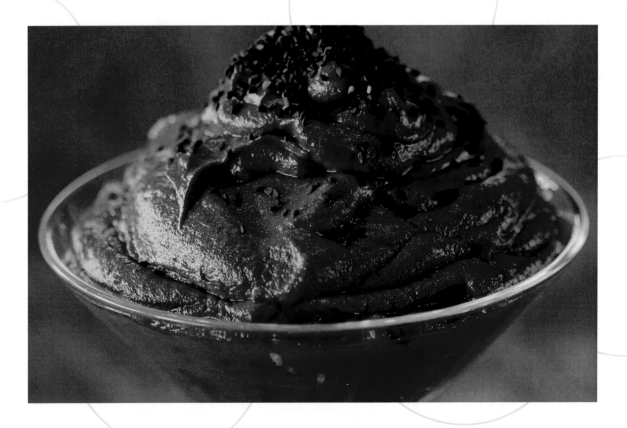

Bessara (Fava Bean Hummus)(E)($)

Per serving (30g ~2 Tbsp) 88 Calories, 2.7g Fat, 11.6g Carbs, 5g Fiber, 5g Protein

Ingredients:

1 1/2 cups (about 8 oz. or 200 g) cooked fava beans
3 cloves garlic
2 Tbsp EVOO
1/4 cup lemon juice
2 Tbsp (or more) reserved cooking liquid
1/2 tsp salt
fresh ground pepper
1 tsp ground cumin
1 tsp turmeric
1/2 tsp cinnamon
1/2 tsp sweet paprika
1/2 tsp hot paprika or cayenne pepper
pinch ground cloves

Directions:

Blend as you would for Hummus.

Note:
I do this in two batches. One I leave a little chunky and the other smooth, then I mix them together.

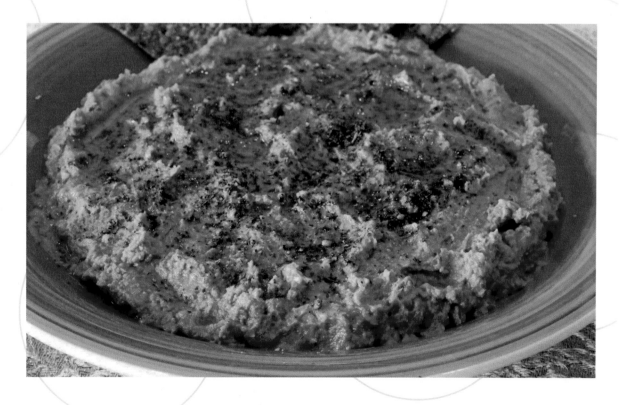

Spinach Basil Parsley Pesto (R)(E)($)
Makes ~ 1 cup
Per serving (¼ cup): 53 Calories, 5.3g Fat, 1.3g Carbs, 0.6g Fiber 0.9g Protein

Ingredients;

1 cup each of spinach, , basil and parsley
1/4 cup lemon juice
2 Tbsp pine nuts
2 cloves garlic
1 Tbsp nutritional yeast
¼ cup EVOO

Directions:

Blend and enjoy over your favorite pasta, as a dip for vegetables or over any simple vegetable dish.

NOTE:
Cannot be frozen.

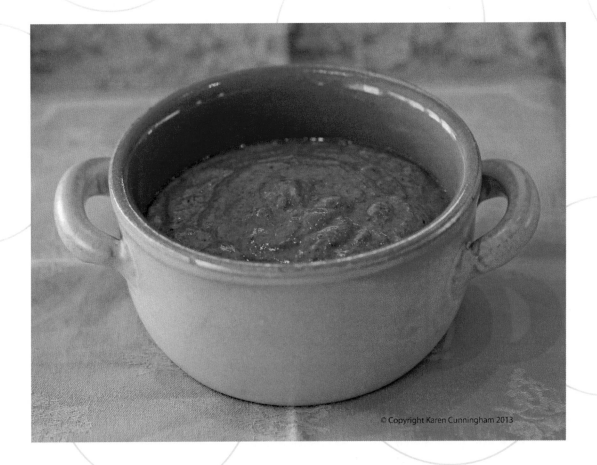

Walnut Pesto (R)(E)($)

Makes ~ 1 cup

Per serving (¼ cup): 95 Calories, 9.6g Fat, 1.3g Carbs, 0.8g Fiber, 2.5g Protein

Ingredients:

1 cup raw walnuts
1 cup fresh basil
1 cup fresh spinach
zest of 1 lemon
2 Tbsp lemon juice
2 (or more or less) garlic gloves
1/4 cup olive oil
extra water to help blending or make a thinner pesto
for pouring

Directions:

Blend and enjoy over raw or cooked pastas, as a topping for an appetizer or over any vegetable.

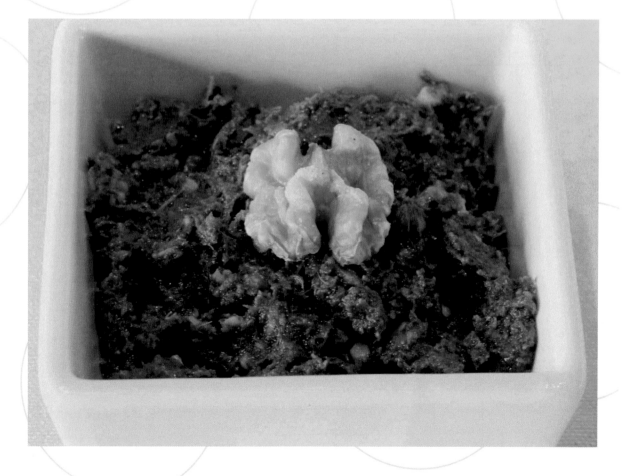

Teriyaki Sauce (E)($)
Per ¼ cup: 54 Calories, 0.8g Fat, 11.6g Carbs, 2.9g Protein

Ingredients:

1/2 cup wheat free Tamari sauce
1 cup orange juice
1 tsp pomegranate concentrate
1 Tbsp minced garlic
1 Tbsp minced ginger
1 tsp sesame oil

Directions:

Mix and use for stir fry's

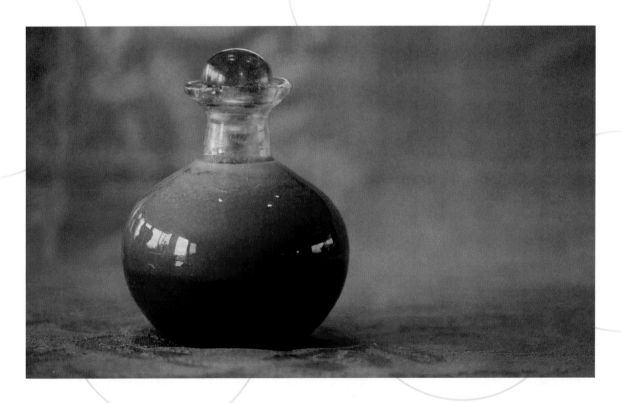

Lemon Dill Sauce (E)($)(R)

Serves: 8
Per serving: 66 Calories, 4.8g Fat, 3.8g Carbs, 2.1g Protein

Ingredients:

1/2 cup cashew cheese (without pimentos)
3 Tbsp lemon juice
2 tsp apple cider vinegar
1/4 tsp ground pepper white of black
3 Tbsp water
3 Tbsp finely chopped fresh dill (or 1 Tbsp dry dill–
you will need to let the recipe sit for 1/2 hour if you
use dried dill)
2 cloves crushed garlic
salt to taste

Directions:

Mix and adjust any of the ingredients to your taste.

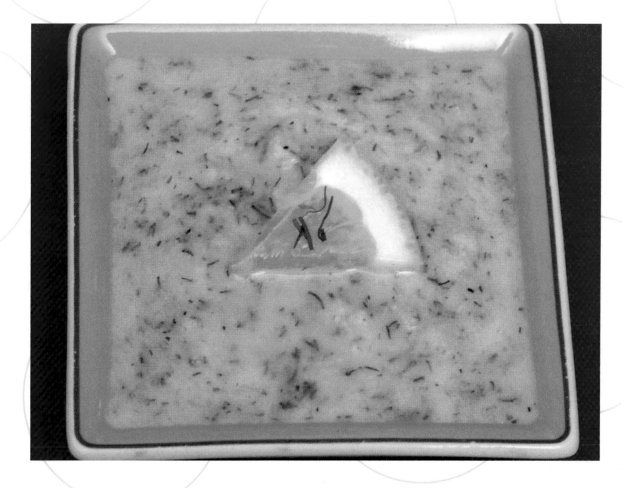

Pumpkin Seed Sauce (E)($)

Makes: ~ 2 cups
Per serving (1/4th recipe): 219 Calorie, 21g Fat, 5.2g Carbs, 0.8g Fiber, 5.3g Protein

Ingredients:

1 bunch cilantro
1/2 cup cashew sour crème (see page 238)
1/2 cup raw pumpkin seeds
2 Tbsp EVOO
2 cloves garlic
1 1/2 tsp mineral salt
1 serrano chile - seeded and inner ribs removed
1 jalapeno chile - seeded and inner ribs removed
1/2 cup of water

Directions:

Blend cilantro, cashew sour crème, EVOO, garlic, mineral salt and chiles in a food processor.

In a medium sauté pan over medium heat, toast the pumpkin seeds until they pop and turn slightly golden, 8 to 10 minutes; do not let them brown.

Set aside briefly to allow to cool.

Add pumpkin seeds and water to the mixer and blend to a smooth paste.

*Great served over your favorite vegetables or serve as a dip.

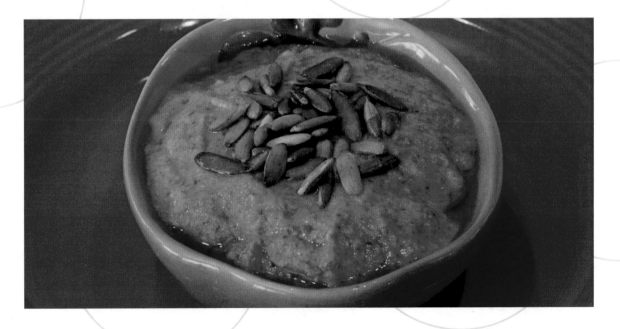

Cilantro Garlic Dipping Sauce (E)($)

Per serving: 102 calories, 8g fat, 6.2g Carbs, 0.6g fiber, 2.8g protein

Ingredients:

1/2 Wildwood Garlic Aioli
1/8 cup water
1/2 cup cilantro

Directions:

Blend and use liberally over veggies.

Note:
This is a Vegan dish but has some calories.

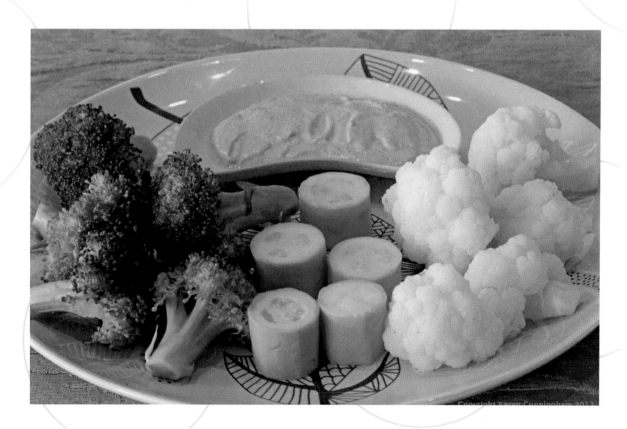

Artichoke and Olive Pesto (E)(Q)

Serves: 3
Per serving: 81 Calories, 2.4g Fat, 12.2g Carbs, 5.6g Fiber, 2.8g Protein

Ingredients:

1 23 oz jar of artichoke hearts in water
5 cloves of garlic (less if you are not a garlic lover)
1/2 cup of mixed, pitted olives - try to use olives that
are fresh – red, black and green
1/4 cup EVOO
3 Tbsp Meyer lemon juice*
1 tsp date purée (see page 304)
salt and pepper to taste

*Meyer lemons are naturally sweeter but a regular
lemon will work

Directions:

Chop all ingredients finely mix and serve over your
favorite pasta.

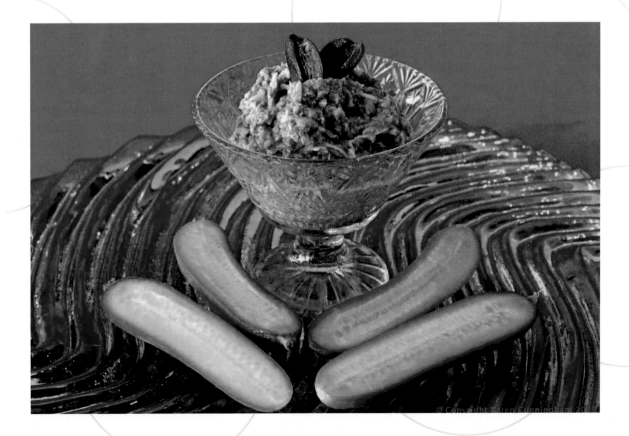

Korean Barbecue Sauce (E)($)(Q)

Serves: 6

Per serving (~2 Tbsp) 37 Calories, 0.5g Fat, 7.4g Carbs, 0.6g Fiber, 0.8g protein

Ingredients:

1 tsp ginger - minced
1 clove garlic, - pressed
1 tsp chile pepper - minced
1/4 cup tamari sauce
1 Tbsp apple cider vinegar
1 Tbsp date purée (see page 304)
2 Tbsp water
1/3 cup unsweetened apple sauce
1/8 tsp red pepper flakes
1/4 tsp sesame oil
1 tsp toasted sesame seeds

Directions:

Place all ingredients except the sesame seeds into a small saucepan and bring to a boil over medium-high heat.

Reduce the heat to very low and simmer until partially reduced, about 15 minutes.

Remove from heat and add sesame seeds. Sauce should thicken as it cools.

To use, warm slightly and serve over vegetables and tofu.

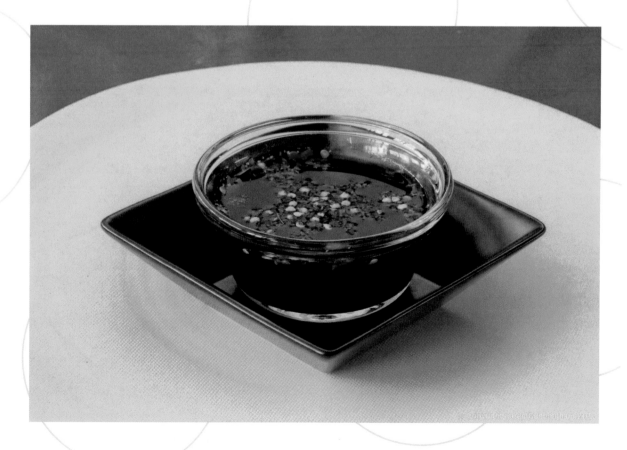

Spicy Almond Sauce (E)($)(Q)
Per Tbsp (~10g) 48 Calories, 5g Fat, 0.8g Carbs, 0.4g Protein

Ingredients:

1 cup toasted almond slices, plus extra for garnish
2 cloves garlic
1 Tbsp sambal oelek
1 tsp Bragg's Liquid Amino
Juice of 3 limes
1/2 packed cup Thai basil leaves
1 cup EVOO
Water to thin, if needed
mineral salt and freshly ground black pepper

Directions:

In a sauté pan over medium heat, toast almond slices just until aromatic, about 3-5 minutes, flipping pan to distribute almonds.

Remove almonds to a sheet of parchment paper.

In a blender, combine garlic, sambal, lime juice, almonds, and Thai basil.

Blend at high speed until almost smooth. Drizzle in the oil and season with salt and freshly ground black pepper to taste.

If sauce is too thick, add a touch of water to thin.

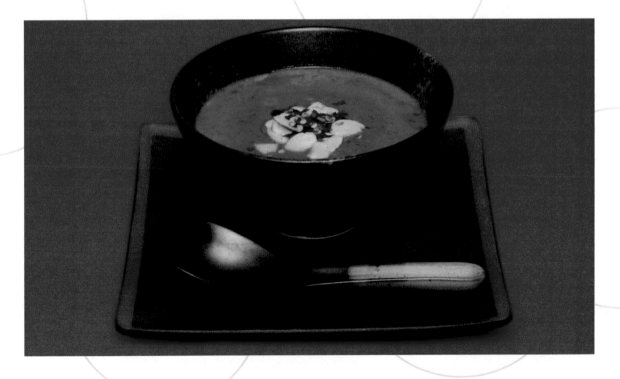

Orange Ginger Stir Fry Sauce (E)($)(Q)(R)
Makes ~ 1 1/2 Cup
Entire sauce: 73 Calories, 0.2g Fat, 43.5g Carbs, 3g Fiber, 1.4g Protein

Ingredients:

1/4 cup Bragg's Amino Acid
2 whole medium oranges - peeled
4 clove garlic
1 inch piece of ginger - peeled
2 pitted medjool date

Directions:

Blend until smooth.

*Can serve as a sauce over stir fry or a dip or as a salad dressing.

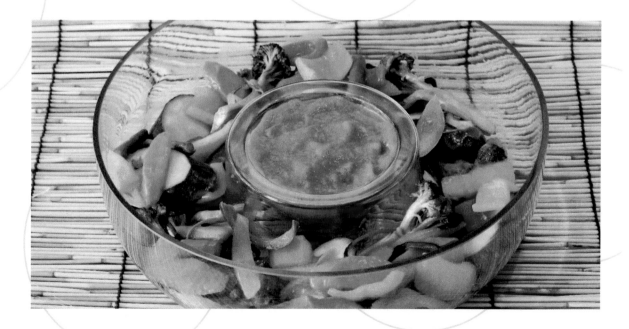

Coconut Chutney (E)(Q)(R)($)

Makes 2 cups

Per serving (1/4 cup): 79 Calories, 6.8g Fat, 4.7g Carbs, 2g Fiber, 0.8g Protein

Ingredients:

Grind together:
1 ½ cups unsweetened desiccated coconut
6-8 chilies or according to your spice level
1 small white onion
1" piece of fresh ginger

For Seasoning:
1 Small white onion - sliced
2 dry red chilies- ground
½ tsp mustard seeds
3 curry leaves (or 1 tsp mild curry powder)
1 Tbsp coconut oil

Directions:

Grind coconut, chilies, small onion and ginger to a coarse paste - adding little water if needed.

Heat oil in a pan, when hot add mustard seeds and allow to splutter.

Add small onion and stir fry until brown.

Add red chilies, curry leaves and fry for a minute.

Lower the heat and add ground coconut mixture and salt.

Stir and heat the mixture until hot, but do not boil.

Turn off the heat and serve.

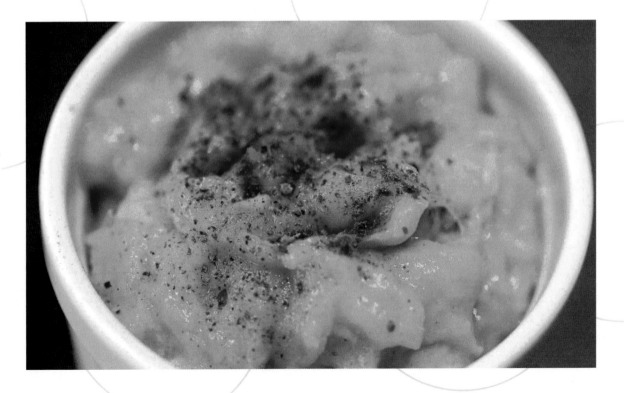

Mango Chutney (E)(Q)(R)($)

Per serving: 73 Calories, 0.7g Fat, 18g Carbs, 2.2g Fiber, 0.7g Protein

2 firm ripe medium mangoes
2 pinches of salt
2 tsp lemon juice
1 tsp apple cider vinegar
2 tsp minced fresh ginger
1 tsp ground cumin

Chop one mango and set aside.
Blend all remaining ingredients in a high-power blender.
Add the diced mango to the blender and blend on low for a few seconds.

Nectarine Chutney (E)(Q)(R)($)

per serving (~2 Tbsp) 42 calories, 1.4g fat, 7.7g Carbs, 1.3g fiber, 0.8g protein

Ingredients:

6 nectarines or peaches or a mix cut into 1 inch chunks
1/2 tsp ground cinnamon
1/8 tsp chipotle chili powder
1 tsp onion flakes
1/8 tsp smoked paprika
1 Tbsp peanut or grapeseed oil to coat the fruit

Directions:

Arrange on a baking dish and roast at 350 degrees for about 20 minutes

Serve over everything – rice, vegetables, tempeh, beans

Parsley Nut Crème Spread (E)(Q)(R)($)

Per Tbsp: 24 Calories, 2.2g Fat, 0.3g Carbs, 0.6g Protein

Ingredients:

1/2 cup brazil nuts
1/4 cup sunflower seeds
handful of fresh parsley
clove garlic
lemon juice
salt, pepper
(water)

Directions:

Blend brazil nuts and seeds, add lemon juice, garlic clove , salt and pepper.

Blend until smooth.

If you like, you can also throw in the parsley. This will lend the spread a light green color. Alternatively, you can finely chop the parsley and mix it in with a spoon.

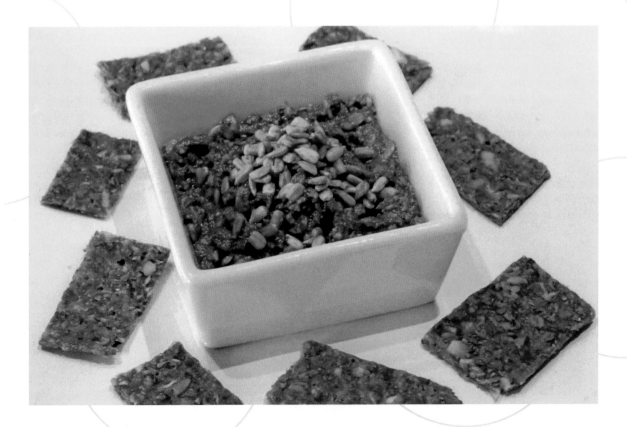

Chestnut Purée (Gravy) (E)

Per serving (~1/2 cup) 105 Calories, 4.2g Fat, 15.4g Carbs, 0.7g Fiber, 1.7g Protein

Ingredients:

1 small onion - diced
1 cup carrots - finely chopped
1/2 stick celery - finely chopped
2 Tbsp EVOO
8 oz vacuum-packed whole roasted chestnuts (1 1/2 cups)
1 1/2 cups organic Low Sodium vegetable broth
1 tsp fresh thyme (1/4 tsp dried)

Directions:

Sauté first three veggies over low heat until lightly browned in EVOO (~ 10 min)

Add the chestnut and stock and simmer gently for 8-10 minutes

Purée and serve as a gravy or add more stock and have as a soup.

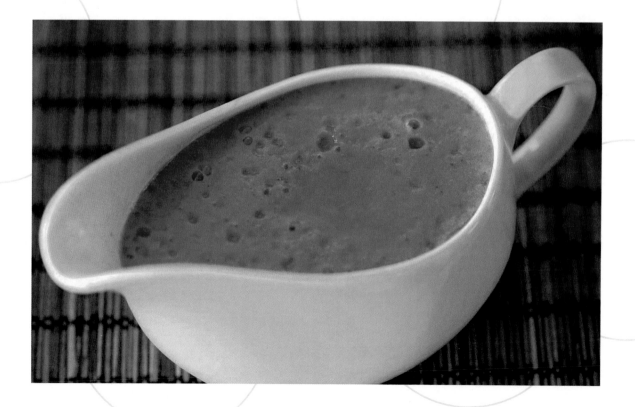

No Bean Hummus (E)(Q)(R)($)
Per 3 tbsp: 115 Calories, 10g Fat, 4g Carbs, 1.6g Fiber, 2.6g Protein

Ingredients:

2 zucchini - peeled and chopped
3/4 cup raw tahini
1/2 cup fresh lemon juice
1/4 cup EVOO
4 garlic cloves
1 tsp sea salt
1/2 tsp ground cumin

Directions:

Blend and enjoy.

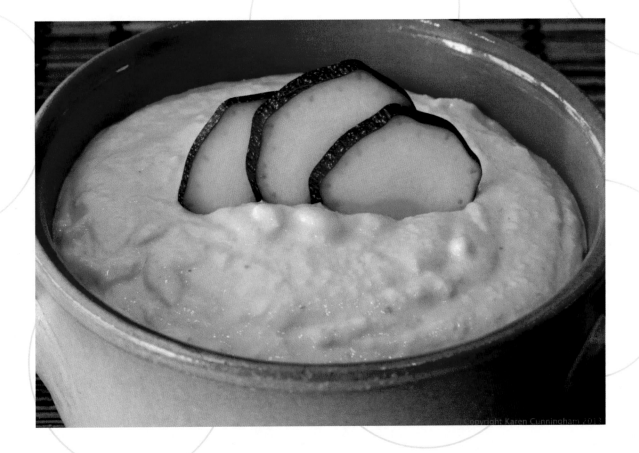

White Bean Alfredo (E)(Q)(R)($)
Per 1/2 cup: 268 Calories, 9g Fat, 35g Carbs, 9g Fiber 13.7g Protein

Ingredients:

1/4 cup EVOO
2 cloves garlic - minced
2 cup cooked white beans - rinsed and drained
1 to 1-1/2 cup unsweetened almond milk
Salt and pepper to taste
Parsley and/or spinach (optional)

Directions:

In a saute pan over low heat, add EVOO. Add the garlic and cook for 2 to 3 minutes.

Transfer the mixture to a blender or food processor; add the white beans and 1 cup of almond milk.

Blend until completely smooth. If the sauce is too thick, add the remaining almond milk until you reach the desired consistency.

Pour the sauce back into the pan over low heat, season with salt and pepper to taste.

Add fresh vegetables and herbs, such as parsley and spinach, if desired.

Warm and serve.

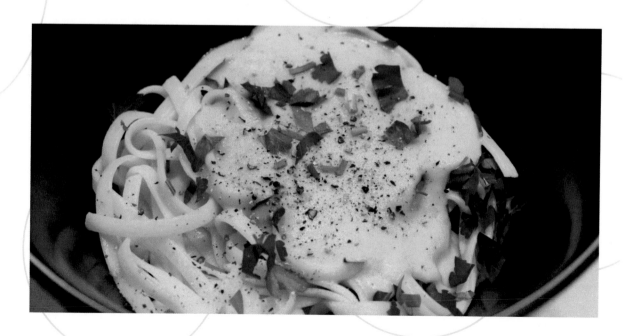

Sweet Tomato Sauce (E)(Q)(R)($)
Serves:2
Per serving: 131 Calories, 1.1g Fat, 29.3g Carbs, 8.1g Fiber, 6.8g Protein

Ingredients:

2 fresh tomatoes
1 orange -peeled
4-5 fresh basil leaves
1 garlic clove
pinch of mineral salt
fresh pepper to taste

Directions:

Place orange, garlic and tomatoes into your food processor and blend until completely smooth.

Add in spices and basil and pulse.

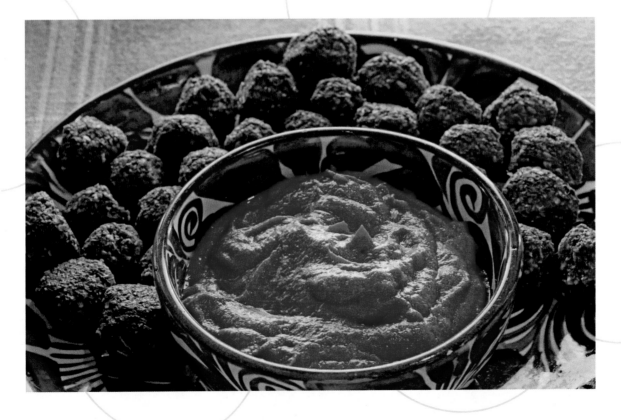

Mango Habañero Barbecue Sauce (E)(Q)(R)($)

Entire recipe: 416 Calories, 16.2g Fat, 75.8g Carbs, 8.8g Fiber, 3.3g Protein

Ingredients:

2 ripe mangoes – peeled and sliced
2 tsp garlic – minced
1 Tbsp – EVOO
¼ tsp mineral salt
1 small habañero pepper – deseeded and chopped finely or ¼ - ½ tsp habañero powder

Directions:

Blend all ingredients and enjoy with your favorite burgers, patties or drizzled over steamed vegetables.

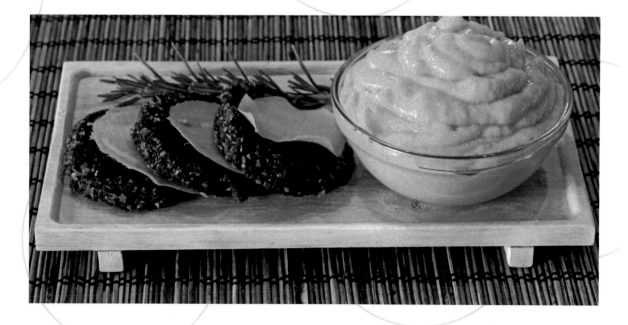

Alfredo Sauce (E)($)
Per serving (~ 1/8th recipe): 71 Calories, 5.1g Fat, 4g Carbs, 1g Fiber, 3g Protein

Ingredients:

2 cloves garlic - minced
1 tsp EVOO
2 cups cauliflower - roughly chopped
1 cup parsnip - roughly chopped
½ cup roughly chopped parsley root, or additional parsnip
1 Tbsp apple cider vinegar
1½ cups non-dairy milk
½ cup nutritional yeast
2 tsp gluten-free Dijon mustard
1 Tbsp fresh lemon juice
Freshly ground pepper, to taste
Sea salt, to taste

Directions:

Add minced garlic and EVOO to a medium saucepan and saute on medium/high heat for 1 minute. Add chopped cauliflower, parsnip and parsley root.

Continue to cook for 1 minute.

Add apple cider vinegar, continue to cook for 2 minutes.

Add non-dairy milk, cover and bring to boil. Reduce heat and simmer covered for 6-7 minutes, until vegetables are soft.

Pour cooked vegetable mix into the bowl of your food processor or blender. Add remaining ingredients and purée until ultra smooth, about 2 minutes.

NOTE:
If you do not have access to parsnips or parsley root, I'm sure additional cauliflower could be used.

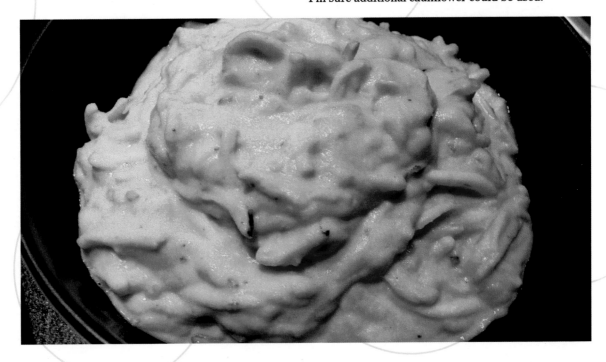

Ketchup (R)($)(E)

Per Tbsp: 35 Calories, 3g Fat, 2.5g Carbs, 1.3g Fiber, 0.3g Protein

Ingredients:

1 1/2 cups of diced tomatoes
3 Tbsp dates (do not soak)
1/4 cup EVOO
1 tsp mineral salt
1 Tbsp apple cider vinegar
1 cup sun dried tomatoes

*Variation – add 1.2 tsp smoked paprika for a smoky
sauce or ½ - 1 tsp chili peppers for a spicy sauce

Directions:

Blend in a high speed blender.

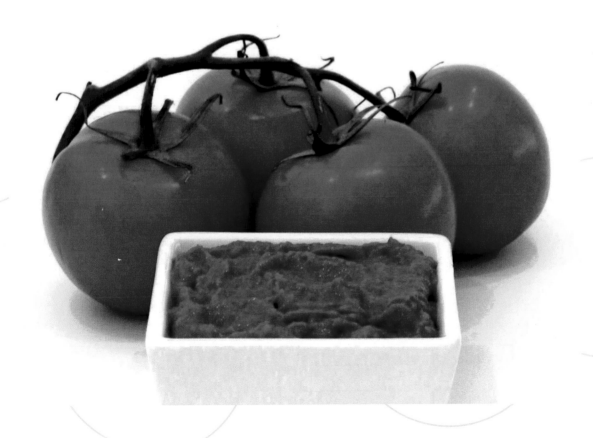

Spicy Peanut Ginger Sauce (E)(Q)(R)($)

Entire recipe: 815 Calories, 70g Fat, 34g Carbs, 5.3 Fiber, 18g Protein

Ingredients:

3 cloves of garlic - crushed
2 Tbsp sesame oil
1/3 cup peanut butter
1 Tbsp fresh ginger - grated
3 Tbsp of lemon or lime juice
1 Tbsp of tamari
2 medium soft dates - pitted
1 tsp of water
¼ tsp Smoked Paprika
Powdered or wet chile spice to suit your taste

Directions:

Blend.

Spicy Almond Ginger Sauce (E)(Q)(R)($)

Per Tbsp: 48 Calories, 5g Fat, 0.8g Carbs, 0.4g Protein

Ingredients:

3 cloves of garlic - crushed
2 Tbsp sesame oil
1/3 cup almond butter
1 Tbsp fresh ginger - grated
3 Tbsp of lemon or lime juice
1 Tbsp of tamari
2 medium soft dates - pitted
1 tsp of water
¼ tsp Smoked Paprika
Powdered or wet chile spice to suit your taste

Directions:

Blend

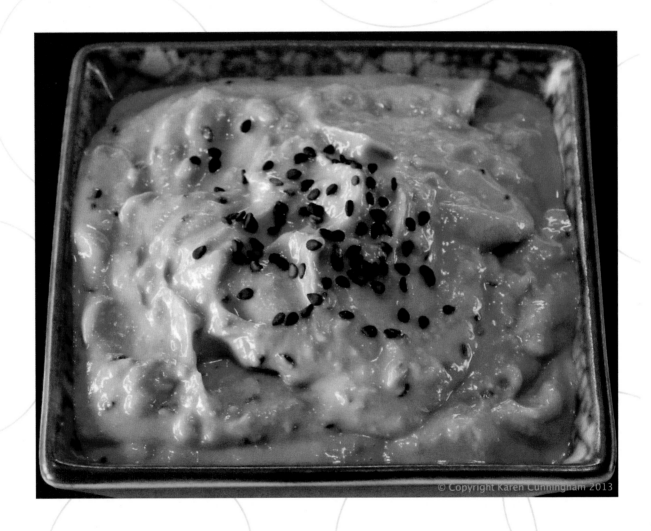

Romesco Sauce (E)(Q)(R)($)

Makes: 2 1/1 cups
Per serving (1/4 cup): 127 Calories, 11.3g Fat, 6.4g Carbs, 1.1g Fiber, 1.5g Protein

Ingredients:

4 medium-size ripe tomatoes (1-3/4 lb. total) - chopped
1 head garlic - sliced in half crosswise
2 Tbsp plus 1/3 cup EVOO
1/4 cup blanched almonds
1/4 cup peeled hazelnuts
1 dried ancho chile - cored, seeded, slit, and opened so it lies fairly flat
1 tsp Mineral salt
2 to 3 Tbsp lime juice
2 Tbsp Pomegranate concentrate

Directions:

Heat the oven to 375°F. Put the tomatoes and one half of the garlic head in a baking pan.

Drizzle about 1 Tbsp. of the olive oil into the cored tomato wells and on top of the garlic half. Roast until the tomatoes and garlic are well caramelized but not burnt, about 90 minutes.

From the remaining half head of garlic, coarsely chop 1 Tbsp garlic and put it in a food processor.

While the tomatoes roast, heat about 1 Tbsp. of the olive oil in a small sauté pan over medium heat. Toast the almonds and hazelnuts in the pan, shaking the pan or stirring so they don't burn, until golden brown, 5 to 6 minutes. Cool the nuts on a paper towel and then put them in the food processor.

Sear chili in the same small pan over medium-high heat (keep it flat with a spatula or a fork) until a smoke wisp appears, about 10 seconds per side. Soak it in 1 cup hot tap water until soft, about 15 minutes. Drain and put the chile in the food processor.

Start with the toasted nuts, chile, and tomatoes to get the purée underway.
Pour in olive oil slowly to create an emulsified sauce, add lime juice and then taste the romesco before making adjustments.

When the tomatoes and garlic are caramelized, let them cool. Pinch off the tomato skins (discard them) and squeeze out the garlic pulp. Put the tomatoes and garlic pulp in the processor. Add the salt and start the processor, pouring in the remaining 1/3 cup olive oil in a slow, steady stream. Then add the Pomegranate concentrate. Add salt to taste. Process the romesco until it comes together as a sauce but not so much as to lose its coarse, nutty texture. The sauce should be thick and creamy. If it seems too thick, add 1 or 2 Tbsp. red wine. If it's too thin, add bread, pulsing a few more times.

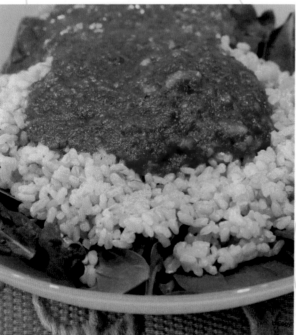

Zucchini Salsa (E)(Q)(R)($)
Per serving: 32 Calories, 0.3g Fat, 6.8g Carbs, 1.8g Fiber, 1.3g Protein

Ingredients:

1 cup seeded tomatoes - chopped
1/2 cup zucchini – small dice
1 stick celery – chopped small
1/2 cup sweet red bell pepper - chopped
1 small onion – small dice
½ cup parsley – roughly chopped
2 tsp lime juice
2 tsp apple cider vinegar
1 tsp seeded jalapeno pepper – fine dice
1 garlic clove - minced
1/2 tsp ground cumin
1/8 tsp mineral salt
1/8 tsp ground black pepper

Options: any vegetable that you like can be added –
just chop the pieces quite small so that they will
absorb all the flavors here

Directions:

Mix gently

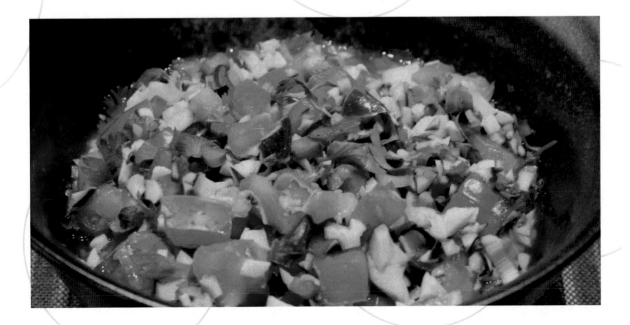

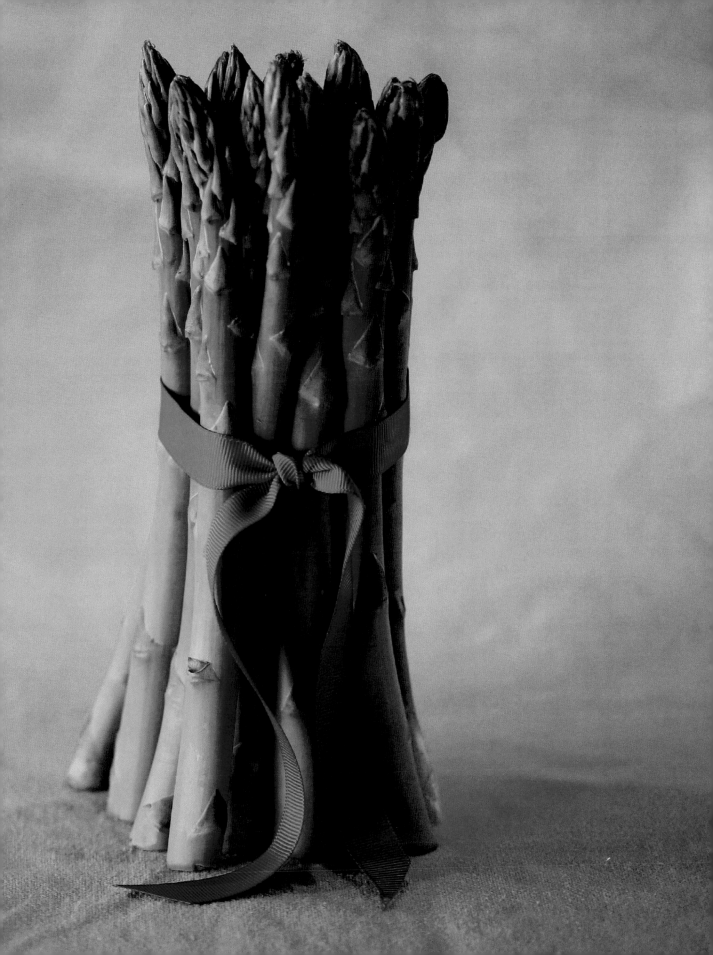

Emmett's Salsa (E)(Q)(R)($)
Serves: 4
Per serving: 96 Calories, 7.5g Fat, 7.9g Carbs, 4.4g Fiber, 1.7g Protein

Ingredients:

2 medium sized tomatoes - chopped
1/2 small red onion - chopped
1 avocado – peeled, seeded and chopped
½ cup cilantro – finely chopped
1 Tbsp lime juice
2 Peppers (optional) Jalapeno or Habañero

Mix and enjoy!

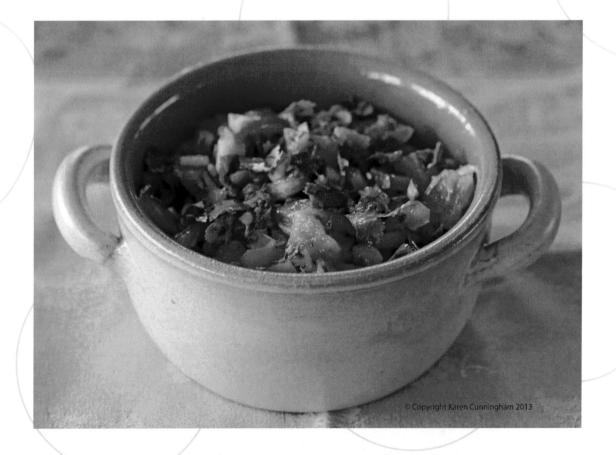

© Copyright Karen Cunningham 2013

Classic Salsa Verde (E)(Q)($)
Per serving (1/6 recipe): 51 Calories, 1.3g Fat, 10g Carbs, 3g Fiber, 1.5g Protein

Ingredients:

1 1/2 lbs tomatillos
½ medium red onion - chopped
1-2 jalapeño chile peppers, or 2-3 serrano chili peppers (include the seeds if you want the heat, remove them if you don't want the heat), stems discarded - chopped
2 (or more) cloves garlic – chopped
1 Tbsp fresh Oregano – chopped (or 1 tsp dried)
½ tsp ground cumin
¼ tsp mineral salt
1 tsp date purée (see page 304)
2 Tbsp lime (or lemon) juice
¼ cup cilantro – chopped fine

Directions:

Remove the papery husks from the tomatillos and rinse well.

Cut the tomatillos in half and place them cut-side down on lined roasting pan.

Broil for 5-7 minutes until blackened in spots.

Let cool enough to handle.

Place the tomatillos, any juice they have released, chili peppers, garlic, salt, lime juice, onion and date purée in a blender, and pulse until well blended.

Stir in the cilantro and enjoy

** Can be frozen

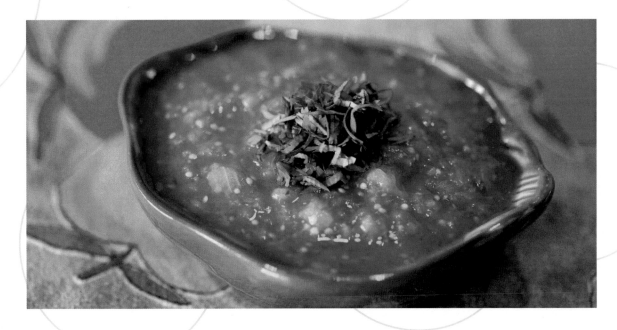

Cucumber Habañero Salsa (E)(Q)(R)($) - Contributed by of Aura Cardona

Serves: 3-4
Per serving: 53 Calories, 0.1g Fat, 12.2g Carbs, 3.5g Fiber, 1g Protein

Ingredients

2 medium Persian cucumbers
1 habañero - finely chopped
1 small red onion finely dices
¼ tsp mineral salt
2-3 Tbsp lime juice

Directions:

Mix gently.

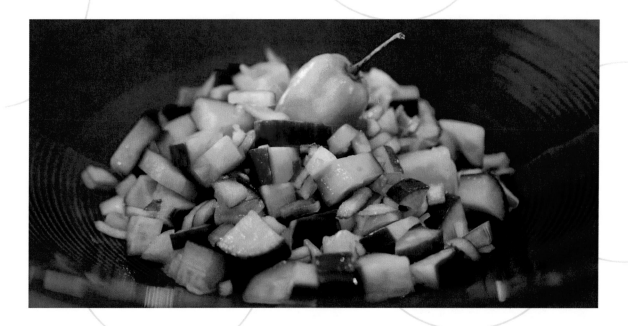

Egyptian Tomato Sauce (E)($)(Q)

Serves: 4

Per serving: 108 Calories, 3.7g Fat, 17g Carbs, 3.9g Fiber, 3.4g Protein

Ingredients:

1 can crushed tomatoes
1 can tomato paste
2 medium onions - chopped finely (diced)
6 garlic cloves - diced very small
2 tsp apple cider vinegar
EVOO
salt
pepper
2 tsp hot chili flakes (to taste)

Directions:

*The key is a long slow low temperature cooking.

Sauté onions until soft.

Add garlic and fry till pale brown

Add paste, salt, pepper, chili and vinegar

Add crushed tomatoes stirring often.

Simmer on low heat until sauce darkens ½ to 1 hour – if the sauce looks too dry.

Add a little water until it is to your liking.

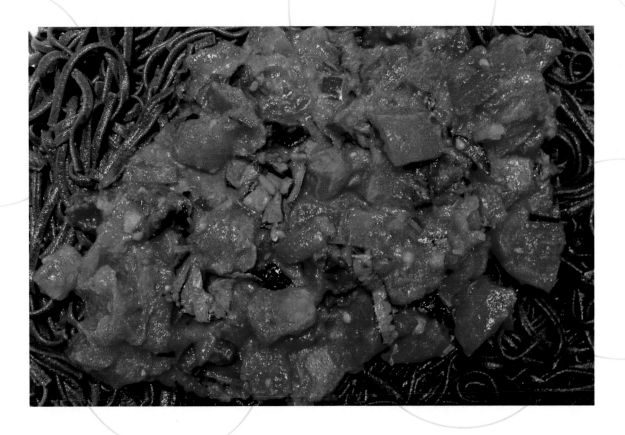

Citrus Vinaigrette (E)(Q)(R)($)

Per serving (1 tbsp): 72 Calories, 6.4g Fat, 5g Carbs, 1.1g Fiber, 0.4g Protein

Ingredients:

Juice from:
1 lemon
1 lime
1 orange
1 medium date - pitted
¼ cup EVOO
Add salt, pepper and dry mustard to your taste.

Directions:

Mix together.

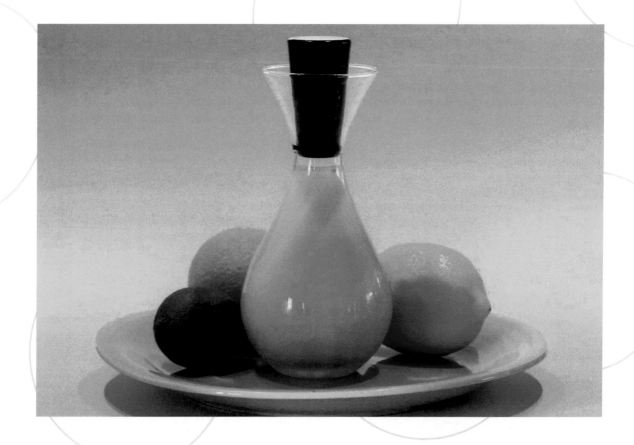

Avocado Basil Pesto (E)(Q)(R)($)
Per serving (1/2 cup): 149 Calories, 15.7g Fat, 3.2g Carbs, 2.4g Fiber, 1g Protein

Ingredients:

2 cups fresh basil leaves
1/4 cup + 1 Tbsp EVOO
1/4 cup toasted pine nuts
1 avocado
2 Tbsp lemon juice
mineral salt & cracked pepper

Directions:

Blend the Pesto ingredients.

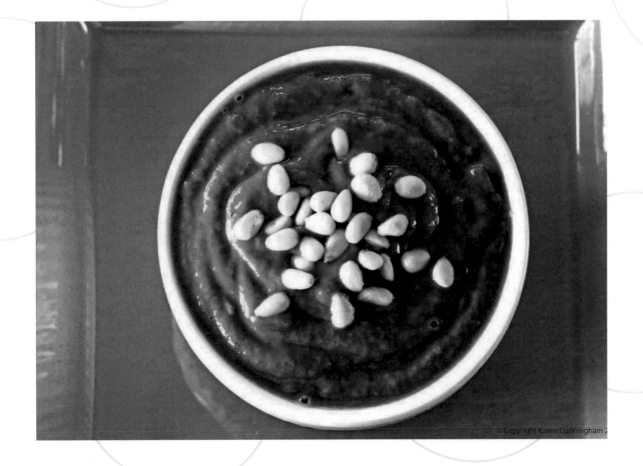

Ginger Crème* (E)(Q)(R)($)

Per serving (1/8th recipe): 140 Calories, 11.4g Fat, 9.2g Carbs, 0.6g Fiber, 2.7g Protein
*Often paired with Chocolate Torte (see page for recipe)

Ingredients:

1 cup cashews
2 Tbsp coconut oil/butter
2 Tbsp date purée (304)
1 Tbsp fresh ginger
Pinch ground clove
2 tsp vanilla
Water as needed

Directions:

Place all ingredients in processor and blend.

Strawberry Crème* (E)(Q)(R)($)

Entire recipe: 59 Calories, 0.2g Fat, 12.3g Carbs, 2.7g Fiber, 1.3g Protein
*Often paired with Chocolate Torte (see page for recipe)

Ingredients:

1 cup strawberries
2 Tbsp lemon juice
1/2 tsp cinnamon
1/4 tsp nutmeg

Directions:

Place all ingredients in processor and blend.

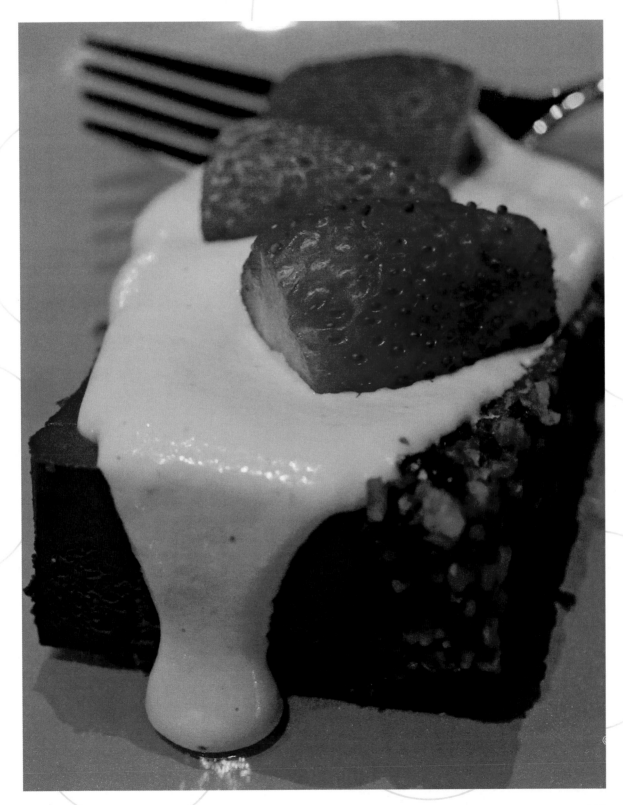

Asian Inspired Marinade (E)(Q)($)

Entire recipe: 572 Calories, 57g Fat, 8g Carbs, 1.7g Fiber, 9g Protein

Directions:

Tempeh or Tofu Marinade
1/4 cup tamari
1/4 cup sesame oil
2 tsp freshly grated ginger
2 tsp sesame seeds

Directions:

Marinate Tempeh or Tofu strips for about an hour or more

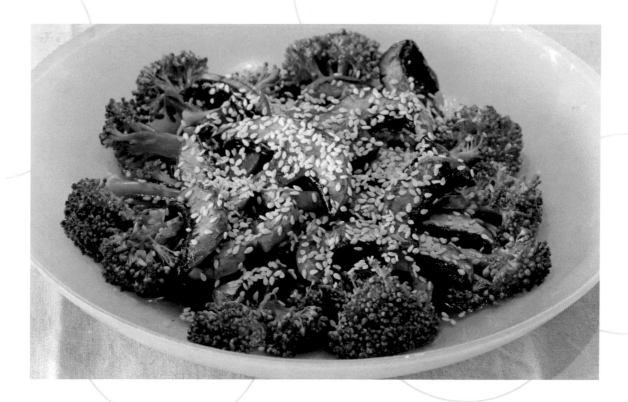

Pomodoro Sauce (Q)(E)($)

Serves: 4
Per serving: 189 Calories, 10g Fat, 24g Carbs, 3.7g Fiber, 4.2g Protein

Ingredients:

2 Tbsp grapeseed oil
2 cloves garlic, peeled and minced
1 small onion - finely chopped
2 tsp olive oil
1 can (28 oz) diced plum tomatoes
3 Tbsp tomato paste
1 tsp Bragg's Apple Cider vinegar
1 tsp dried oregano
1 tsp dried basil
1/2 tsp red pepper flakes
½ cup chopped parsley leaves
Fresh basil – as much as you love

Directions:

Sauté garlic and onion in grapeseed oil in medium saucepan over medium heat 5 minutes.

Add remaining ingredients except fresh basil and cook, stirring occasionally, for 30 minutes.

Lower heat if sauce begins to boil.

Power over noodles and garnish with basil.

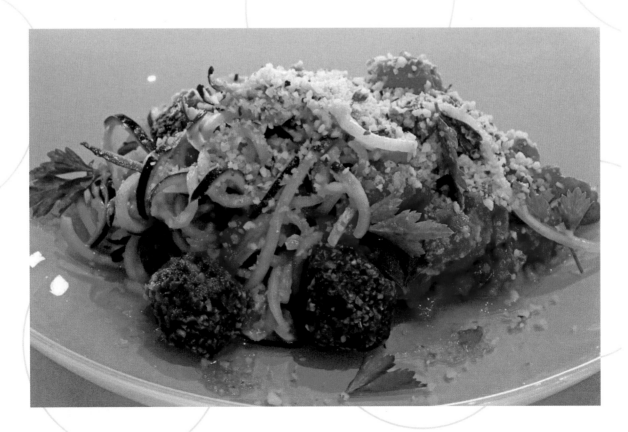

Spinach Parsley Pesto (R)(E)($)(Q)

Makes ~1 cup
Per serving (¼ cup): 69 Calories, 6.9g Fat, 1.6g Carbs, 0.7g Fiber 1.2g Protein

Ingredients:

1 cup baby spinach and parsley
1-2 small green chilies
1/4 cup lemon juice
2 Tbsp pine nuts
2 cloves garlic
1 Tbsp nutritional yeast
3 Tbsp EVOO

Directions:

Blend and enjoy over your favorite pasta, as a dip for vegetables or over any simple vegetable dish.

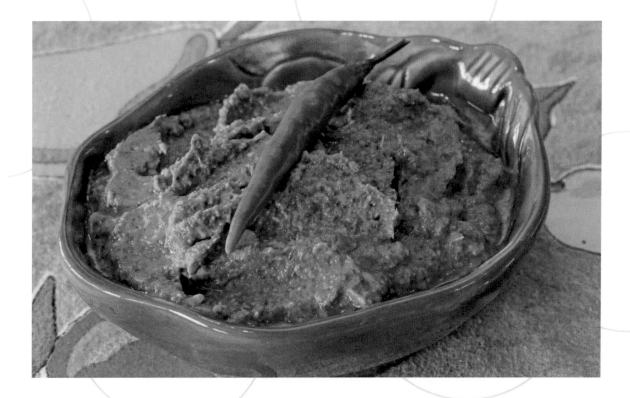

Coconut Topping (E)(Q)(R)($)

Serves: 8
Per serving: 121 Calories, 11.1g Fat, 18.6g Carbs, 2.8g Fiber, 1.4g Protein

Ingredients:

1/4 cup + 2 Tbsp coconut milk
1+1/2 Tbsp Bragg's Liquid Aminos
1/2 tsp dried crushed chili
1/4 tsp ground coriander
1/2 cup dry shredded coconut, unsweetened
1 fresh red chili, minced, OR 1/2 tsp dried crushed chili (add more or less to taste)
1 clove garlic - minced
1 spring (green) onion - chopped fine
1 tsp grated galangal OR ginger
1 tsp grated lime zest
1 tsp date purée (see page 304)
1 Tbsp lime juice

Directions:

Mix and enjoy

NOTE:
Keeps for about a week in the fridge
Freeze friendly

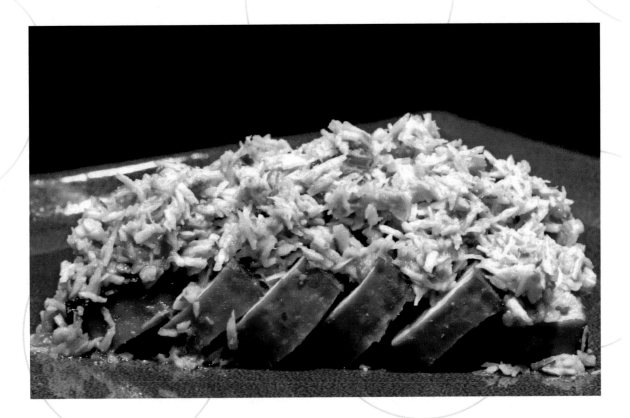

Herbed Yoghurt Sauce (E)(Q)($)

Serves: 6

Per serving: 33 Calories, 0.7g Fat, 6.1g Carbs, 1.1g Fiber, 1.5g Protein

Ingredients:

6 oz non dairy yoghurt
½ cup mint - chopped
½ cup parsley - chopped
2 (or more) garlic cloves - chopped
2 Tbsp lemon juice
1 Tbsp Lime juice
pinch mineral salt and pepper

Directions:

Blend and enjoy over lots of different recipes.

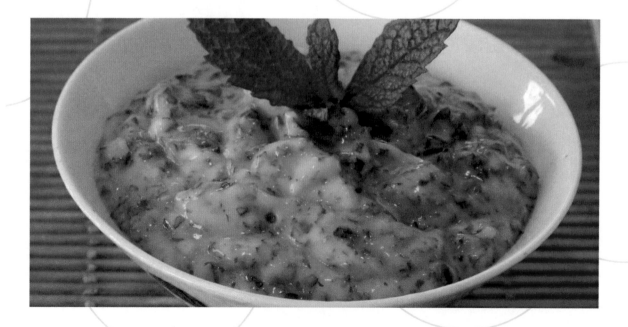

Radish Pesto (E)(Q)(R)($)

Per serving (1/4th recipe): 44 Calories, 3.7g Fat 2.4g Carbs, 1g Fiber, 1.5g Protein

Ingredients:

radish leaves
2 cloves garlic
1 inch strip of lemon zest
1 Tbsp lime juice/
1 Tbsp nutritional yeast
1 Tbsp EVOO spiked with chili

Directions:

Blend.

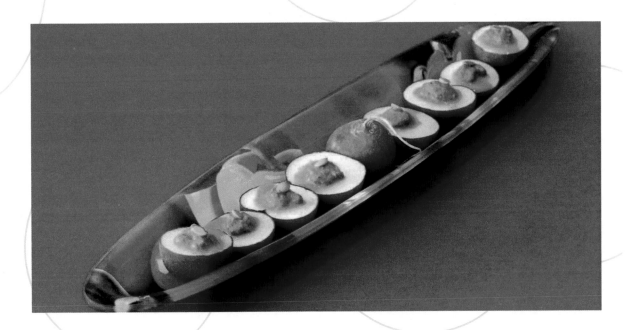

Yoghurt Mango Dressing (E)(Q)($)

Makes 1 cup

Per serving*: 65 Calories, 1.8g Fat, 11.5g Carbs, 1g Fiber, 0.9g Protein

*Analyzed using coconut yogurt, not cashew yogurt

Ingredients:

1 ripe mango – peeled and flesh removed from seed
½ cup plain coconut yoghurt (or homemade cashew yoghurt - see page 240)
¼ tsp ground black pepper
½ tsp cayenne pepper (or to taste)
¼ tsp Mineral salt

Directions:

Blend.

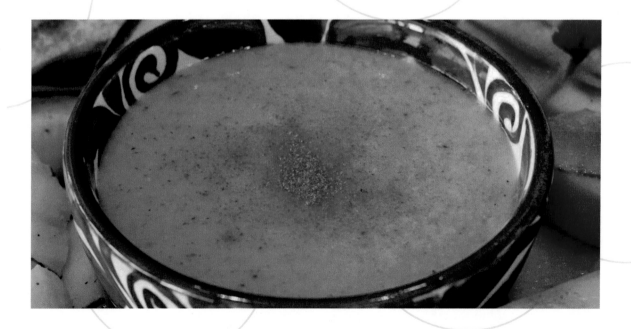

Spicy Pumpkin Dip (E)(Q)($)
Per serving (1/6th recipe): 120 Calories, 10.2g Fat, 5.8g Carbs, 4g Fiber, 3.5g Protein

Ingredients:

1 cup cooked pumpkin or butternut squash
½ cup lightly toasted pumpkin seeds
1 cup cooked garbanzo beans
1 clove garlic
2 tsp dried rosemary
pinch mineral salt
½ habañero chili (this could be left out)
2 Tbsp EVOO
¼ cup vegetable stock

Directions:

Blend and enjoy

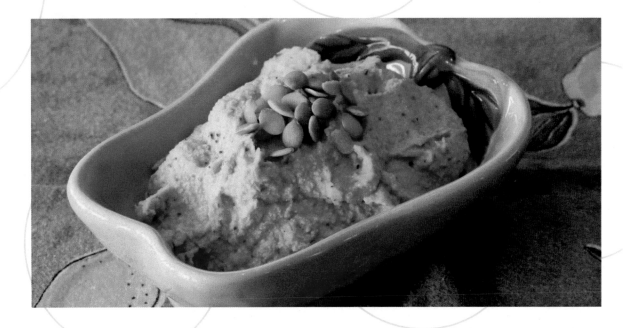

Ranch Dressing (E)(Q)(R)($)
per 2 Tbsp: 123 Calories, 13.8g Fat, 0.4g Carbs, 0.1g Protein

Ingredients:

½ cup Grapeseed Oil
¼ cup unsweetened almond milk (more if you like a runnier dressing)
2 tsp apple cider vinegar
1-2 tsp garlic powder
1 tsp mineral salt
1 tsp onion powder
½ - 1 tsp ground black pepper
1 tsp dried dill (or 1 Tbsp fresh dill – chopped)
1 tsp dried parsley (or 1 Tbsp fresh parsley - chopped fine)
½ tsp dried chives

Directions:

Put almond milk and vinegar in the blender and let sit for 10 minutes to curdle.

Blend the rest of the ingredients into the milk/vinegar mixture.

Adjust seasonings to your taste.

NOTE:
This is a high fat dressing so use sparingly

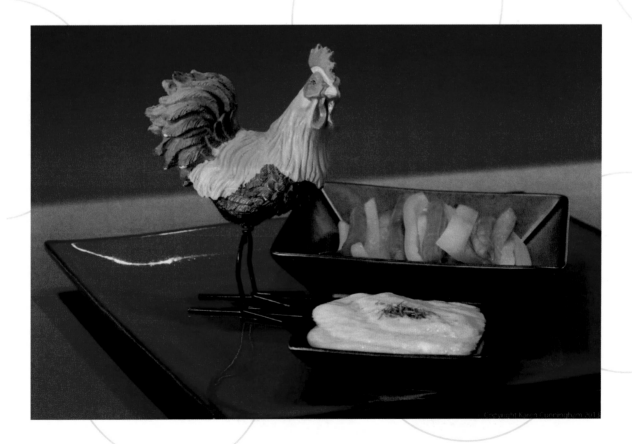

Buffalo Bites Sauce (HOT) (E)(Q)($)

Per serving (1/6th recipe): 191 Calories, 18g Fat, 5g Carbs, 0.8g Fiber, 0.7g Protein

Ingredients:

1 tsp HOT cayenne pepper, or to your taste (I rate this at about a 7)
1/2 cup of water
1 medium onion - chopped
4 cloves garlic - crushed
1 medium tomato - chopped
1 cup of apple cider vinegar
½ cup grapeseed oil
4oz bottle of Louisiana Hot Sauce (you know, that very popular sauce that we can't name – starts with a T), or similar
2 Tbsp lemon or lime juice
1 tsp of maple syrup
1/4 cup of tomato paste

Directions:

Add the Cayenne and 1/2 cup of water, 1/2 cup of vinegar, Hot Sauce and salt to your blender Blend on high for twenty seconds. Allow to sit in the blender

Place Grapeseed oil in a pan over a medium flame. Add the chopped onion, garlic, tomato and cook for about five minutes, stirring occasionally.

Pour this mixture into blender with the percolated cayenne pepper sauce. Blend on high for two minutes. Add the lemon juice, Maple syrup and tomato paste, and blend again for a few seconds.

Pour back into the pan where you sauteed the onion, and let it gently simmer for 15-20 minutes.

This is a sauce that is generally served over Buffalo Bites (see page for recipe).

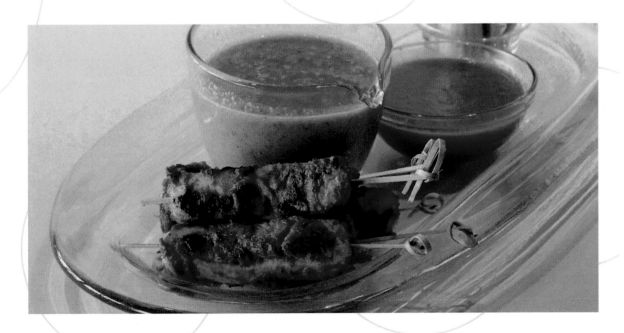

Roasted Bell Pepper Pesto (E)(Q)(R)($)
Per serving: 139 Calories, 12g Fat, 6.4g Carbs, 1.8g Fiber, 4.6g Protein

Ingredients:

3 roasted red bell peppers, peeled and deseeded
2 cloves garlic
2 Tbsp cup EVOO
1 1/2 cups toasted walnuts, chopped into small pieces
1 Tbsp lemon juice
1 Tsp chia seeds
2 Tbsp ground flax meal
1 clove garlic, crushed
1 Tsp ground cumin
1 Tsp pomegranate concentrate

Directions:

Blend.

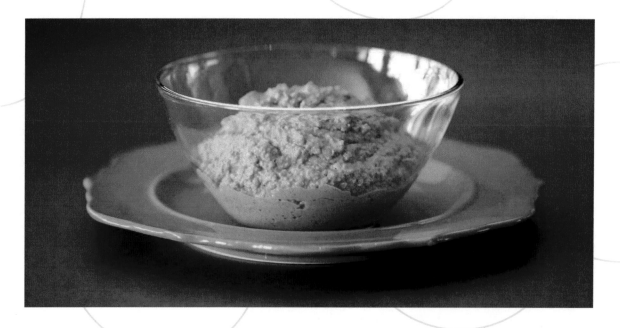

Japanese Salad Dressing (E)(Q)(R)($)
Per serving: 137 calories, 13.7g fat, 4g Carbs, 2.7g fiber, 0.3g protein

Ingredients:

1/2 cup vegetable oil
1/4 cup tamari sauce
1/2 small onion - chopped
1/2 rib celery - chopped
1/2 lime - juiced
2 Tbsp fresh ginger - minced
1 Tbsp maple syrup
1 Tbsp chipotle ketchup (see page 227)
1/2 tsp black pepper

Directions:

purée all ingredients in a blender until smooth.

Refrigerate at least 1 hour before serving.

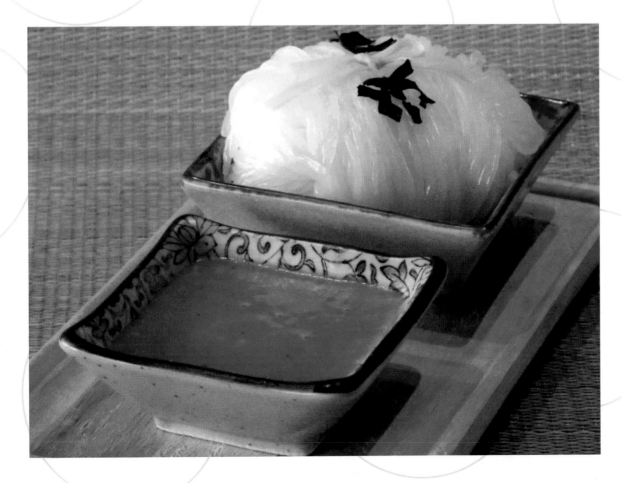

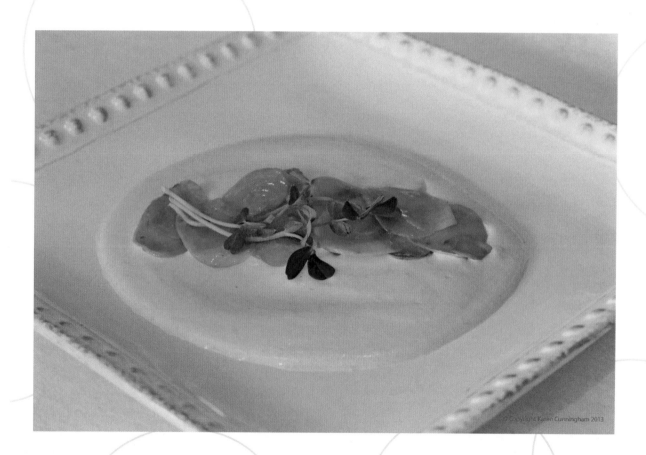

Pine Nut Sauce (E)(Q)

Makes ~ 4 cups
Per serving: 288 Calories, 29g Fat, 5g Carbs, 1.5g Fiber, 5g Protein

Ingredients:

4 cups pine nuts - soaked 1 hour or more
1/2 cup EVOO
2 medium shallots, peeled and diced
Zest of 1 lemon
1/2 cup lemon juice
4 tsp nutritional yeast
2 1/2 tsp sea salt
Freshly ground black pepper

Directions:

Process all ingredients in a food processor until as smooth as possible.

Rosemary-Crème Sauce (E)(Q)

Per serving: 3 Calories, 0.5g Carbs, 0.1g Protein

Ingredients:

1 tsp minced rosemary
1 Tbsp freshly squeezed lemon juice
3/4 cup filtered water
Pinch of sea salt
1 clove garlic, peeled
Freshly ground black pepper

Directions:

purée all the ingredients in a high-speed blender until smooth.

Zhug (E)(Q)(R)($)
Per serving (1/12th recipe): 88 Calories, 8.6g Fat, 3.5g Carbs, 0.7g Fiber, 0.8g Protein

Ingredients:

3 bunches cilantro
4 cloves garlic - minced
8 small hot red peppers - stems removed
2 Tbsp lime juice
1 tsp ground cardamom
1 tsp ground cumin
1/2 tsp mineral salt
1/2 tsp ground black pepper
1/2 cup EVOO

Directions:

Blend and enjoy.

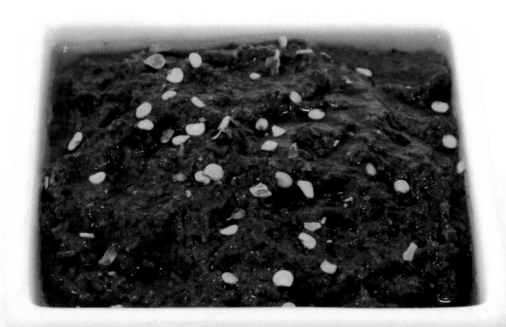

Horseradish Cranberry Sauce (E)(Q)(R)($)

Entire recipe: 37 Calories, 0.1g Fat, 9.6g Carbs, 1.4g Fiber, 0.4g Protein

Ingredients:

1 small medjool date
1 Tbsp unsweetened cranberry sauce
1 Tbsp prepared horseradish sauce

Directions:

Mix.

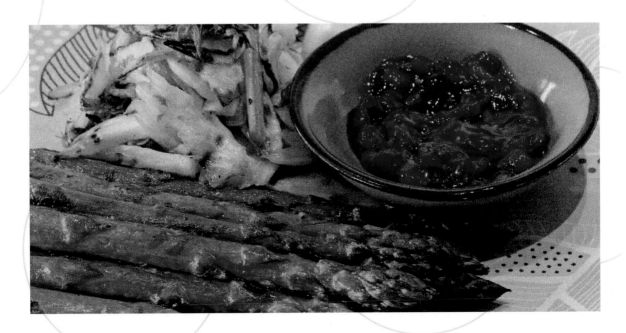

Spicy Pineapple Sauce (E)(Q)(R)($)
Entire recipe: 203 Calories, 0.5g Fat

Ingredients:

1/2 fresh pineapple (14 oz unsweetened pineapple)
1 serrano chili

Directions:

Mix.

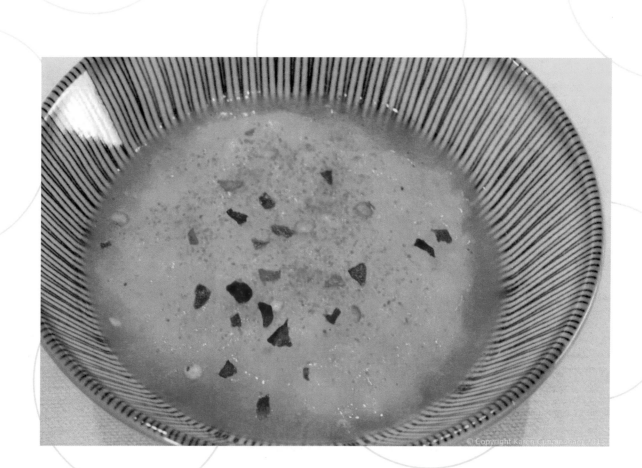

Chipotle Ketchup (E)(Q)(R)($)

Makes ~ 1 cup
Entire recipe: 294 Calories, 15g Fat, 38g Carbs, 8.4g Fiber, 9.3g Protein

Ingredients:

1 cup sundried tomatoes
1 dried chipotle pepper
1 small red tomato
1 Tbsp EVOO

Directions:

Soak the sundried tomatoes and the chipotle pepper for about 8 hours.

Drain .

Open the chipotle pepper and remove the seeds unless you like it really hot.

Roughly chop the tomatoes and blend the 4 items together.

You can make this really smooth or leave it a little chunky.

Store in the refrigerator.

NOTE
Can be frozen.

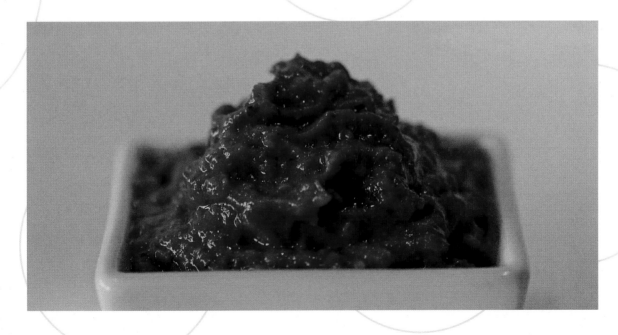

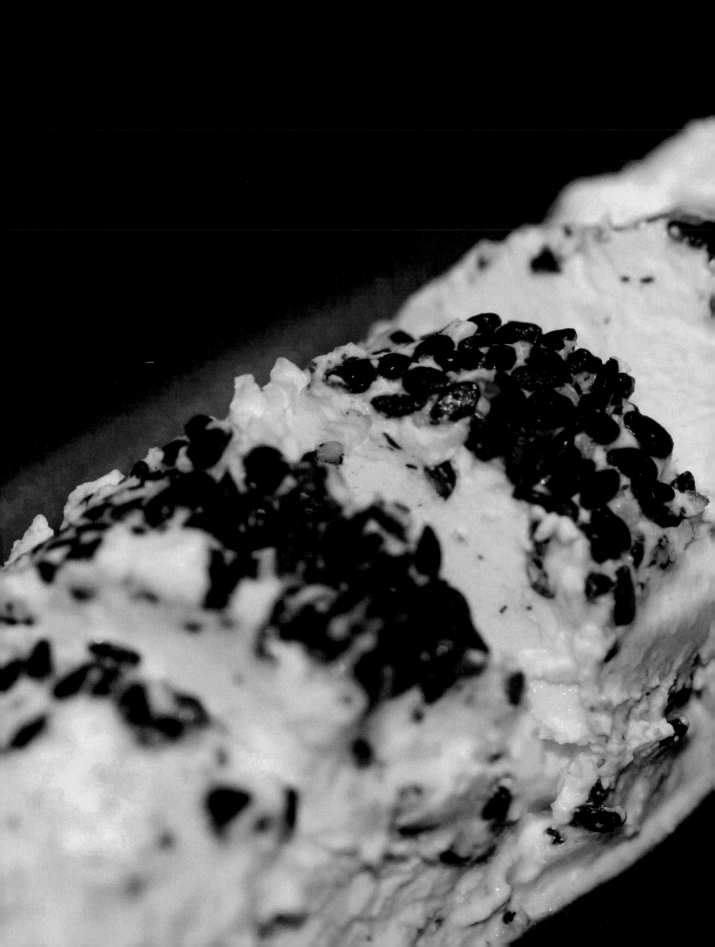

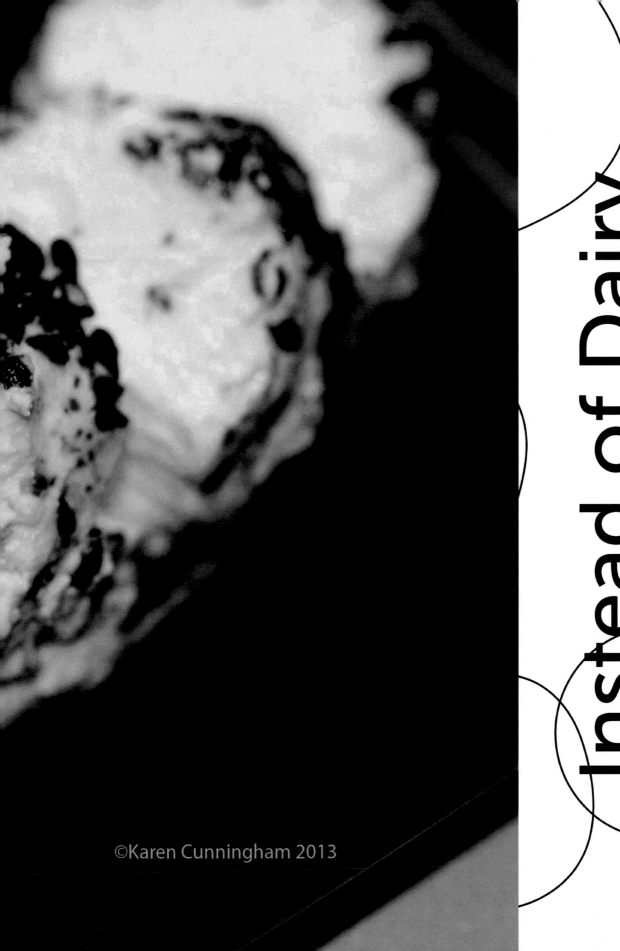

Instead of Dairy

Crème Cheese (E)(R)

Makes 1 cup
Per serving (1 Tbsp): 63 Calories, 5g Fat, 3.6g Carbs, 1.7g Protein

Ingredients:

1½ cups raw cashew - soaked for 2 hours
¼ cup apple cider vinegar
2 Tbsp fresh lemon juice
2-3 Tbsp water
12 inch square of cheesecloth + string to tie it

Directions:

Blend all ingredients in high speed blender until as smooth as you can make it. You may have to stop the process and scrape down the side a couple of times.

Scrape mixture into the cheesecloth and tie into a ball with the string.

Suspend mixture so that it can drip for 24 hours.

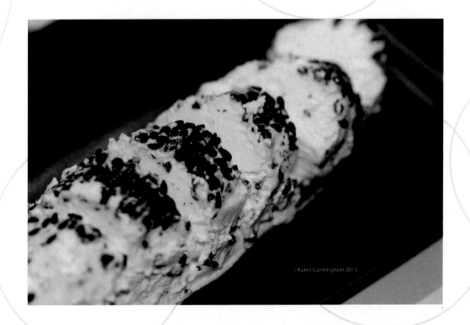

©Karen Cunningham 2013

Cashew Cheese (E)(R)
Per ¼ cup: 158 Calories, 12g Fat, 9.8g Carbs, 1.8g Fiber, 5.3g Protein

Ingredients:

2 cups cashews (raw is best, roasted is still great, and try flavored cashews too)
1/2 cup water
1 large red bell pepper (roasted)
1/4 cup yeast flakes
2 garlic cloves
1 Tbsp lemon juice
2 tsp Bragg's Liquid Aminos
1 Tbsp sesame oil
1 tsp sea salt (optional) if the cashews are unsalted – TASTE before adding salt

Directions:

Blend and enjoy. You can add more water for a runnier consistency

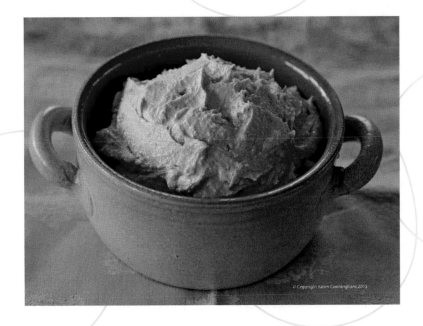

"Tres Leches" Crème Milk (R)
Per serving (1/8 recipe): 202 Calories, 16g Fat, 11g Carbs, 2.7g Fiber, 5.4g Protein

Ingredients:

1 cup fresh coconut flesh*
1 cup raw cashews soaked for 20 minutes
1 cup peeled almonds – you can soak your own for 1 hour and the skins will slip off
1 Tbsp maple syrup
1 Tbsp vanilla
2 pitted large dates - chopped into very small pieces
1 Tbsp arrowroot or tapioca starch

* If you can't find it soak 1/2 cup unsweetened desiccated coconut in 1/2 cup coconut milk for 4 hours

Directions:

Soak the nuts as suggested

Then blend the nuts, minus soaking liquid with the wet ingredients*

Finally place the mixture in a bowl and stir in the arrowroot thoroughly.

Place in the fridge to thicken. If your mixture is not thick enough add more arrowroot

*I use a high speed blender to get that real creamy texture. If you do not have a high speed blender your cream will be a little gritty – but still delicious

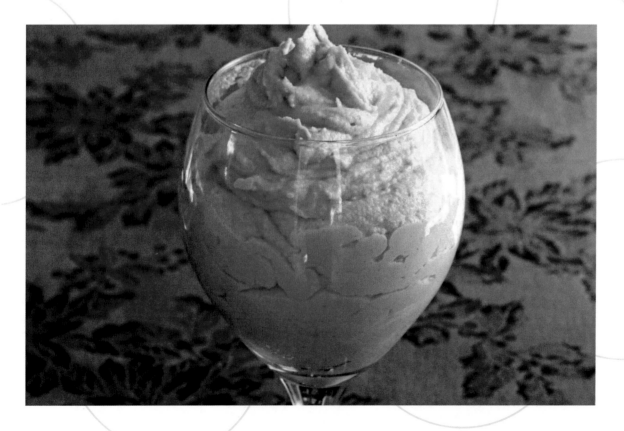

Macadamia Nut Ricotta (R)

Serves: 6

Per serving (1/4 cup): 245 Calories, 25g Fat, 5.2g Carbs, 3.2g Fiber, 3.2g Protein

Ingredients:

2 cups raw macadamia nuts
1 packet of digestion plus
1 cup filtered water.
1 tsp salt
1 Tbsp nutritional yeast

Directions:

Soak nuts in 2 cups filtered water for 4 hours.

Drain soaked macadamia nuts, then add the 1 cup of filtered water and 1 packet of digestion plus

Place all ingredients in a high speed blender and blend until very smooth.

Line a regular colander with several layers of cheesecloth.

Place the nut cheese mixture in the colander and place a small plate over the top so it presses the nut cheese – add a little more weight so that the nut cheese can drain.

Leave to drain and ferment for 24 hours.

Add salt and nutritional yeast – stir thoroughly and then put it a container in the fridge.

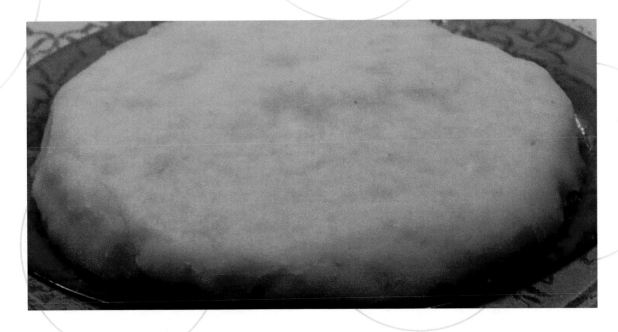

Pine Nut Parmesan (R)*
Per serving: 38 Calories, 3.3g Fat, 1.7g Carbs, 1.2g Protein
*You will need a food processor and a dehydrator to make this recipe

Ingredients:

1 cup raw pine nuts, soaked for 2 hours or more
1 cup raw cashews, soaked for 2 hours or more
1/2 cup filtered water
1/4 cup lemon juice
4 Tbsp nutritional yeast
1 clove garlic, minced
1/2 tsp sea salt

Directions:

Blend all ingredients together in a food processor.

Using a spatula, spread the mixture onto lined dehydrator sheets.
Dehydrate at 115 degrees F for about 8 hours.

Flip the sheets over and remove the liners.

Dehydrate an additional 8 hours or until crisp.

Break the cheese up into small pieces and store in an airtight container.

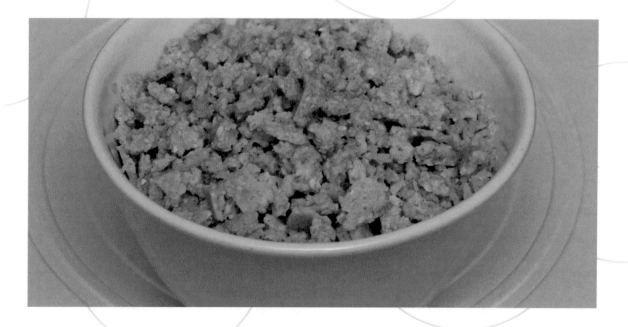

Brazil Nut Parmesan (R)

Serves ~16
Per serving (~9g): 55 Calories, 5.4g Fat, 0.2g Carbs, 1.2g Protein

Ingredients:

2 cups Brazil nuts – soaked in water 8-24 hours
3 Tbsp nutritional yeast
2 Tbsp lemon juice
1 tsp salt

Directions:

Drain and dry the Brazil nuts.

Chop all ingredients except for the lemon juice in a food processor until they resemble breadcrumbs.

Place in a mixing bowl and stir in the lemon juice.

Put mixture on a cookie sheet or dehydrator sheet

Dehydrate for 3 hours at 105 degrees
Or
Leave mixture to air dry in a warm place for 24 hours

This is delicious over vegetables or grains and pasta.

One of my favorites mixed with cooked millet over Asian Style Kale salad (see page 41)

*Brazil nuts have anti-cancerous compounds in them

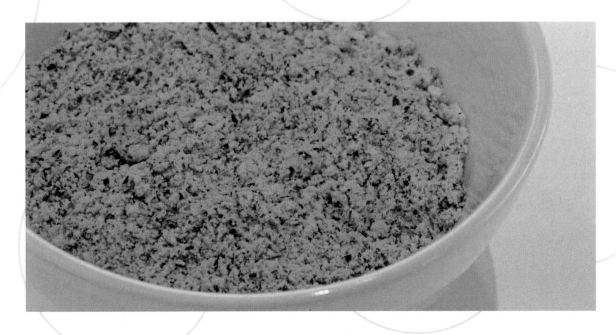

364 Days of Healthy Eating (because nobody is perfect)

Vanilla Cashew Crème (E)(R)
Per serving (¼ cup): 100 Calories, 8g Fat, 5.7g Carbs, 2.6g Protein

Ingredients:

1/2 cup raw cashews
1/2 tsp vanilla
1/4 – 1/2 cup water

Directions:

Blend and pour on all your sweet treats.

Walnut Parmesan (E)(R)
Per ¼ cup: 192 Calories, 15g Fat, 7.4 g Carbs, 4.4g Fiber, 11g Protein

Ingredients:

1 cup walnuts - soaked 4 hours - then drained and dried well or dried in the oven at 105 degrees for an hour or so
1/3 cup nutritional yeast
1 tsp mineral salt and pepper - or more to taste

Directions:

Process walnuts into a rough floury mix; add in other ingredients until you have a crumbled Parmesan cheese texture.

Taste and add other things according to your palate.

Coconut Crème Fraiche (R)
Per serving: 95 Calories, 9g Fat, 4.1g Carbs, 2.4g Fiber, 0.9g Protein

Ingredients:

2 cups coconut meat from young coconuts or 1 cup unsweetened dried desiccated coconut soaked in coconut water for 8 hours – then squeezed to remove most of the liquid
Add 1/4 tsp mineral salt,
1 Tbsp lemon juice

Directions:

In a high speed blender blend all ingredients to a yogurt like consistency – you will have to scrape down the sides of the bowl several times.

If the mixture is too thick add a little coconut milk or water.

Chill in the refrigerator.

NOTE: Can be frozen – I usually divide this into small amounts and freeze

236

Cashew Ricotta (R)

Serves: 4
Per serving: 152 Calories, 10.9g Fat, 10.3g Carbs, 2g Fiber, 6g Protein

Ingredients:

1/2 cup raw cashew pieces (approximately 4 ounces)
1/4 cup fresh lemon juice
2 cloves fresh or roasted garlic
1 pound firm organic tofu - drained and crumbled
1 1/2 tsp dried basil
1 1/2 tsp salt

Directions:

In a food processor, blend together the cashews, lemon juice, EVOO, and garlic until a thick creamy paste forms.

Add the crumbled tofu to the food processor, working in two or more batches if necessary, until the mixture is thick and well blended.

Blend in the basil and salt.

Cashew Cheese #2 (E)(R)

Per ¼ cup: 158 Calories, 12g Fat, 9.8g Carbs, 1.8g Fiber, 5.3g Protein

Ingredients:

2 cups cashews (raw is best, roasted is still great, and try flavored cashews too)
1/2 cup water
1 large red bell pepper (roasted)
1/4 cup yeast flakes
2 garlic cloves
1 Tbsp lemon juice
2 tsp Bragg's Liquid Aminos
1 Tbsp sesame oil
1 tsp sea salt (optional) if the cashews are unsalted –
TASTE before adding salt

Directions:

Blend and enjoy.

*You can add more water for a runnier consistency

Vegan Heavy Crème (Crème Fraiche Substitute)* (E)(R)

Makes 2 cups
Per serving (2 Tbsp): 123 Calories, 13.8g Fat, 0.2g Carbs, 0.1g Protein
*using a high speed blender will produce a thicker smoother crème

Ingredients:

¾ cup almond or hemp milk
1 Tbsp lemon or lime juice
1 cup grapeseed oil or sunflower oil
½ tsp maple syrup
¼ tsp mineral salt

NOTE
To make sweetened heavy cream just add - 1 Tbsp maple syrup

Directions:

Blend almond milk and lemon juice.

While blending separately mix other ingredients together.

Add the second mixture very slowly to the blender mixture in one thin stream, while still blending on high, and keep blending until it gets really thick. (It should get thick as you get to the end of the oil).

Vegan Sour Crème (E)(R)
Per serving: 36 Calories, 3.7g Fat, 0.2g Carbs, 04.g Protein

Ingredients:

1 12 oz (1 1/2 cups) soft organic Tofu
3 Tbsp EVOO
2 Tbsp lemon juice
2 tsp apple cider vinegar
3/4 tsp finely ground salt

Directions:

Drain the Tofu for about an hour and then blend all of the ingredients.

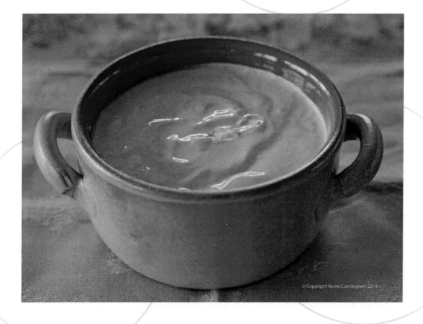

Simple Cashew Crème (E)(R)

Serves:
Per serving: 157 Calories, 12.7g Fat, 9g Carbs, 0.8g Fiber, 4.2g Protein

Ingredients:

1 cup raw cashews – soaked 20 minutes and then drained
1 cup filtered water
pinch mineral salt

Directions:

Rinse cashews thoroughly until the water runs clear

Simply blend the cashews salt and water until the mixture is really creamy.

NOTE:
Can be frozen.

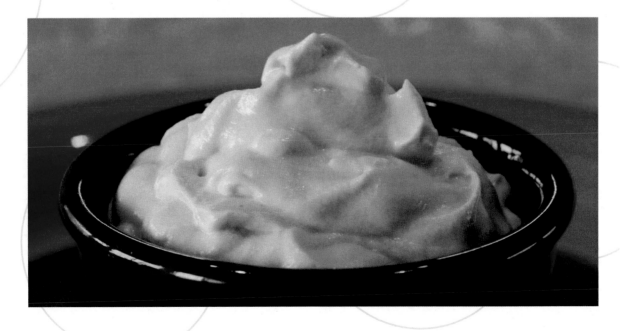

Cashew Yoghurt* (R)

Makes 1 cup
Per serving (1/4 cup): 197 Calories, 15.9g Fat, 11.2g Carbs, 1g Fiber, 5.2g Protein
* You will need a high speed blender and a dehydrator for this recipe

Ingredients:

1 cup cashews
1 cup water
1 package probiotics
1 tsp – 1 Tbsp lemon juice

Directions:

Soak cashews in water for 1 or 2 hours.
Drain and then blend the cashews with water till smooth.
Add the culture and stir well.
Place in a covered small glass container
Place in the dehydrator at 105 degrees for about 8-10 hours
Add 1 tsp – 1 Tbsp lemon juice and stir – add more lemon depending on your taste.
Keeps for up to 5 days in the refrigerator.

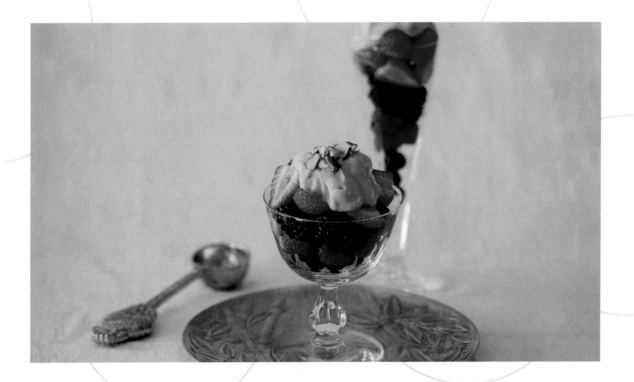

Spiced Cashew Crème with Fruit (E)(R)

Serves: 4

Per serving: 225 Calories, 16g Fat, 17g Carbs, 2.1g Fiber, 5.7g Protein

Ingredients:

1 cup orange pieces
1 cup raw cashews - soaked for 30 minutes in warm water
1 tsp cinnamon
1 tsp vanilla
1 tsp Maple syrup and

Directions:

Blend

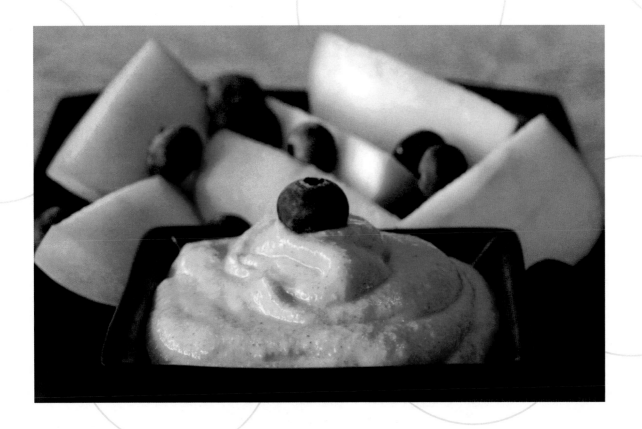

Macadamia Nut Cheese (R)

Serves:
Per serving: 183 Calories, 19g Fat, 4g Carbs, 2.3g Fiber, 2.3g Protein

Ingredients:

2 ¼ cups raw macadamia nuts - soaked for 4 hours
1 cup filtered water
1 tsp high quality probiotics
1 tsp mineral salt
2 tsp nutritional yeast

Directions:

Blend macadamia nuts, water and probiotics in a high-speed blender until smooth.

Place the mixture in a strainer that has been lined with cheesecloth and place a weight on top.

The weight should not be so heavy that it pushes the cheese through the cloth, but heavy enough to gently start to press the liquid out.

Leave to culture for 24 hours in a warm place (not over 85 degrees)

Then stir in mineral salt and nutritional yeast.

Stir together gently and store in the refrigerator

Keeps for about two weeks

NOTE
Not suitable for freezing

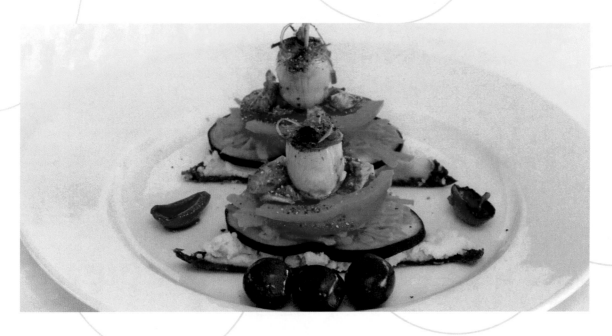

Macadamia Nut Brie (R)

Per serving: 119 Calories, 11.2g Fat, 4.7g Carbs, 1.4g Fiber, 1.7g Protein

Ingredients:

1 cup macadamia nuts* - soaked 4-8 hours in cold water, then drained and rinsed.
1 cup boiling water
2 Tbsp tapioca flour
1 Tbsp pure maple syrup
1 Tbsp yellow miso
2 Tbsp tahini
1 Tbsp apple cider vinegar
1 tsp dry mustard
1 tsp mineral salt
1 Tbsp EVOO
1/2 package Pamona's Pectin

*Last time I made this I used 1/2 macadamias and 1/2 cashews and I liked it even better.

Directions:

Lightly oil a small round bowl set aside. Measure out half of the dry pectin, about 4.5 tsp.

Combine calcium packet from pectin box with 1/2 cup water (not listed in ingredients above) in a small lidded jar and shake until thoroughly combined.

Blend all ingredients except pectin and calcium water in your turbo blender or food processor until completely smooth.

Add dry pectin and half (1/4 cup) of the calcium water and pulse until all combined and thick. Immediately scrape hot brie out into the small round prepared dish.

Refrigerate for a couple hours, turn out on to a plate, brie will be slightly soft (as brie is) but ready to use in this recipe.

Basic Cashew Cheese (E)(R)

Per serving (~1/20th recipe): 84 Calories, 6.4g Fat, 5.6g Carbs, 0.8g Fiber, 2.4g Protein

Ingredients:

2 cups cashews, soaked 20 minutes
1 cup water
1 tsp probiotics
¾ teaspoon salt
2 teaspoons nutritional yeast

Directions:

Blend cashews, water and probiotics in a high-speed blender until smooth.

Place the mixture in a strainer that has been lined with cheesecloth, and place a weight on top. The weight should not be so heavy that it pushes the cheese through the cloth, but heavy enough to gently start to press the liquid out.

Leave to culture at room temperature for at least 24 but no longer than 48 hours. Once culturing is complete, stir or process in the salt and nutritional yeast. Transfer the cheese to a ring mold.

At this point you can either place it in the refrigerator, still in the ring mold as it's not as firm as macadamia cheese, for 24 hours, and then remove the ring mold. Or you can place it in the freezer to set harder for 1 to 2 hours; then remove the ring mold and place the whole thing in the dehydrator at 105°F for 24 hours to get a rind.

Not Butter (R)

Makes 1 cup (215 grams), or the equivalent of 2 sticks vegan butter
Per serving (1 Tbsp): 94 Calories, 10.8g Fat, 0.2g Carbs, 0.1g Protein

Ingredients:

¼ cup + 2 tsp almond milk
1 tsp apple cider vinegar
¼ + 1/8 tsp Mineral salt

½ cup + 2 Tbsp + 1 tsp refined coconut oil, melted
1 Tbsp sunflower oil

1 tsp liquid sunflower lecithin

Directions:

Place the almond milk, apple cider vinegar and salt in a small cup and whisk together with a fork.

Let it sit for about 10 minutes so the mixture curdles.

Melt the coconut oil in a microwave so it's barely melted and as close to room temperature as possible.

Measure it and add it and the sunflower to a food processor.

Making smooth vegan butter is dependent on the mixture solidifying as quickly as possible after it's mixed. This is why it's important to make sure your coconut oil is as close to room temperature as possible before you mix it with the rest of the ingredients.

Add the almond milk mixture and sunflower lecithin to the food processor.

Process for 2 minutes, scraping down the sides halfway through the duration.

Pour the mixture into a mold and place it in the freezer to solidify. An ice cube mold works well.

The vegan butter should be ready to use in about an hour.

Store it in an airtight container in the refrigerator for up to 1 month or wrapped in plastic wrap in the freezer for up to 1 year.

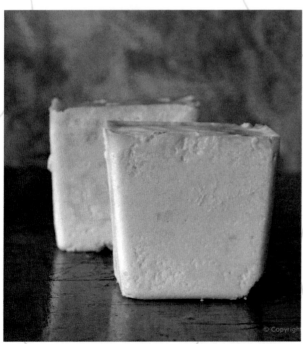

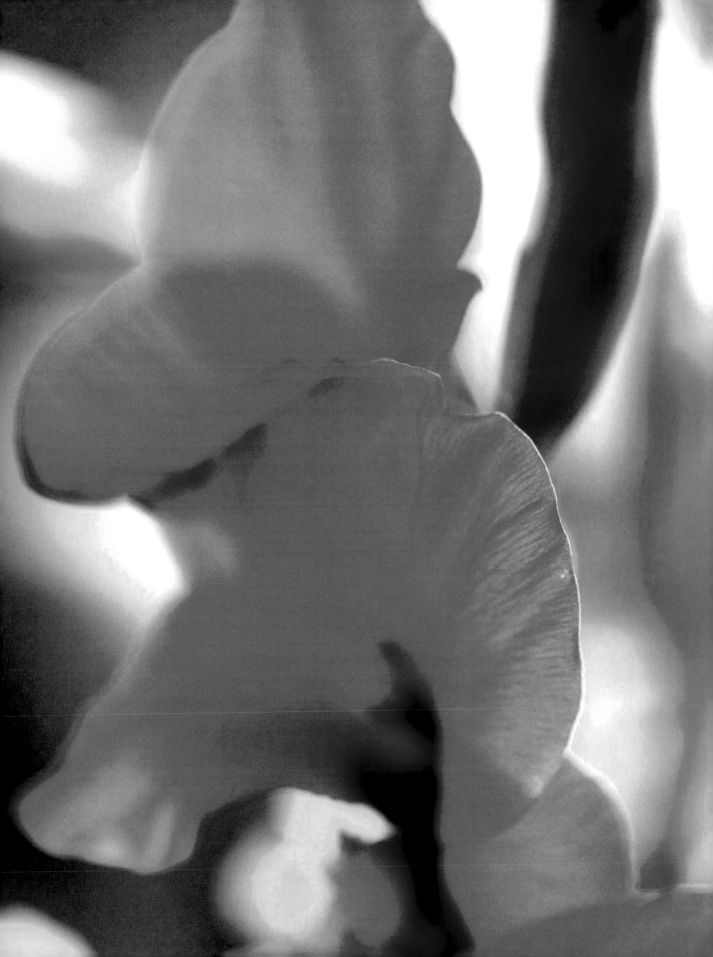

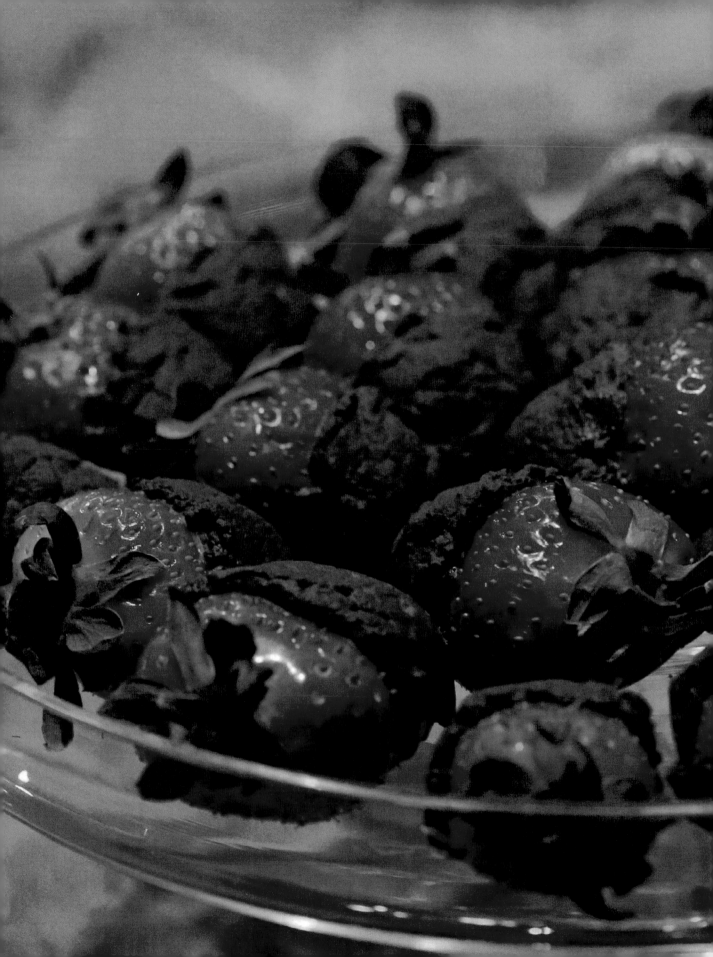

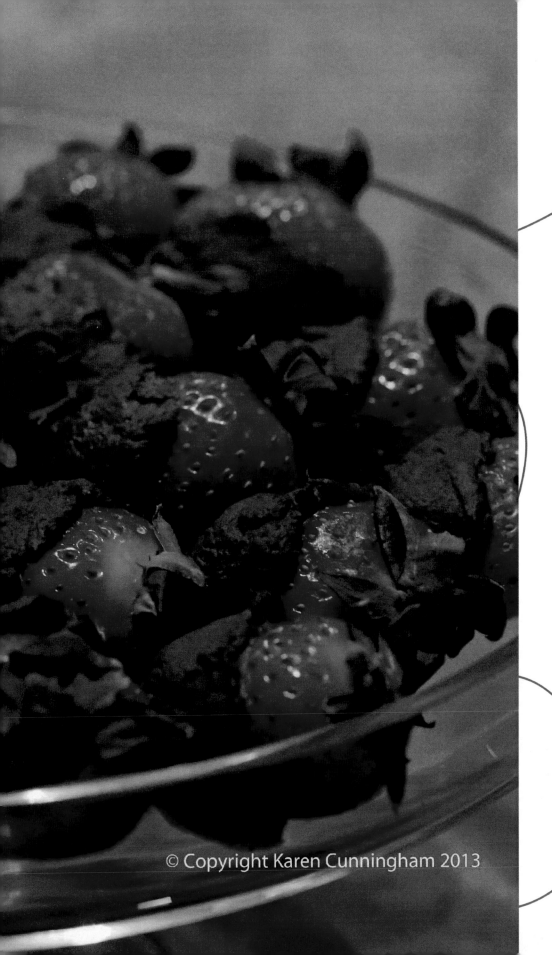

Desserts

Vanilla and Chocolate Protein Truffles (E)(R)

Serves: 30
Per truffle: 102 Calories, 7g Fat, 1.3g Sat. Fat, 7g Carbs, 1.3g Fiber, 3g Protein

Dry Ingredients:
1 cup cranberry-rice-yellow pea protein powder
1/2 cup raw sunflower seeds
1/2 cup cranberries – roughly chopped
1/2 cup desiccated unsweetened coconut
1 cup organic brown rice crisps

Wet Ingredients:
1/2 cup organic almond butter
2 Tbsp melted organic coconut oil
1 Tbsp vanilla essence
3 Tbsp organic maple syrup

For the Coating:
3 Tbsp organic fair trade cocoa powder
3 Tbsp organic carob powder

Directions:

Mix all dry ingredients in one bowl

Mix all wet ingredients in another bowl

Then combine the two with gloved hands and form into 1 inch balls pressing well until you have the right pressure to keep them solidly together.

If your mixture seems to dry, add a little extra maple syrup or coconut oil.

Now place truffles on a separate plate

In a wide small container add the carob and cocoa powders – then one at a time roll until well coated in the carob cocoa mixture

Put finished truffles in small paper cups and refrigerate for several hours

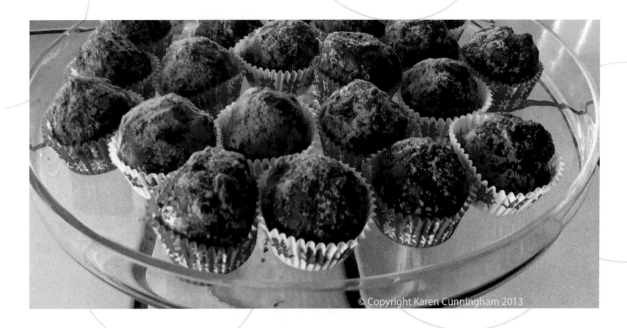

Apple Crisp (E)($)

Serves: 8
Per serving: 194 Calories, Fat: 3.7g Carbs: 39g, Fiber: 4g, Protein 2.5g

Ingredients:

4 cups sliced peeled green apples
1 cup GF rolled oats
1 Tsp ground cinnamon
pinch of ground nutmeg
1/4 Tsp ground allspice
¼ cup unsweetened desiccated coconut
2 Tbsp coconut oil
pinch of salt

Directions:

Preheat Oven to 375 degrees F (190 C)

Place apples in a greased 8-in. (20 cm) square baking dish.

In a bowl, combine the rest of the ingredients. Cover top of crisp with foil or other cover and bake at 375 degrees for 25-30 minutes or until apples are tender.

Uncover crisp and re-bake for 5 minutes or so until the topping is just crisp. Serve warm with your favorite topping if desired.

Note:
I have an apple slicer-cutter from Williams-Sonoma that makes slicing apples a few minute project.

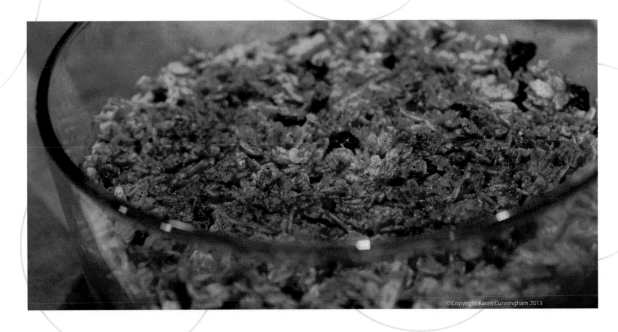

Chocolate Torte (R)

Per serving (~1/14 cake): 340 Calories, 27.1g Fat, 9.5g Sat Fat, 27g Carbs, 6g Fiber, 6.3g Protein

*Often paired with Ginger Crème (see page 196) or Strawberry Crème (see page 196)

Ingredients:

CRUST:
1 ½ cups raw pecans chopped in food processor (Be careful not to turn it to nut butter, you want it crumbly and some pieces of different sizes.)
¾ cup raisins roughly chopped
1 Tbsp vanilla extract
1 Tsp cinnamon
Pinch salt

FILLING:
2 cups raw cashews, soaked 20 minutes, then drained
1 cup water
2 cups fair trade organic cacao powder
1½ cups grated cacao butter, melted – I place it in a bowl over boiling water. (Do not microwave the cacao butter)
2 Tbsp vanilla extract
½ cup maple syrup
2 Tsp lemon juice

Directions:

CRUST:
Process Pecans and Raisins separately – they do not cooperate together in the food processor.
Mix all the crust ingredients together well in a bowl and by hand (I use gloves).
Press firmly into the bottom of 7" springform pan and place in freezer.

Note: Use the springform base upside down, i.e. so the lip faces downwards. I also cover it with foil for easier removal

FILLING:
Blend the cashews, water, vanilla, maple syrup, and lemon juice in a high speed blender until smooth.
Add cacao butter and cacao powder, and blend again.
Pour chocolate mixture onto base and use a spatula to achieve a level surface.
Place in fridge for 3 hours to set or quick set in freezer for an hour

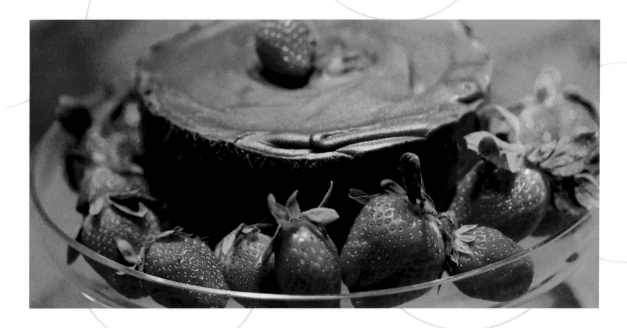

Blueberry Cheesecake (R)

Serves: 12

Per serving: 241 Calories, 15.5g Fat, 23.9g Carbs, 2.9g Fiber, 5.7g Protein

Ingredients:

CRUST:
1 cup walnuts
2/3 cup pitted, packed dates

FILLING:
3 cups blueberries
1 1/2 cups cashews
1/4 cup pure maple syrup
2 Tbsp lemon juice
1 Tsp ground cardamom
(start with less and add more, cardamom can be strong!)
1 Tsp pure vanilla extract
Pinch of salt
4 Tbsp melted cacao butter

Description:

CRUST:
Chop Walnuts into crumbs in a food processor. Be careful not to over process or you will have nut butter. Press the crust into 7 inch spring form pan with pan base lip facing downwards (for easy removal). Or you can use mini silicone muffin cups.
Set in freezer for one hour while making filling.

FILLING:
In a blender, combine all but the cacao butter, until completely smooth and creamy.
Add the butter and blend again to incorporate.
Pour the mixture over the crust(s)
Chill in the fridge or freezer until firm.
Garnish with blueberries, edible flowers, or any other garnish of your choice.

Serve with coconut crème Anglaise

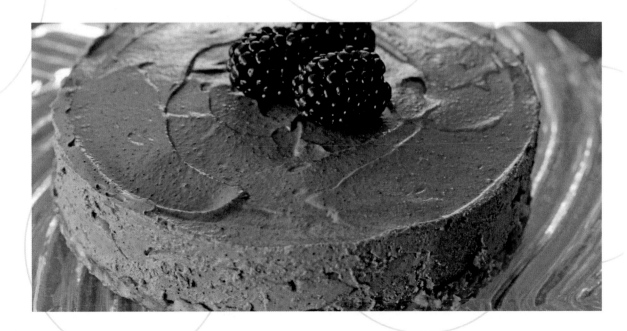

Baked Apple with Vanilla and Orange Cashew Crème (E)($)

Serves: 4
Per apple: 312 Calories, 8.9g Fat, 51.8g Carbs, 6.4g Fiber, 10.9g Protein

Ingredients:

4 medium green apples – cored
1 ½ cups blueberries
½ cup vanilla Pea, cranberry rice protein powder
2 cups fresh squeezed orange juice
½ cup raw cashews – soaked for 20 minutes and drained

Directions:

Bake apples covered with foil for about 30 minutes at 350 degrees until tender but not mushy.

Meanwhile blend the protein, orange juice and cashews until smooth and creamy – place in the refrigerator to chill.

Put each apple in a serving bowl and drizzle with the cashew cream and blueberries.

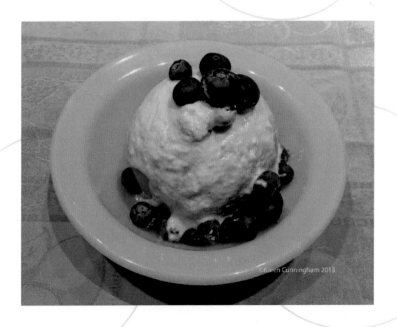

Chocolate Almond Bites (E)($)

Makes 24 bites

Per bite: 60 Calories, 4.8g Fat, 4.2g Carbs, 1.1g Fiber, 1.2g Protein

Ingredients:

1/2 cup cocoa powder
1 cup blanched sliced almonds
1/4 cup unsweetened desiccated coconut
1/4 cup maple syrup
1 Tbsp pure vanilla extract
4 Tbsp melted cacao butter
2 Tbsp melted coconut oil

Directions:

Melt cacao butter and coconut oil over double boiler

Mix all ingredients together

Form into small 1/2 inch balls

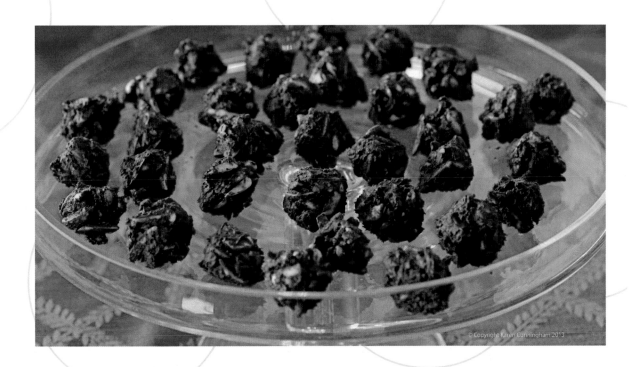

Orange and Carrot Cake (R)

Per serving (1/12th cake with icing): 344 Calories, 26g Fat, 29g Carbs, 4.8g Fiber, 5.2g Protein

Ingredients:

3 cups carrot - finely grated
2 cups pecans - ground in a food processor
¼ cup raisins - roughly chopped
1 tsp ground nutmeg
1 tsp ground cinnamon
¼ tsp ground coriander
¼ tsp ground cardamom
Dash cloves
1 cup soft dates
1/2 cup orange juice
1/4 tsp mineral salt
1/2 tsp grated orange zest
1/2 cup unsweetened desiccated coconut

Directions:

Make a date purée by blending the dates and orange juice.

Thoroughly mix all ingredients together in a large bowl.

Press cake into 9x9 baking dish.

Place on a dehydrator sheet and dehydrate at 115 degrees F for 8 – 12 hours or in your conventional oven at its lowest setting, 125 for three hours

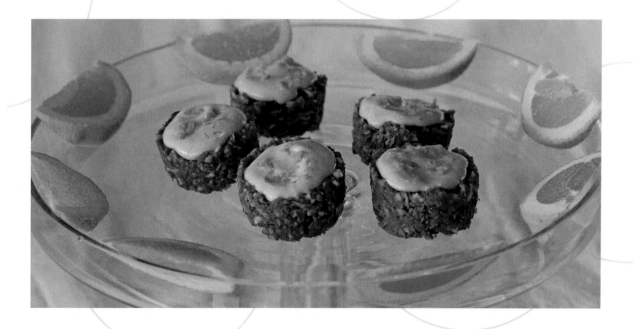

Chocolate Mousse (R)(E)

Serves: 6

Per serving: 150 Calories, 10.3g Fat, 1.7g Sat. Fat, 16g Carbs, 6g Fiber, 2.2g Protein

Ingredients:

6 medium Medjool dates (big soft dates) – pitted
Note: If you do not have access to these dates, use another dry date and soak in hot water for an hour to reconstitute.
1/3 cup water
2 medium avocados in premium condition (not too soft) - peeled and de-seeded
4 Tbsp cocoa powder
2 Tbsp Maple Syrup
2 tsp vanilla essence
Pinch of mineral salt

Directions:

In a high speed blender, blend the dates and water slowly until a paste forms with no lumps left in the mixture.

Add the rest of the ingredients and blend slowly until all ingredients are incorporated – then blend on high to form a creamy mixture.

Remove from blender to a container and refrigerate for at least one hour – will keep in the fridge for a couple of days.

Wonderful with Raw White Chocolate. (see page for recipe)

Not recommended for freezer.

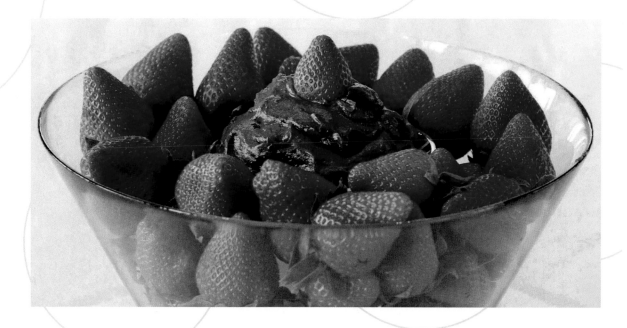

Fruit Cake (E)(Q) - Inspired by Leanne Borghesi
Serves: 8
Per serving: 367 Calorie, 17g Fat, 54.5g Carbs, 7g Fiber, 8.3g Protein

Ingredients:

1 medium sized cold seedless watermelon – cut into the largest rectangle you can manage – use cut pieces for something else – or just eat them
1 can coconut cream - chilled
1 ½ - 2 cups toasted sliced almonds
3 cups mixed berries or other fruit

Directions:

Arrange rectangular sized block of watermelon on a platter

Press the coconut cream evenly over the visible surfaces

Gently pack the almonds around the sides of the melon

Top with colorful berries

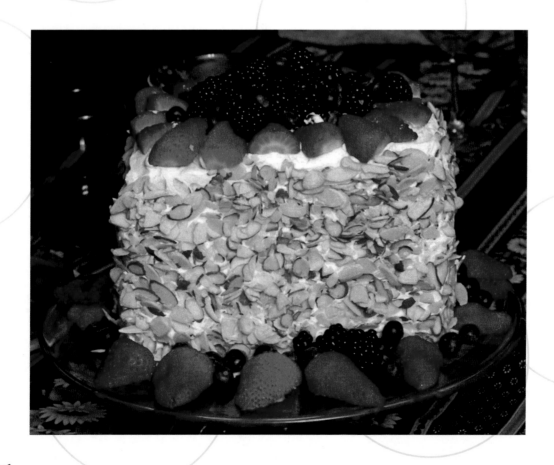

Orange Gelato (E)(R)

Serves: 10

Per serving: 281 Calories, 25g Fat, 17g Sat. Fat, 13g Carbs, 1.6g Fiber, 3.8g Protein

Ingredients:

2 cups cashews
1/2 cup coconut butter/oil
1/4 cup maple syrup
1 tsp vanilla extract
3 cups almond milk
1 cup orange juice
2 tsp orange zest
Pinch of salt

Directions:

Blend all ingredients in a high-speed blender until smooth.

Pour mixture into a rectangular container and place in the freezer to set.

Once set, remove from freezer and re-blend about an hour before you are going to use it – replace to freezer for an hour or less and serve.

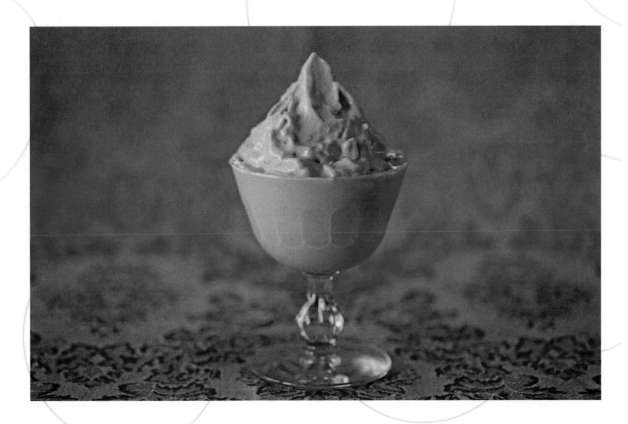

Carrot Cake (R)
Per serving: 263 Calories, 19g Fat, 23g Carbs, 3.3g Fiber, 5g Protein

Ingredients:

2 1/2 cup shredded carrots (about 3-4 large carrots)
1 cup raw walnuts
1 cup pitted dates
1/2 cup unsweetened desiccated coconut
1 tsp cinnamon
1/2 tsp nutmeg
pinch of salt

Directions:

Line an 8×8 square pan with parchment paper so that the edges hang over the sides of the pan.

By hand or in a food processor with the grating attachment, shred carrots. Place in large bowl and set aside.

With the blade attachment, chop walnuts and dates until mostly smooth – some chunks are good. Add coconut, spices, and salt and process together until just combine – do not over process. Add to carrots and mix well until combined.

Spread cake into prepared pan, smooth top, and chill for a couple of hours.

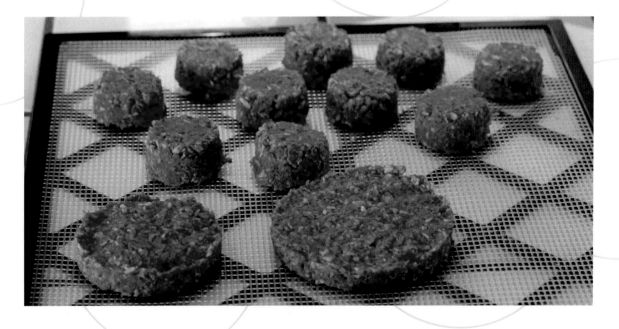

Coconut Macaroons (E)

Per serving: 91 Calories, 8.2g Fat, 4.2 Carbs, 1.4g Fiber, 1.3g Protein

Ingredients:

1/4 cup virgin coconut butter/oil
1 1/2 cup desiccated coconut
1/4 cup date purée (see page 304)
¾ cup finely chopped almonds (almond meal)
1 tsp vanilla extract

Directions:

Cream coconut butter, vanilla and date purée together in a mixing bowl with a spatula.

Add shredded coconut and almond meal to above mixture and combine well.

With a spoon, ice cream scoop or melon baller scoop out a small amount of mixture. Form scooped mixture into a ball. Place on Dehydrator tray fitted with mesh screen. Continue this step until all the batter has been used up.

Dehydrate at 105F for 6-8hours.

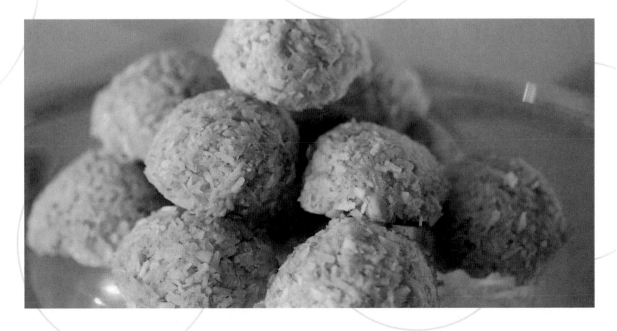

Summer Fruit Torte (Q)(E)(R)

Serves: 8
Per serving: 287 Calories, 22g Fat, 24.7g Carbs, 5.6g Fiber, 3.4g Protein

Ingredients:

CRUST
1 1/2 cups macadamia nuts (or a combination of walnuts and macadamia nuts)
1 Tbsp coconut oil
1/2 cup dates
1/4 cup dried, unsweetened coconut
1 pinch sea salt

TOPPING
2 peaches
2 nectarines
2 plums
2 apricots
½ cup raspberries
1 cup blueberries

Directions:

Pulse all the crust ingredients together in a blender and then press mixture fairly firmly into the base of a 9 inch spring with the base upside down – lip is facing downwards – place in the freezer for a couple of hours or more- if you freeze this it is fine

When you are ready to serve. Remove the base from the freezer and take of spring form, but leave crust on the base.

Decorate with the sliced fruits and enjoy

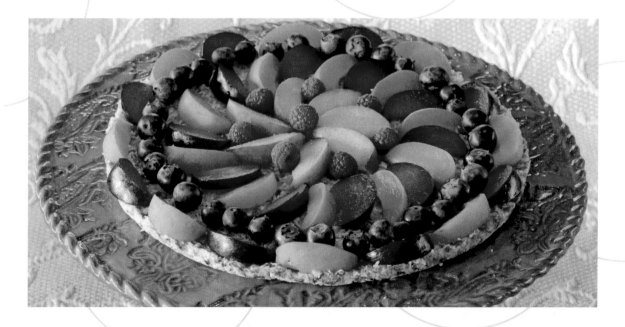

Strawberry Pistachio Macaroons (R)(E)

Makes 8 sandwiches
Per sandwich: 124 Calories, 7.2g Fat, 13.6g Carbs, 2.7g Fiber, 3.6g Protein

Ingredients:

1 cup raw pistachios, soaked for 1 hour
⅔ cup strawberries - stem trimmed off
½ cup Dates - pitted
pinch of mineral salt

Directions:

Place all of those ingredients into a food processor with an s-blade.

Pulse or run it until the ingredients start clumping together and creating a dough. You may need to scrape down the sides a couple of times to get an even texture.

You can leave them a little chunky or make them totally smooth.

Next, take roughly 2 large tablespoons of the "dough" and shape them into circles that are 3/8" thick. Do this onto parchment paper or paraflexx sheets for your dehydrator.

Once all of the dough is used, place the cookies in the dehydrator and set the temperature to 115°F.

Dehydrate for 5 hours, then carefully peel them off of their sheet and turn them over onto the mesh tray.

Dehydrate for another 5 hours, or until the cookie is to your desired consistency. I like my raw cookies pretty dry, so I dehydrated them for around 12 hours, total.

Make little sandwiches with ½ tsp raw white chocolate* and a slice of fresh strawberry .

*see page for recipe

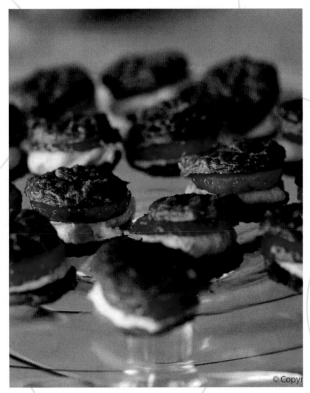

Banana Coconut Crème Pie (R): Vanilla and Chocolate Versions
Vanilla Version- Per Serving (1/12 recipe): 461 Calories, 35g Fat, 36g Carbs, 6g Fiber, 5g Protein
Chocolate Version - Per serving (1/12 recipe): 464 Calories, 36g Fat, 36.8g Carbs, 6.4g Fiber, 5.3g Protein

Ingredients:

CRUST:
1 cup macadamia nuts
1 1/2 cups desiccated coconut
1/8 tsp mineral salt
8 soft medjool dates - pitted and chopped
2 cups sliced bananas

FILLING:
2 cups sliced bananas
1/2 cup raw cashews (soaked for at least 4 hours in filtered water and drained)
1 1/2 cups young coconut meat*
1/3 cup plus 1 Tbsp maple syrup
1/4 tsp mineral salt
2 tsp pure vanilla extract
1/3 cup raw coconut oil - warmed to liquid state
Optional: 3 Tbsp Cacao powder – for a chocolate infused filling

CRÈME FILLING:
3/4 cup raw cashew pieces - soaked 4 hours and drained
1/4 cup coconut water
1 cups fresh young coconut meat (or additional soaked cashews if not available)
3 Tbsp maple syrup
1/4 tsp mineral salt
1 Tbsp pure vanilla extract
1/4 cup raw coconut oil - warmed to liquid
1/2 cup large flake coconut

*available frozen in most Asian markets

Directions:

For the crust, combine the nuts and coconut in a food processor until mixture is crumbly. Add the salt and dates and process until the mixture starts to come together when squeezed. Press into the bottom and up the sides of a 6-inch spring form pan, with the bottom of the pan turned lip down. Layer the 2 cups of sliced banana over base. Freeze while you prepare the filling.

For the filling, combine 2 cups bananas, coconut, coconut water, maple syrup, mineral salt, and vanilla in a food processor and process until smooth. With the motor running, slowly add the coconut oil and process for a minute. If you choose the chocolate version, divide the mixture into 2 bowls, then place one back in the food processor and add cacao powder. Process until combined.

Pour the chocolate filling mixture over the prepared crust, then top with sliced bananas, then pour the plain filling over the second layer of bananas. Place in the freezer to set for about 2 hours or overnight. If making the non-chocolate version, pour half of the mixture over the crust, then add the second two cups of sliced bananas, then add the remaining mixture and freeze for 2 hours minimum.

Meanwhile, to make the topping, combine the cashews, coconut water, mineral salt, maple syrup and vanilla and process until smooth. Add the coconut oil slowly with the motor running. Once the pie in the freezer has set, pour crème over the top of the pie and sprinkle with the flaked coconut. Store in the freezer until 1 hour before serving. Remove from spring form pan.

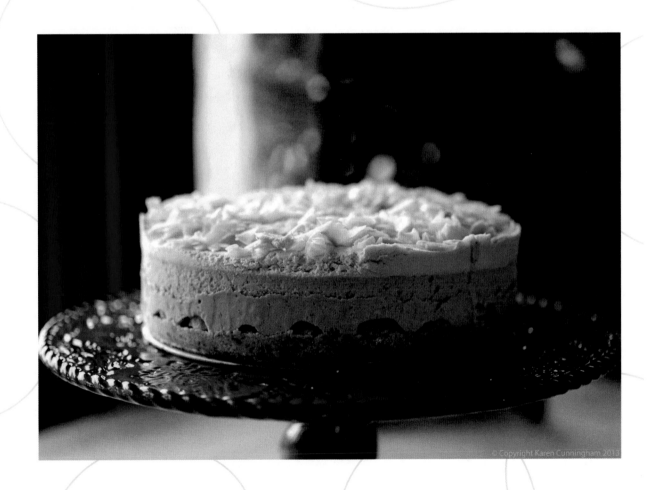

© Copyright Karen Cunningham 2013

White Chocolate (R)

Per serving (¼ cup): 135 Calories, 11g Fat, 8.1g Carbs, 0.7g Fiber, 3.2g Protein

Ingredients:

2 cups cashews
½ cup water
2 tsp lemon juice
½ cup cacao butter - grated or chopped small then melted
¼ cup maple syrup
Pinch salt

Directions:

Blend all ingredients in a high-speed blender until smooth

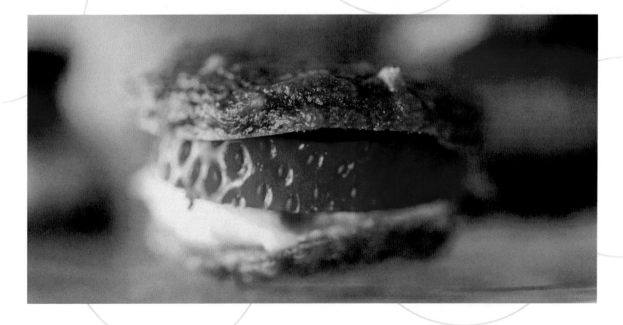

Power Cookies (E)($)

Makes: 24 cookies
Per cookie: 76 Calories, 2.1g Fat, 13.2g Carbs, 2.8g Fiber, 1.9g Protein

Ingredients:

3 large mashed bananas
2 cups gluten free oats
1 scoop soluble fiber
1 Tbsp organic cold milled ground flax
1/2 cup raisins
1/2 cup walnuts - chopped
3 large moist dates (medjool) - finely chopped
3 Tbsp orange juice
1 tsp vanilla
1 tsp cinnamon
pinch mineral salt

Directions:

Using an ice cream scoop make cookies into mounds on a lined cookie sheet.

Bake at 350 degrees for 20-25 minutes..

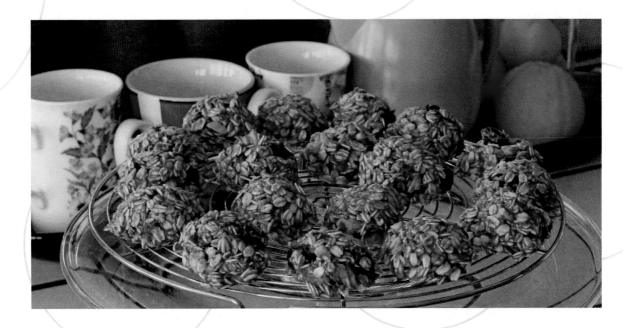

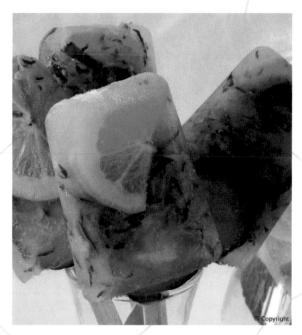

Cucumber Lemonade Pops

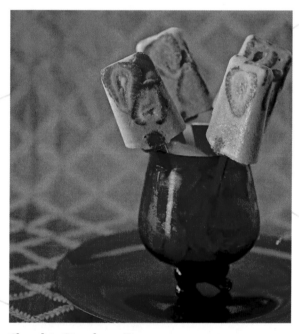

Chocolate Strawberry Pops

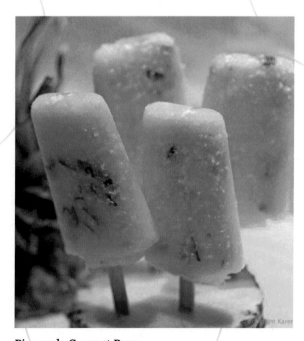

Pineapple Coconut Pops

Cucumber Lemonade Pops (E)($)

1 long Persian cucumber – ½ grated – ½ sliced into
¾ inch thick rounds
6 slices lemon
½ cup lemon juice
1 Tbsp Maple syrup
2 tbsp spearmint – sliced thin
½ cup water
6 popsicle sticks and containers

Mix the maple syrup, mint, grated cucumber, lemon
juice, and water together and divide evenly among
popsicle containers
Slide in a slice of lemon
Skewer the remaining cucumber slices on popsicle
sticks as shown in photograph and secure them into
the popsicles – freeze.

Per popsicle: 19 Calories, 0.2g Fat, 4.1g Carbs, 0.7g
Fiber, 0.3g Protein

Chocolate Strawberry Pops (E)($)

2 scoops chocolate pea, rice and cranberry protein
powder
1 cup strawberries for blending
¼ cup sliced strawberries for the popsicle containers
8 oz water or your favorite milk – almond, hemp, rice

Blend all ingredients except for the sliced berries until
smooth. Place the sliced berries evenly in the popsicle
containers and then fill to ¼ of the top of the
containers with the chocolate strawberry blend.

Per popsicle: 39 Calories, 0.4g Fat, 3.2g Carbs, 0.7g
Fiber, 5.5g Protein

Pineapple Coconut Pops (E) ($)

1 cup fresh pineapple
1 cup coconut milk
2 Tbsp spearmint leaves – finely chopped

Blend the pineapple and coconut milk together
Stir in the sliced mint and pour into popsicle
containers.

Freeze.
Per popsicle: 25 Calories, 0.8g Fat, 4.9g Carbs, 0.7g
Fiber, 0.2g Protein

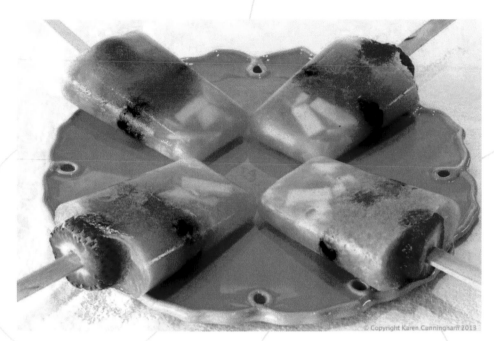

Mixed Fruit Pops

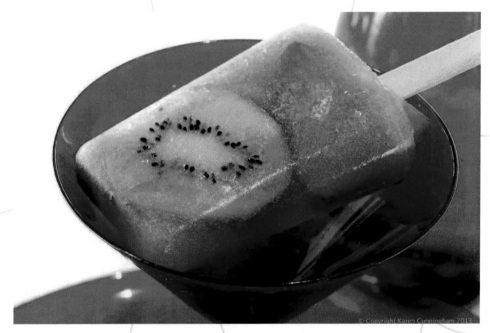

Kiwi Pops

Mixed Fruit Pops (E)($)

1 ripe mango – peeled and cut into small pieces
½ cup blueberries
12 strawberries
2 cups watermelon purée (simply blend watermelon
in a food processor or high speed blender popsicle
sticks and popsicle containers)

Add a few pieces of fruit to each popsicle container.

Skewer six strawberries as you see in the photo.

Place popsicle stick in the container and the fill to ¼
inch from top of containers with watermelon juice and
freeze.

Per popsicle: 49 Calories, 12.2g Carbs, 1.4g Fiber, 0.7g
Protein

Kiwi Pops (E)($)

3 cups watermelon purée (seedless if possible)
1/2 cup fresh blueberries
1/2 cup chopped fresh strawberries
1 kiwi, peeled and sliced
1 peach or nectarine, diced small
handful fresh cherries, pitted and chopped

Cut the watermelon into chunks and then purée it in a
blender until smooth. Set aside.

Set out about 1 dozen popsicle molds (amount needed
will vary depending on size of molds). Fill each one
with the chopped fresh fruit. Then pour in the
watermelon purée until each mold is full to the top.
Place a popsicle stick into each one. Place into your
freezer and freeze for about 6 to 8 hours.

When ready to serve, run the popsicle molds under
warm water for a few seconds and then pull each one
out.

Per popsicle: 25 Calories, 0g Fat, 6.3g Carbs, 0.7g
Fiber, 0.5g Protein

Poached Pears (E)($)(Q)

Serves: 4

1 pear with sauce: 181 Calories, 0.5g Fat, 46.8g Carbs, 7.1g Fiber, 1.7g Protein

Ingredients:

4 firm pears – peeled
2 cups fresh squeezed orange juice
2 Tbsp lemon or lime juice
½ cup water
¼ tsp ground cardamom
1 tsp cinnamon

Directions:

In a saucepan that can accommodate the 4 pears, stand the pears in the pan.

If they are not steady, gently cut a little of the bottom of each pear to make a flat surface.

Mix the remaining ingredients except for the cinnamon and pour over pears.

Simmer covered, gently for about 20 minutes until pears are soft but not mushy – during the cooking time spoon the juice over the top of the pears every few minutes to infuse the flavor.

Remove from heat, take pears out of the simmer liquid and let cool a little

Sprinkle each pear with cinnamon and serve with a little of the simmer liquid over the top.

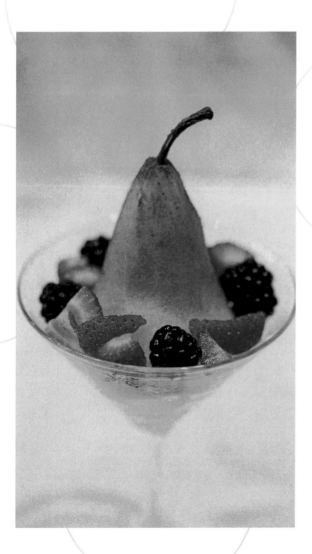

Mango Sorbet (E)($)

Serves: 3-4

Per serving: 277 Calories, 16.4g Fat, 32g Carbs, 3g Fiber, 5.8g Protein

Ingredients:

1 cup raw cashews – soaked 20 minutes - then drained
2 cups fresh mango
1 Tbsp maple syrup (optional)

Directions:

Blend ingredients together and then place in ½ cup amounts in the freezer.

When everything is frozen, and just when you are ready to serve. Put the frozen pieces into the blender and blend till just creamy

Serve immediately

Can be refrozen

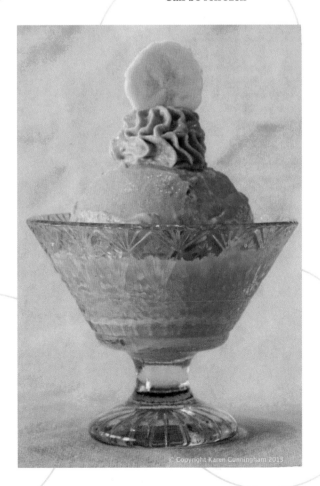

Lemon Delights (E)(R)

Per serving (1/8th recipe): 159 Calories, 11g Fat, 6.7g Sat. Fat, 10.3g Carbs, 5.7g Fiber, 3.2g Protein

Ingredients:

1 1/2 cup almond flour
1/ cup coconut flour
¼ tsp mineral salt
1 medjool date
finely grated zest of 1 of the lemons
6 Tbsp lemon juice
2 tsp vanilla
1/4 cup coconut oil

Directions:

Blend date and lemon juice

Add the remaining ingredients and process until smooth

Remove from processor and roll into small 1 inch balls or press onto cookie sheet and cut into small square 1 1 ½ inches.

Leave as is or roll in coconut, nuts, seeds or dried fruits and refrigerate

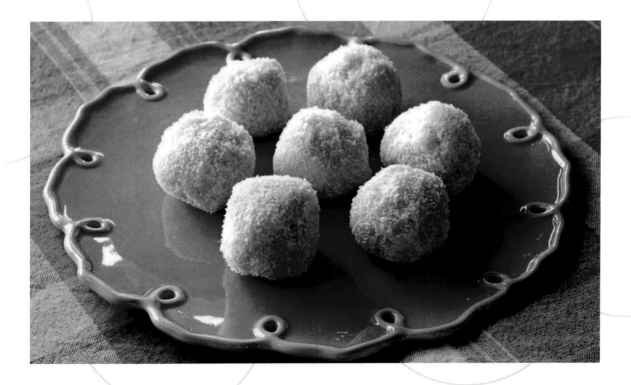

Chocolate Banana Ice Crème (E)(Q)

Serves: 6
Per serving: 192 Calories, 12.5g Fat, 15g Carbs, 3.1g Fiber, 9.2 Protein

Ingredients:

2 scoops chocolate – cranberry, pea and brown rice protein powder
¼ cup cocoa powder
2 frozen bananas
10 oz coconut (or other non dairy) milk

Directions:

Blend and enjoy.

NOTE:
Can be refrozen.

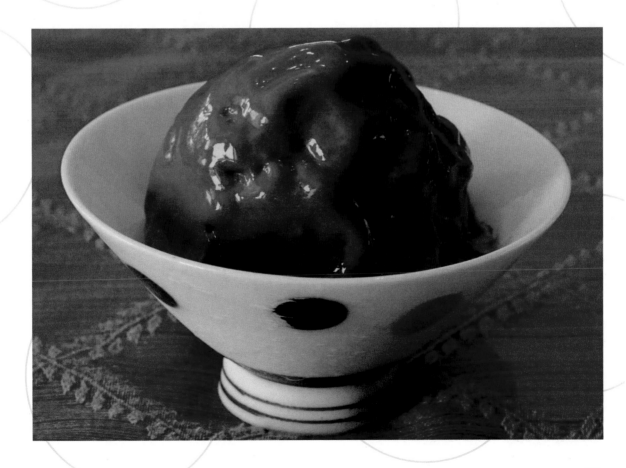

Banana Strawberry Ice Crème (E)(Q)

Serves: 6
Per serving: 203 Calories, 12g Fat, 16g Carbs, 4g Fiber, 10g Protein

Ingredients:

2 Scoops vanilla – cranberry, pea, brown rice protein
Powder
2 frozen bananas
2 cups frozen strawberries
10 oz coconut (or other non dairy) milk

Directions:

Blend and enjoy.

** Can be frozen.

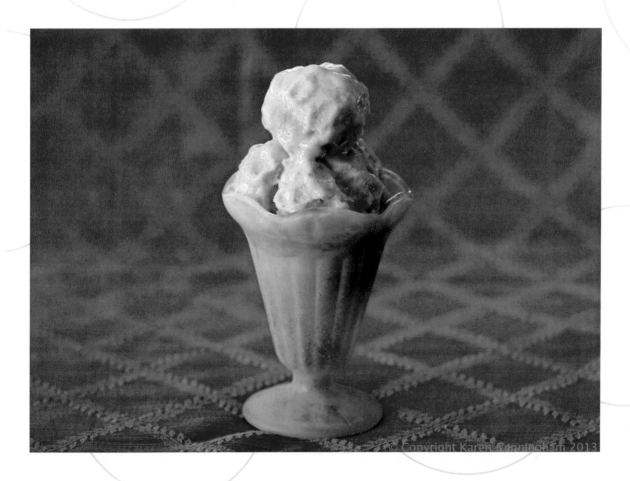

Watermelon Cupcakes** (E)(Q)($)
Makes 8-10
1 cupcake: 44 Calories, 2.9g Fat, 4.7g Carbs, 0.7g Protein
** can be frozen to make popsicles

Ingredients:

1 small yellow seedless watermelon
1 small red seedless watermelon
½ cup coconut cream

Ingredients:

Cut the watermelons into a large square – use the cut of bits for juice for watermelon pops.

Slice the watermelon into 1 inch slices.

Using a 2 inch cookie cutter, make cookie slices from your one inch slices.

Simple stack the watermelon slices and add a 1 tsp dollop of coconut cream to each slice and secure with a small skewer.

Now you can add a popsicle stick and freeze them to make popsicles.

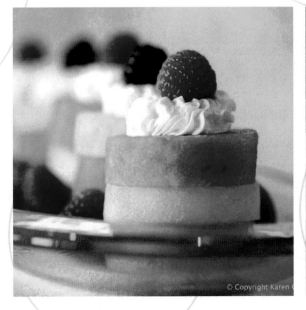
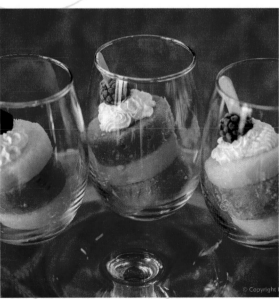

Mixed Berry Crumble (E)(Q)

Serves: 10
Per serving: 177 Calories, 14.5g Fat, 13.1g Carbs, 3.9g Fiber, 1.8g Protein

Ingredients:

1x9 inch glass casserole dish
4 cups mixed berries
1 cup strawberries
1 cup blueberries
1 cup blackberries
1 cup raspberries
½ cup orange juice
1 tsp orange blossom water (optional)

TOPPING
1 cup GF oats
1 cup unsweetened desiccated coconut
2 Tbsp coconut oil
½ tsp cinnamon
1/8 tsp ground nutmeg
¼ tsp cardamom
½ cup raisins
Mix all topping together

Directions:

Layer the berries in the glass casserole.

Place the mixed crumble topping over the berries.

Cover the dish and bake for 40 minutes, uncover the dish and bake another 10 minutes or so to lightly brown the topping.

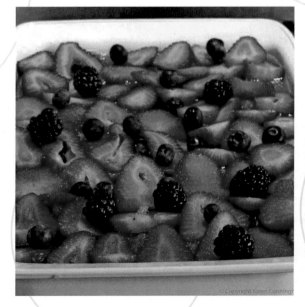
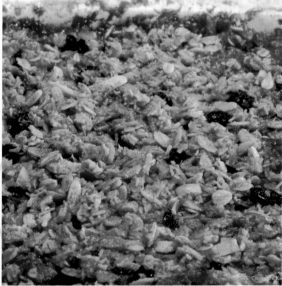

Raw Brownies (R)(E)(Q)

Cut into 24 squares
Per square: 57 Calories, 3.7g Fat, 6.9g Carbs, 1.4g Fiber, 0.8g Protein

Ingredients:

1 cup pecans (you can use walnuts in a pinch, but pecans are much better!)
1 cup Medjool dates
5 Tbsp raw cacao (cocoa) powder
4 Tbsp shredded unsweetened coconut
1/4 tsp mineral salt

Directions:

Place pecans in your food processor and process until the pecans become small and crumbly.

Add dates and process until mixture sticks together

Add the remaining ingredients and process again until the mixture turns a dark chocolate brown. Do not over process. You still want to see some texture in the mix.

Press mixture into a 9x9 brownie pan and refrigerate.

Cut into pieces once cold – it is much easier to cut this when the mix is cold. Then they can be stored at room temperature.

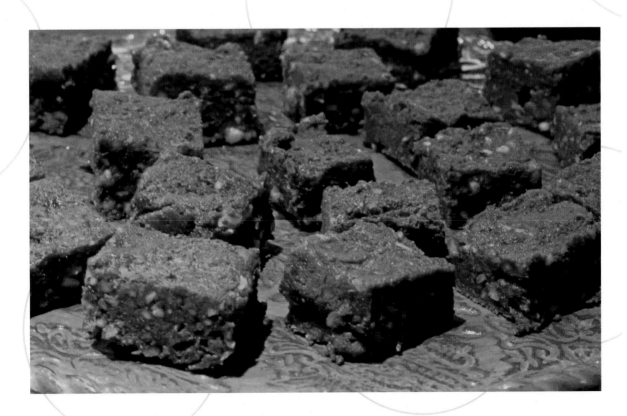

Raspberry Apple Crumble (E)(Q)

Serves: 10
Per serving: 177 Calories, 14.5g Fat, 13.1g Carbs, 3.9g Fiber, 1.8g Protein

Ingredients:

2 Cups cooked unsweetened green apples
2 cups raspberries

Topping:
1 1/2 cups macadamia nuts (or a combination of walnuts and macadamia nuts)
1 Tbsp Coconut Oil
1/2 cup dates
1/4 cup dried, unsweetened coconut
1 pinch sea salt

Directions:

Heat the oven to 350 degrees.

Place the apples in an oven proof glass pan and top with the raspberries.

Mix the topping together and crumble over the berries – cover the pan with foil.

Bake for about 30 minutes and then remove the foil and bake for a further ten minutes or so until the coconut is browned a little.

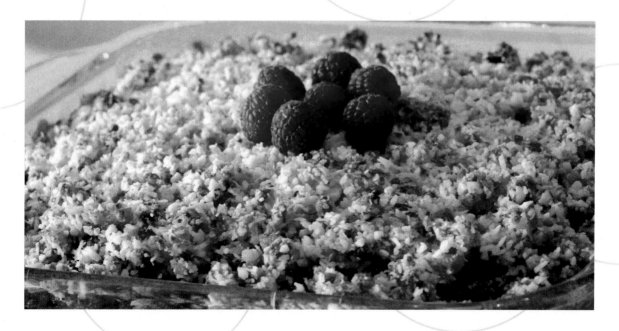

Grilled Aussie Bananas (E)(Q)

Serves: 1
Per serving: 201 Calories, 6.5g Fat

Ingredients:

1 large ripe banana
3 Tbsp chocolate banana ice crème (see page for recipe)

Directions:

Wrap the banana in foil if using indoor griddle or leave as is if barbecuing .

Make a slit on the upside of the banana.

On high heat cook/barbecue the banana until it starts to blacken and the banana inside seems cooked – about 5-10 minutes.

Remove to a serving plate.

Open the slit and put the chocolate ice cream inside and serve immediately.

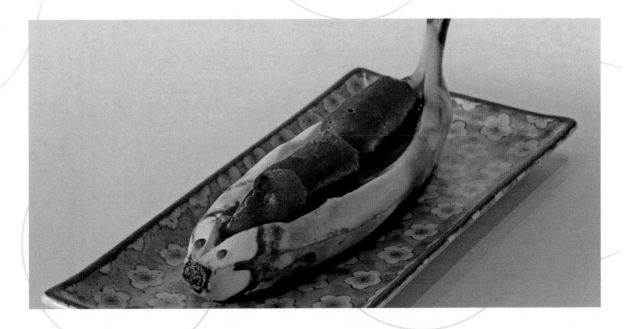

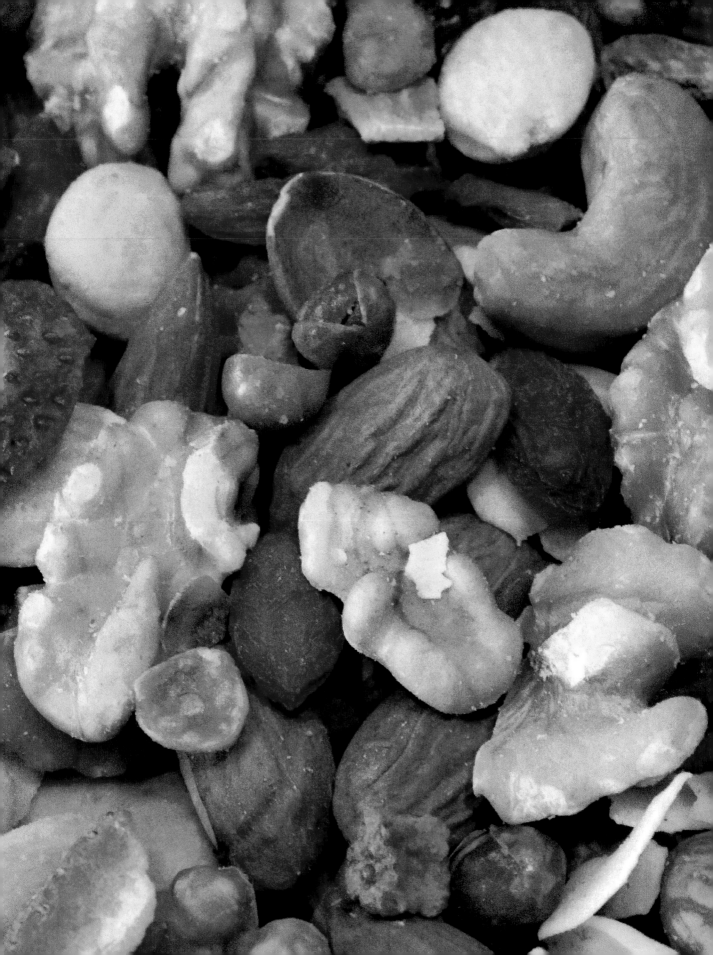

Snacks

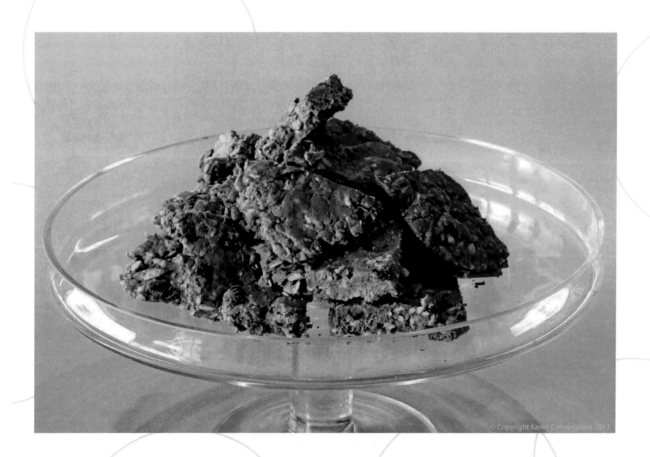

Chocolate (or Vanilla) Brown Rice Protein Bars (E)(Q)
Makes: 16
Per serving: 314 Calories, 20g Fat, 22.5g Carbs, 4g Fiber, 17g Protein

Ingredients:

5 scoops chocolate or vanilla cranberry-rice-yellow pea protein powder
2 cups nut butter (almond, peanut, sunflower, cashew) or a mix
2 Tbsp dried blueberries
2 Tbsp flax seeds
2 Tbsp sunflower seeds
4 dates blended smooth (blend with some nut butter)
1/2 cup maple syrup
1-2 Tbsp grapeseed oil
4 cups brown rice crisps

Directions:

Mix all ingredients in a bowl except rice crisps.

When ingredients are combined mix in rice crisps by hand (Mixer will crush them).

Press into a pan and chill in the refrigerator, cut into small pieces and enjoy .

Coconut Flax Protein Bars (E)(Q)
Makes: 16
Per serving: 159 Calories, 7g Fat, 15g Carbs, 2.2g Fiber, 11g Protein

Ingredients:

1 cup cranberry-rice-yellow pea protein powder
1 cup brown rice crisps
3/4 cup gluten free oats
3/4 cup maple syrup
1/3 cup almond butter
1/3 cup sunflower butter
2 Tbsp whole flax seeds
2 Tbsp unsweetened desiccated coconut (optional)

Directions:

In a hot glass bowl add maple syrup, butters and protein – mix well
Add rice crisps and oatmeal – mix well
Spoon into 8x8 tray – pressing mixture into the tray
Sprinkle flax seed and coconut over the top and press well
Refrigerate two hours or until set.
Cut into pieces.

Note:
Can be frozen

Karen Cunningham's Protein Bars (E)(Q)
Per serving: 216 Calories, 13g Fat, 19.6g Carbs, 3.4g Fiber, 9.2g Protein

Ingredients:

2 cups cranberry-rice-yellow pea protein powder
3 cups gluten free oats
2 cups organic Almond butter
1 cup maple syrup
2 Tbsp flax seeds

Directions:

Pour almond butter and maple syrup in microwavable bowl. Heat for 60-90 seconds until pliable and easy to mix. Combine well.
Mix dry ingredients in a large bowl – would be easiest in an electric mixer on low speed.
Add almond butter and maple syrup mixture – mix slowly until ingredients combined well
Press mixture quite firmly into in a 9x13 pan.
Sprinkle flax seeds over the top and gently press into the mixture (you could use sesame seeds instead)

Refrigerate 1 hour. Cut into 24 squares.

Cheesy Kale Chips * ($)(E)

Per serving (1/6th recipe): 199 Calories, 14.8g Fat, 12.3g Carbs, 3.3g Fiber, 7.9g Protein

*I use my dehydrator for these to avoid losing any nutrients, so mine are considered raw, but as most people do not have a dehydrator, here is the oven version

Ingredients:

3/4 cup cashews
1/4 cup water
1/4 Tsp salt
1 bunch kale, washed and dried and de-stemmed
2 cloves garlic
1 Tbsp sesame tahini paste
1/2 red bell pepper, stem and seeds removed
1 Tbsp tamari sauce
2 Tbsp EVOO
1/3 cup nutritional yeast (not to be confused with Brewer's yeast)
2 Tbsp lemon juice

Directions:

Preheat oven to the lowest heat setting. Line several baking sheets with silpats or unbleached parchment paper.

Soak cashews for about 4 hours and then drain them.

Add everything to your blender and blend to a smooth paste.

In a large bowl, combine kale and cashew paste, making sure kale is evenly coated. Place kale pieces on baking sheets allowing space between each piece so they do not touch or overlap.

Bake kale until crisp and completely dry, between 2 and 4 hours. Check after the first hour and turn leaves over. Check kale periodically. Chips will be ready when crunchy and stiff and topping doesn't feel chewy or moist.

Kale chips will keep in an air tight container for one week.

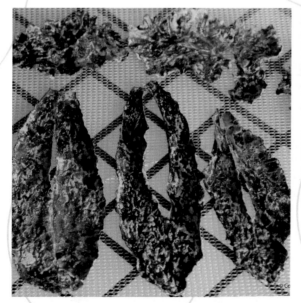

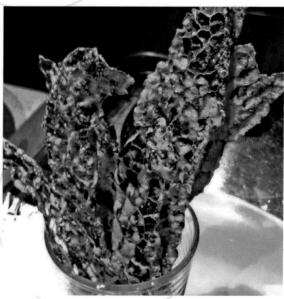

Spiced Almonds ($)(E)
Per serving: 124 Calories, 12.2g Fat, 2.8g Carbs, 1.6g Fiber, 2.5g Protein

Ingredients:

2 cups Raw almonds – soak for 4 hours
½ cup EVOO
½ tsp ground black pepper
1 tsp mineral salt
2 Tbsp dried rosemary

Directions:

After soaking the almonds, drain and slip of their skins

Lay almonds on a paraflexx sheet and dry at 115 degrees for about 10 hours. You could also do this on a lined cookie sheet in your oven at the lowest temperature for about 4 hours or so.

Mix the ingredients together and then roast the almonds at 300 degrees for about an hour.

Taste them. If they are still a little soft inside, bake a little longer until they are crunchy.

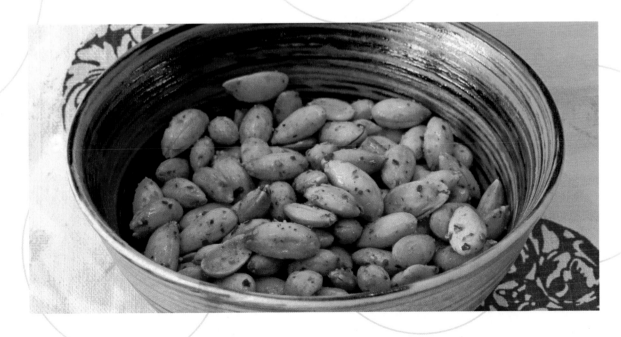

Toasted Tamari Sunflower Seeds (E)(Q)($)

Serves: 4
Per serving: 73 Calories, 6g Fat, 2.8g Carbs, 1.1g Fiber, 3.3g Protein

Ingredients:

1 cup sunflower seeds
2 Tbsp Tamari Sauce

Directions:

These are a great little snack and also taste fantastic over any salad.

In a medium fry pan over medium heat toast sunflower seeds until they just become fragrant and start to change color.

Turn off the heat and add a Tbsp or so of Tamari sauce.

Stir vigorously with a wooden spoon to coat the seeds then remove from fry pan immediately.

NOTE:
Pan will need to be soaked right away as the tamari tends to stick.

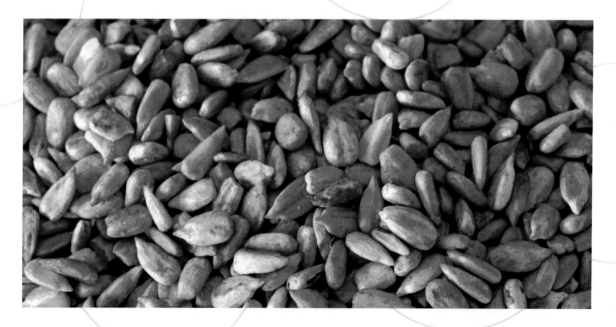

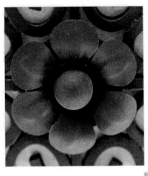
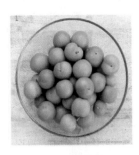
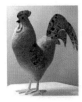
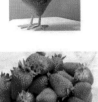

sprout

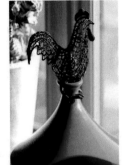

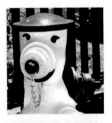
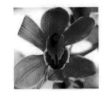

Eat well
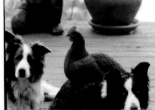
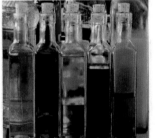
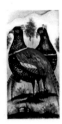

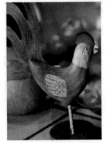
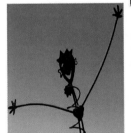
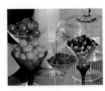
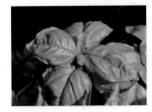
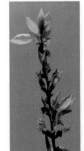

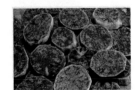

PLAY

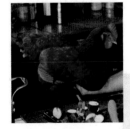

relax

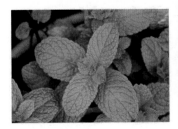
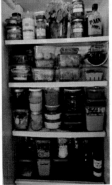

e
x
e
r
c
i
s
e

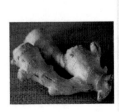
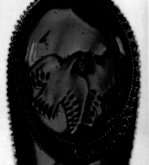

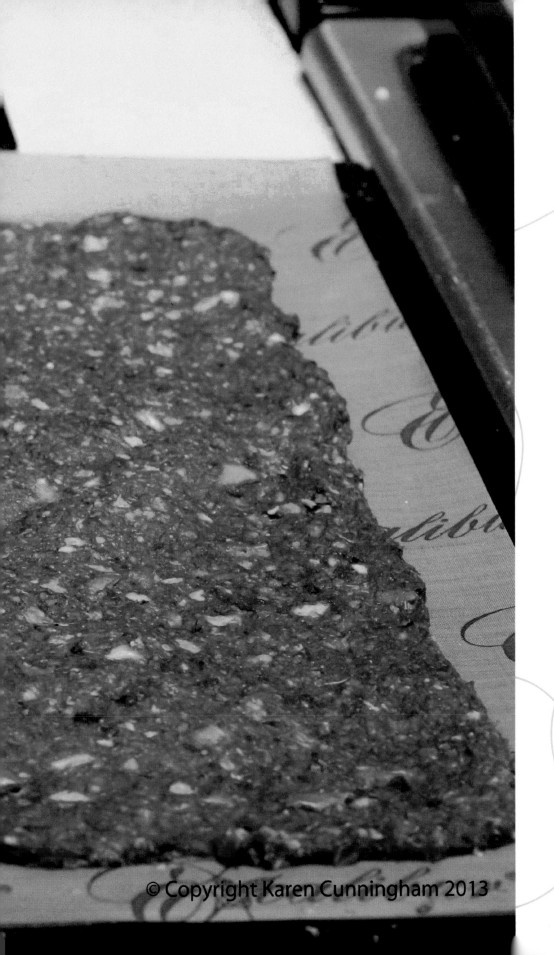

Bread

Onion Bread (R)

Serves: 12
Per serving: 126 Calories, 9.3g Fat, 5.6g Carbs, 5.3g Fiber, 4.7g Protein

Ingredients:

1 yellow onion
1 cup soaked brazil nuts
1/2 cup soaked sunflower seeds
1/2 cup ground flax seeds
1/2 cup soaked almonds
2 Tbsp chia seeds
1 Tbsp date purée (see page 304)
2 tsp EVOO

Directions:

Blend all ingredients in a food processor or blender.

Spread on dehydrator unbleached parchment sheet.

Dehydrate 1 hour at 145 then turn heat down to 105 for 24 hrs

Turn over half way through

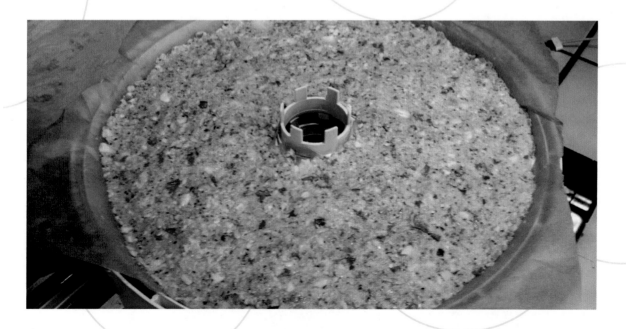

Sundried Tomato Buckwheat Bread (R)*

Makes 18 slices
Per serving (1/20th recipe): 254 Calories, 19g Fat,10g Carbs, 8.5g Fiber, 11.6g Protein

*This recipe requires a dehydrator

Ingredients:

1/2 cup EVOO
1 1/2 cups sun dried tomatoes in oil - drained
3 cups sprouted buckwheat – (see sprouting recipe)
1 cup flax meal
3 1/2 cups peeled zucchini - roughly chopped
2 cups apple - cored and roughly chopped
3 Tbsp lemon juice
2 avocados
1 large onion
1/2 cup minced parsley

Directions:

In a processor grind the olive oil, drained sun dried tomatoes, sprouted buckwheat, zucchini, apple, lemon juice, avocados, onion and herbs until thoroughly mixed.

In a large mixing bowl mix the batter with the flax meal by hand. There will be too much mixture for the food processor to handle.

Divide the mixture in 2 and place on Paraflexx sheets, on dehydrator trays.

Use a spatula to spread the mixture evenly to all 4 sides and corners of Paraflexx dehydrator sheet. If mixture is too sticky you can wet the spatula to make things easier. With a knife score the whole thing into 9 squares.

Dehydrate for 2 hours and then remove the Paraflexx sheets by placing another dehydrator tray and mesh on top and invert so that your original sheet of bread is upside down. That will allow you to peel the Paralexx sheet off and continue to dehydrate the underside of the bread.

Dehydrate for approx 8 hours more (do this overnight so you're not tempted to eat it before it's ready) or until bread feels light in your hand.

If the pieces don't fully come apart where you scored, use a knife to cut them.

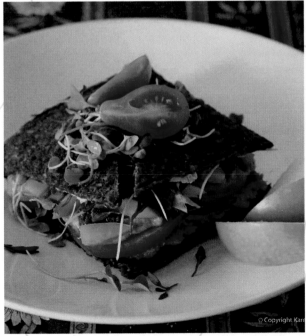

Buckwheat Mungbean Bread (R)

Per serving (1 slice): 145 Calories, 10.3g Fat, 13.4g Carbs, 4.8g Fiber, 3.4g Protein

Ingredients:

2 cups fresh mung bean sprouts
¾ cup almonds
½ cup raw cashew nuts
½ cup pepitas
1 ¼ golden linseed
1/8 cup sun-dried tomatoes
4 fresh dates
4 small gloves of garlic
2 Tbsp fresh ginger
2 small onion
½ cup fresh coriander
2 fresh chilies
1 Tbsp organic olive oil
1/8 cup nutritional yeast
1 tsp mineral salt
5-7 g freshly ground cumin seed
3/4 cup water
cayenne pepper to taste
fresh good water

Directions:

Chop sprouts roughly.

Transfer to same large mixing bowl place dates, soaked tomatoes, strained pepitas and salt in, scrape down walls and add the soaking water from the tomatoes.

Transfer to bowl.

Blend/grind drained almonds and cashews, then add olive oil, nutritional yeast and water, blend till creamy.

Transfer to bowl.

Add the gelatinous linseed to the large mixing bowl and stir until all ingredients are well entwined add cayenne to taste.

Garbanzo Flour Tortillas (E)($)(Q)

Serves: 4
Per serving: 167 Calories, 14.8g Fat, 7.8g Carbs, 3g Fiber, 2.9g Protein

Ingredients:

1 cup Garbanzo Flour
1 cup coconut milk
1/2 tsp salt
3/4 tsp turmeric
1/4 tsp chili powder (or not)

Directions:

Blend all ingredients together until you have a standard consistency pancake batter.

Heat griddle on medium high.

Use a little coconut oil to grease the griddle.

Place approximately 2-3 Tbsp of the batter onto the griddle and spread until taco sized. cook one side until you see some bubbles forming on the top side of the taco. Flip and cook the other side. You want these light brown.

Remove from heat and keep warm until ready to use. These will keep a day or so in the fridge, but are best at the time you make them.

Use as you would a regular tortilla.

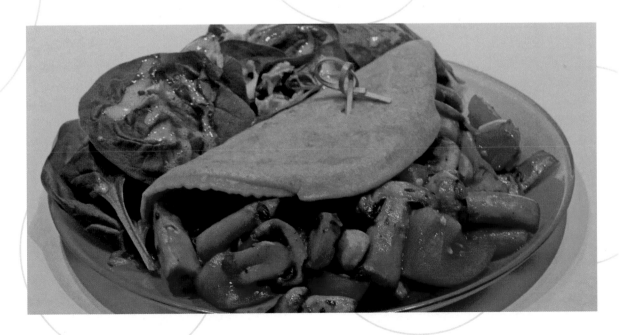

Garbanzo Flour Pie Crust (E)

entire recipe: 597 Calories, 53g Fat, 27g Carbs, 7.5g Fiber, 9g Protein

Ingredients:

1 1/2 cups besan flour
1 tsp salt
1/4 cup EVOO
1/2 cup cold water (up to 1/2 cup)

Directions:

Mix EVOO and water

Place besan flour and salt in a mixer and turn to low speed

Slowly add the oil water mix and process until well blended and the dough becomes a ball.

Turn out onto a rolling board covered with unbleached waxed paper (I use Natural Value paper as it is non-toxic and recyclable).

Place another layer of wax paper on top and roll as thin as you like, say 1/4" or less.

Cut into sizes that will cover your pies.

Bake at 375 alone for a more crunchy crust = 10-15 minutes, or if you cover the pies at this time the crust will end up a little softer = 15-20 minutes

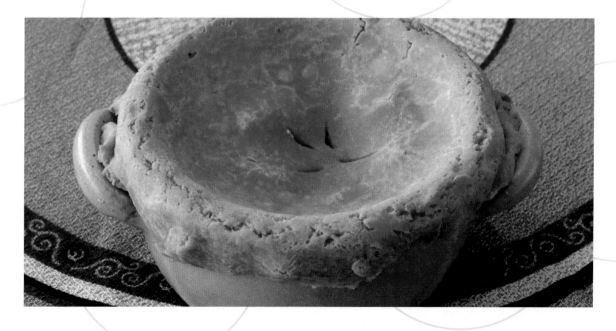

Dosa (Indian Pancakes) ($)(E)

Makes 20-25 pancakes*
Per pancake: 68 Calories, 0.2g Fat, 14g Carbs, 1.7g Fiber, 2.2g Protein

*can be stored in the refrigerator

Ingredients:

3/4 cup of parboiled rice (also labeled Idli rice in Indian stores)
3/4 cup of medium grain rice
1/2 cup whole black gram (urad dal – without husk)
1/2 tsp Fenugreek seeds (methi)
salt to taste (start from 1-1/2 tsp)
grapeseed oil for the pan - just enough for a light coating to prevent sticking

Directions:

Soak the black gram and Fenugreek together in a bowl and the rice separately in another bowl for at least 3 hours.

You need a high speed blender to grind the dosa batter until almost smooth

Pour into a large bowl (this mix will expand to almost twice its volume). Add salt and mix well.

Set this aside to ferment overnight somewhere fairly warm, or cover and place in a dehydrator at 90 degrees.

Next day, mix the batter well. Heat an iron skillet or crepe pan and, grease with little oil. I use a cut onion to spread the oil - this prevents the batter from sticking.

Drop ½ cup of batter onto the hot griddle and spread it around into a thin crepe

Let it cook for 2-3 minutes until you see the edges turning up. You will be easily able to place a spatula under it. Also if you have spread it thinly, you will be able to see the bottom cooked when you start seeing reddish-brownish color from the surface.

Turn and cook for another 1-2 min.

Fold and serve hot.

NOTE: These are best served as soon as they are made. The number of side dishes enjoyed along with this is endless. Enjoy it with coconut chutney (see page 186).

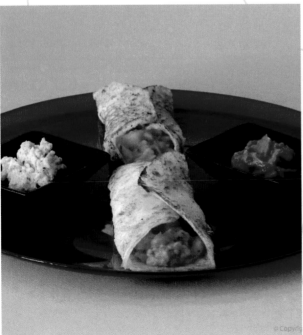

Besan Pancake ($)(E)
Makes 5-6 pancakes
Per serving: 31 Calories, 1.1g Fat, 4.4g Carbs, 0.8g Fiber, 1g Protein

Ingredients:

1 cup besan (garbanzo flour)
1 cup water
½ tsp mineral salt
1 Tbsp potato or tapioca starch
grapeseed oil for the griddle

Directions:

Mix all ingredients and let sit for about 10 minutes

Heat the griddle and lightly grease the surface

Drop about a ½ cup measure of batter onto the hot griddle and cook until browned on one side. Flip and brown. Remove from the griddle and keep on a plate until ready to use. These keep well for a few days in the fridge

Options: You can add spinach, onion, tomato or just about any vegetable

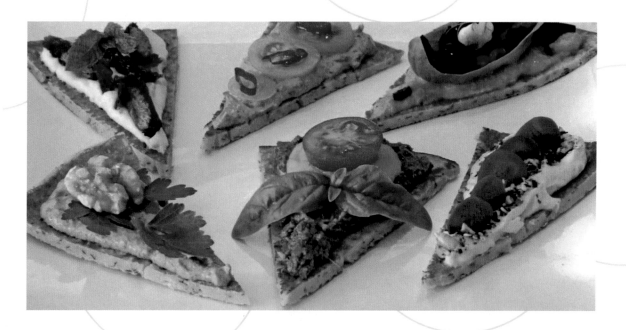

Socca - Provencal Garbanzo Bean Pancake ($)(E)

Makes 3

Per serving (1/4th pancake): 124 Calories, 11.1g Fat, 6g Carbs, 1.7g Fiber, 1.7g Protein

Ingredients:

1 cup Garbanzo flour flour
1/2 tsp mineral salt
1/2 tsp ground pepper
1 cup warm water
3 Tbsp grapeseed oil
1/2 medium onion - sliced
1/2 Tbsp fresh rosemary leaf – minced

Directions:

In a medium skillet heat 1 Tbsp oil and gently fry the onion until soft and lightly browned

(option 1)Heat large skillet to medium-high heat.

OR

(option 2) lightly grease 3 4 1/2 inch mini cake pans

In a large bowl, sift flour, salt and pepper together. Add rosemary

Whisk in warm water and 2 Tbsp Grape Seed oil.

Cover the bowl and allow the batter set for at least 30 minutes, which should have the consistency of thick cream. Stir sliced onion into the batter.

(Option 1) Add 1 Tbsp Grape Seed oil to the hot pan, pour batter onto pan and bake for 12-15 minutes or until the pancake is firm and the edges are set (top may not be browned).
Set socca a few inches below your broiler for 1-2 minutes, just long enough to brown it in spots. Cut into wedges and serve hot, with toppings of your choice.

(Option 2) OR preheat oven to 450 degrees and bake them for 30 minutes until set and slightly browned on top

Set socca a few inches below your broiler for 1-2 minutes, just long enough to brown it in spots. Cut into wedges and serve hot, with toppings of your choice.

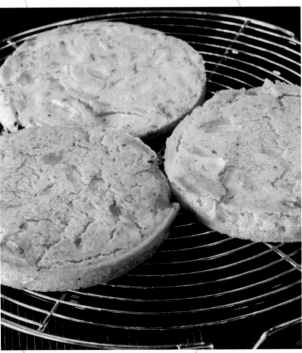

Ethiopian Injera (X)($)
Makes 30 Injera
Per Injera: 34 Calories, 0g Fat, 6.6g Carbs, 1.2g Fiber, 1.2g Protein

Ingredients:

For the starter:
Takes five days. If you want to have some starter left over to make injera again, wait seven days.
3/4 cup water - room temp. (70 degrees)
1/2 cup teff flour
A pinch active yeast (about 1/8 tsp)

For the Injera:
1/4 cup teff starter
1-3/4 cups water - at room temperature
1-3/4 cups teff flour
1/4 tsp Mineral salt

Directions:

Day 1:
Combine ingredients for the starter in a bowl.

Loosely cover the starter with the lid/cloth and ferment for two days on the counter or someplace that is about 70 degrees. You should see some rising in about four hours. Let alone for 2 days.

Day 3:
Stir the starter. This is when the "stinker" effect starts. The starter has a very yeasty and grassy smell. You will also notice that small bubbles on the surface now.

Feed the starter 1/3 cup teff flour and 1/2 cup water and loosely cover with the lid. Let alone for 2 days.

Day 5:
Starter should have separated into distinct layers. You would think that something has gone wrong with it - what with watery layer on top and dense muddy flour at the bottom! But that's exactly what we are looking for :) Stir starter, it should be slightly fizzy and have a very strong gassy aroma.
Feed with 1/3 cup teff flour and 1/2 cup water. Loosely cover and allow to sit alone for at least 4 hours before using to make Injera. You should have about 2 cups of starter by now.

Now lets go to the Injera recipe Uses only 1/4 cup of the starter. If you want to use all the 2 cups of the starter increase the flour, salt and water accordingly

Place the starter in a bowl. Pour the water over the starter and stir to dissolve.

Add the teff flour and mix until the batter is smooth. It will have the consistency of thin pancake batter.

Ferment. Cover and let stand for 5 to 6 hours at room temperature. Reserve 1/4 cup of the starter for the next batch.

Add the salt and stir to dissolve.

Heat a 10- or 12-inch skillet over medium heat (you'll also need a tight-fitting lid). Using a paper towel, wipe the skillet with a thin layer of vegetable oil.

Ethiopian Injera (cont.)

Pour about 1/2 cup (for a 10-inch skillet) or 3/4 cup (for a 12-inch skillet) of batter in the center of the skillet.

Tilt and swirl the skillet immediately to coat evenly.

Let the bread cook for about 1 minute, just until holes start to form on the surface.

Cover the skillet with the lid to steam the injera.

Cook for about 3 minutes, just until the edges pull away from the sides and the top is set.

The first 1-2 Injera's might not be fabulous – but then the first pancake or 2 is never great either.

Just cook it on one side. It does not get the spongy texture immediately. But let it rest for 3-5 minutes and it suddenly gets that amazing texture.

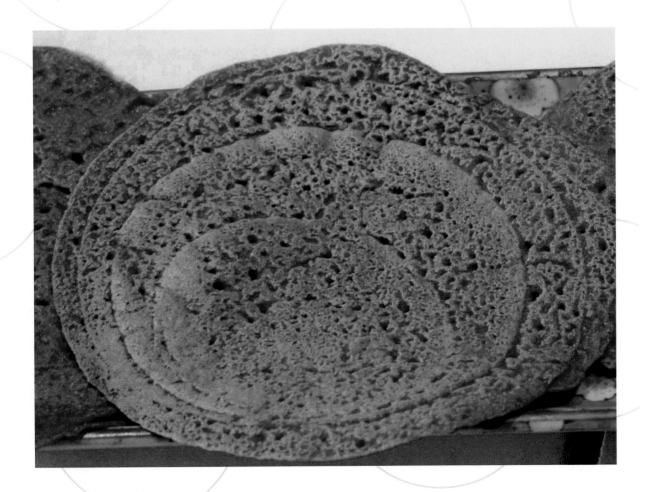

Pizza Crust (R)(E)*

Serves: 6
Per serving: 307 Calories, 14g Fat, 23.3g Carbs, 19g Fiber, 15.2g Protein

*This recipe requires a dehydrator.

Ingredients:

5 medium carrots - grated
2 cups whole GF oats – made into flower in your food processor
1 1/2 cups flax seeds – ground in high speed blender or by hand
2/3 cups water

Directions:

Mix all prepared ingredients in a large bowl and let sit for one hour.

Form your pizza crust on a Paraflexx sheet.

Dehydrate at 105 degrees for 3 hours.

Using a second dehydrator tray, place over the pizza and turn over.

Remove the Paraflexx sheet and continue to dehydrate for another 6-8 hours

Top with your favorite raw pizza toppings.

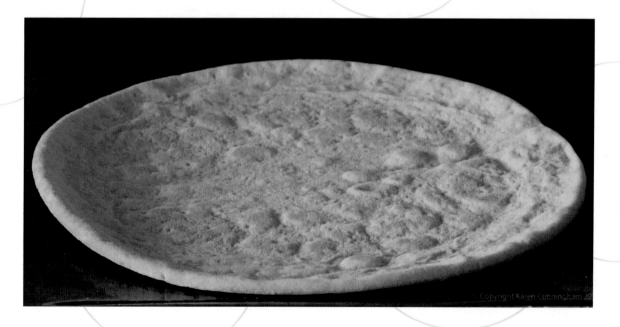

Cauliflower Pizza Crust (E)($)

Serves: 6
Per serving: 116 Calories, 7.7g Fat, 8.6g Carbs, 4.4g Fiber, 6.1g Protein

Ingredients:

3 cups ground cauliflower
1 cup and 2 T. almond flour
4.5 flax eggs
4 Tbsp nutritional yeast
1 tsp sea salt
1 tsp dried rosemary
1 tsp garlic powder
freshly ground pepper to taste

Directions:

Process the cauliflower in the food processor until it resembles ground rice.

Mix all ingredients in the food processor. It will be a sticky dough.
Separate into 6 pieces and flatten to 6 inch circles.
Bake un-topped for 20 minutes.

Remove bases and top with your ingredients and re-bake for another 15 minutes or so

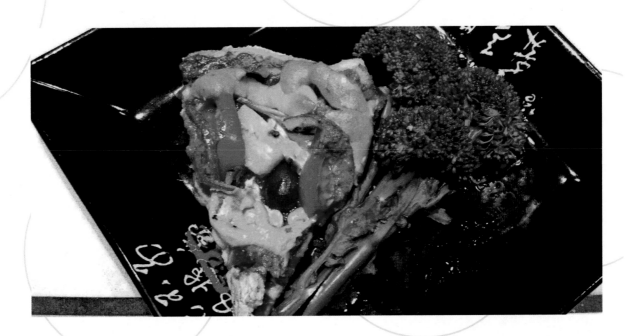

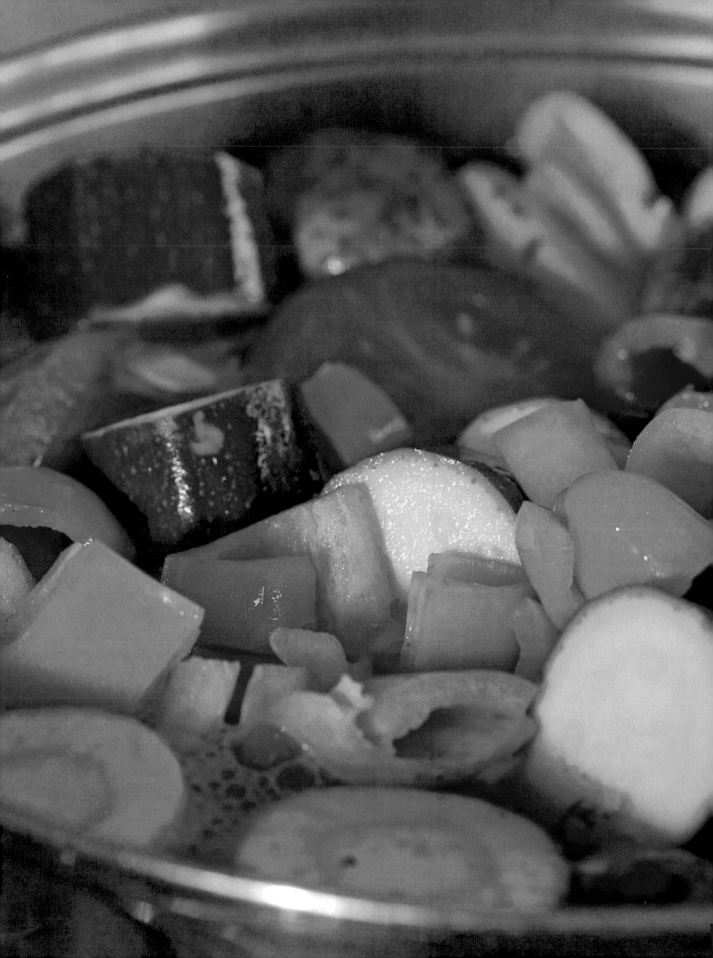

Broths, Stocks and Others

Date Purée (E)(Q)

Per 1/4 cup: 56 Calories, 0.1g Fat, 14.8g Carbs, 1.6g Fiber, 0.5g Protein

Ingredients:

2 cups soft pitted medjool or other high quality dates.

Directions:

Cover the dates with water and soak overnight.

purée in a high speed blender and then freeze in ice cube containers.

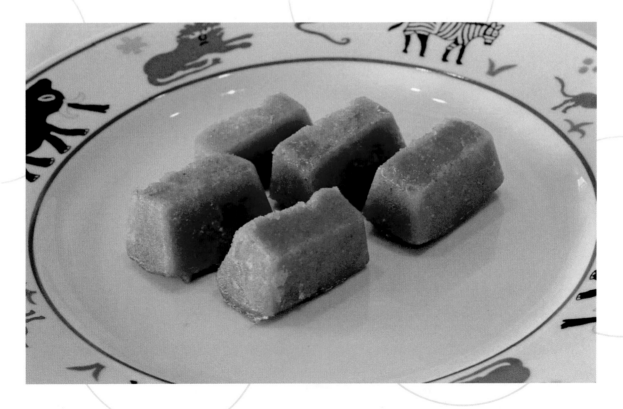

Alkalizing Broth (E)(Q)($)

Per cup: 23 Calories, 0g Fat, 5g Carbs, 1g Fiber, 0.5g Protein

Ingredients:

4 qt. Spring water
3 medium sweet potatoes - diced
4 carrots - cubed
2 medium onions - chopped
2 small beets - diced
3 stalks of celery - chopped
1 bunch of parsley - chopped
1 bunch of kale or other leafy vegetable
2 cloves of garlic - minced or pressed
2 tsp dried, flaked dulse (seaweed) or 1 sheet nori or kombu
Pinch of sage

NOTE:
Add dandelion greens or any other root or orange vegetables that you enjoy to the broth.

For a little spice, add a hot pepper

For a little sweeter flavor, add lemon or orange

Directions:

Wash and scrub all vegetables. Do not peel unless you cannot find an organic vegetable. Bring water to a boil. Add vegetables and bring the water back to a boil. Once boiling, turn heat down to simmer. Cover the pot.

Simmer the vegetables for several hours. Remove 2/3 cup of vegetables, blend in blender, and mix with some broth to make purée to eat with meals or mix to thicken other soups. It is full of fiber.

Strain the broth. It is alkaline and rich in minerals, especially potassium, which can be flushed out of the body when taking extra liquids.

Sip broth between meals and enjoy a healthier, more alkaline gut!

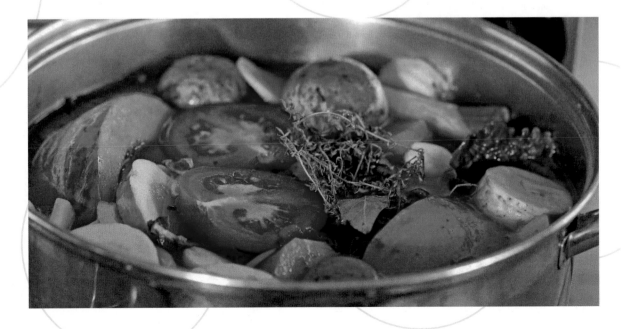

Fermented Vegetables* ($)
Makes 2 quarts
Per serving (1/2 cup): 22 Calories, 0.2g Fat, 4.5g Carbs, 1.5g Fiber, 1g Protein

*Use sterilized mason jars

Ingredients:

½ large super fresh white cabbage – the cabbage has the required friendly bacteria to start this process
1 head garlic
2 cups parsley
2 jalapeno chilies
2 Habañero chilies
1 red bell pepper
2 cups baby kale
6 radishes
1 large red onion
1 whole bunch of celery - juiced
2 tsp salt per jar

Directions:

Chop the vegetables and pack into jars

Mix required salt with the celery juice and pour over the vegetables

Put lids on loosely – so the fermenting vegetables gasses can leave the jars.

Place jars in a warm place undisturbed for 3 days – then taste and see if you like the flavor adjust seasonings –leave for a few more days – still with the lids loosely attached. Check again. If a white mold appears on top of the vegetables, this is harmless – just scoop it off and throw it away.

Reserve some of the juice as this is now a vegetable probiotic starter.

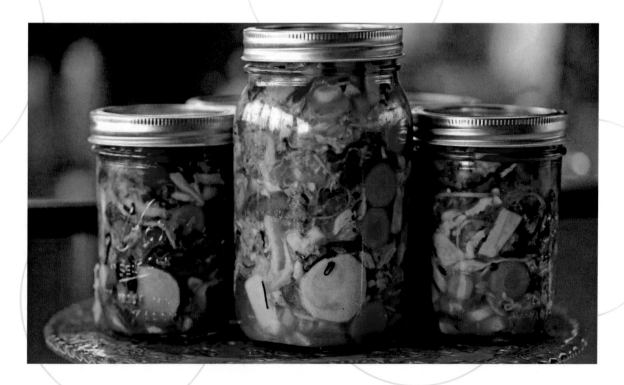

Dashi - Japanese Stock ($)
Makes 4 cups
Per 1 cup: 65 Calories, 0.1g Fat, 13.3g Carbs, 2.6g Fiber, 2g Protein

Ingredients:

4 cups cold water
6 inch piece kombu (kelp, find in Asian market)
3 whole shiitake mushrooms
Pinch dried wakame (kelp, similar to kombu but with different minerals and flavor)
2 Tbsp best cooking Sake
2 Tbsp Mirin (sweet rice wine)
2 1/2 Tbsp Tamari

Directions:

In a pot of the water, soak the Kombu and shiitake mushrooms for about an hour.

Bring to a boil and add the wakame and Tamari – boil 5 minutes.

Turn off the heat and add the Mirin and Sake.

Remove the solids from the stock.

Use what you need for today and freeze the rest in 1 Tbsp containers or ice cube trays.

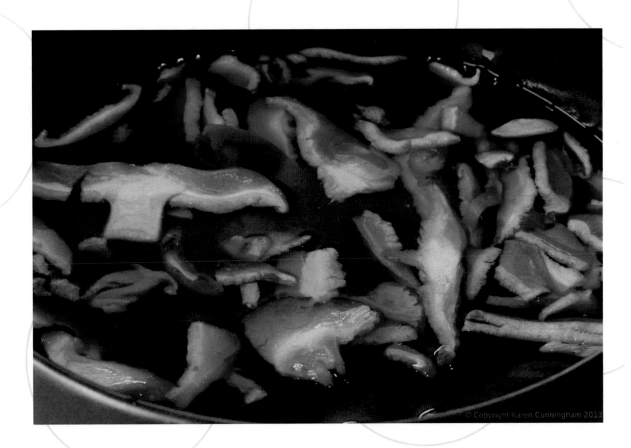

© Copyright Karen Cunningham 2013

Hearty Vegetable Broth ($)(Q)(E)

Per serving (1 cup): 108 Calories, 3g Fat, 18g Carbs, 5.3g Fiber, 2.5g Protein

Ingredients:

1 gallon water
1 pound celery – chopped with leaves
1 1/2 pounds sweet onions
1 pound carrots - cut into 1 inch pieces
1 pound tomatoes - chopped
1 pound green bell pepper - cut into 1 inch pieces
1/2 pound turnips - cubed
2 Tbsp Grapeseed oil
3 cloves garlic
3 whole cloves
1 bay leaf
6 whole black peppercorns
1 bunch fresh parsley - chopped

Directions:

Heat oven to 350 degrees
Toss the celery, onions, carrots, tomatoes, peppers and turnips with the oil and place on a roasting pan in the oven. Roast for about 45 minutes.

Remove from the oven and pour some of the water into the pan to loosen the juices from the bottom of the pan

After a few minutes – put all ingredients into a large stock pot with the water and the remaining ingredients and simmer until the volume is about halved.

Use in your favorite dishes
Can be frozen

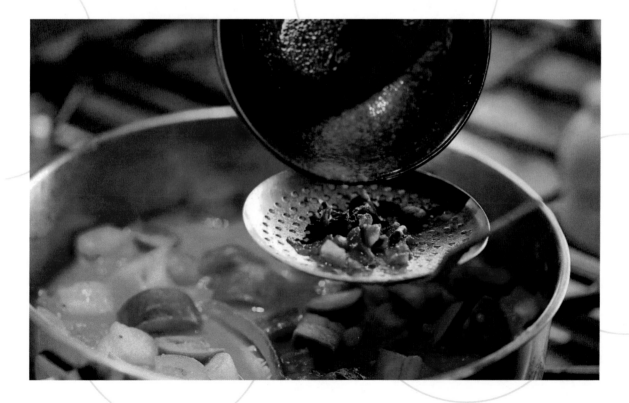

Socca Tower ($)(E)

Serves: 3
Per serving: 306 Calories, 26.3g Fat, 16g Carbs, 3.8g Fiber, 4g Protein

Ingredients:

socca pancakes (see page 297)
1 large turnip – peeled and sliced into three pieces
1 meyer lemon (they are sweet – use regular lemon if not available) – sliced
1 red onion – sliced
2 Tbsp EVOO
¼ tsp
3 Tbsp cilantro
3 Tbsp cashew sour crème (see page 238)
2 Tbsp of your favorite Tomato sauce (I like romesco - see page 198)

Directions:

Heat over to 350 and place the onion lemon slices and turnip slices on a non stick sheet on a cookie sheet.

Drizzle with 1 TBSP of the EVOO and sprinkle with the salt

Roast until the vegetables are cooked – you want the lemon and the onion to caramelize – about 20 – 30 minutes

Meanwhile blend the cilantro wit the remaining EVOO and set aside

Heat the tomato sauce.

When the vegetables are ready build your tower: Socca topped with tomato sauce - then turnip – cilantro sauce – sour crème – lemon and finally the onion

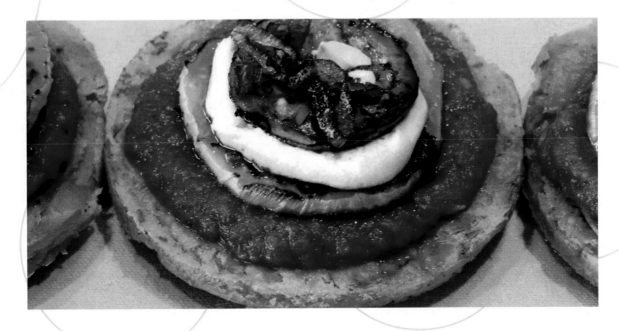

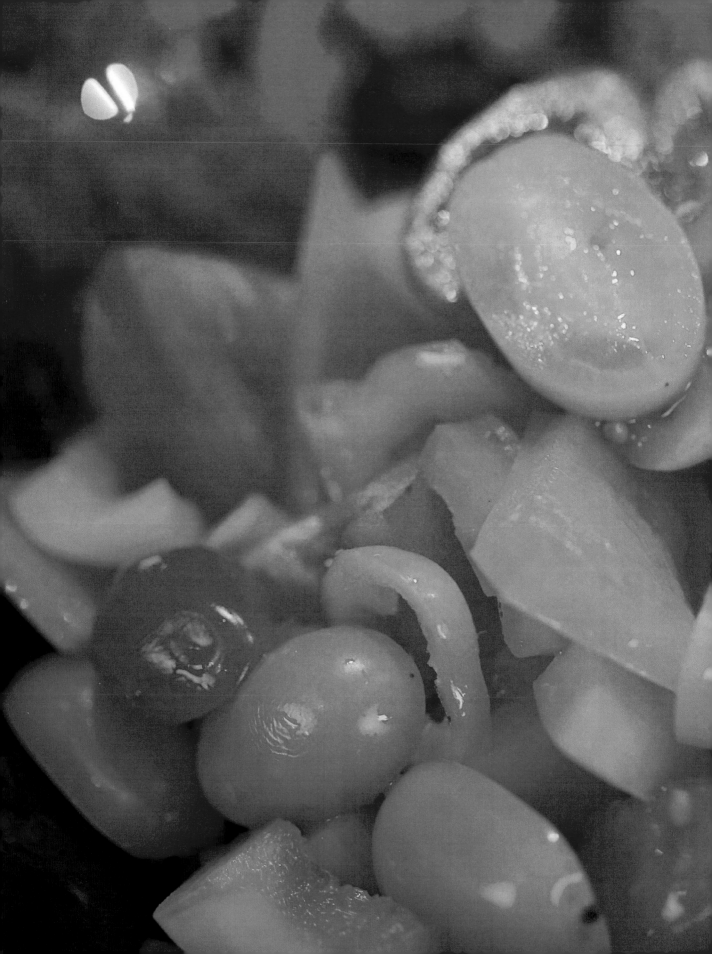

Naked Vegetables

Lemon Asparagus ($)(E)(Q)
Per serving (4): 41 Calories, 3.6g Fat, 2.7g Carbs, 1.1g Fiber, 0.9g Protein

Ingredients:

1 bunch asparagus washed and woody stems remove (hint: hold 1/3 towards the end of the asparagus and the end and bend. It will snap at the woody part. Use woody ends in stock pot or discard.)
zest of 1 lemon
juice of 2 lemon
salt and pepper
EVOO

Directions:

Heat griddle or fry pan to high heat

Rub asparagus with a little EVOO and salt and pepper

Place asparagus on the griddle and cook for just a couple of minutes until the asparagus turns bright green and has a couple of brown spots from grilling.

Remove from the grill and place on a serving platter

Cover with the lemon zest and lemon juice and serve immediately

NOTE:
This dish is also great at room temperature or the next day alone or with a salad

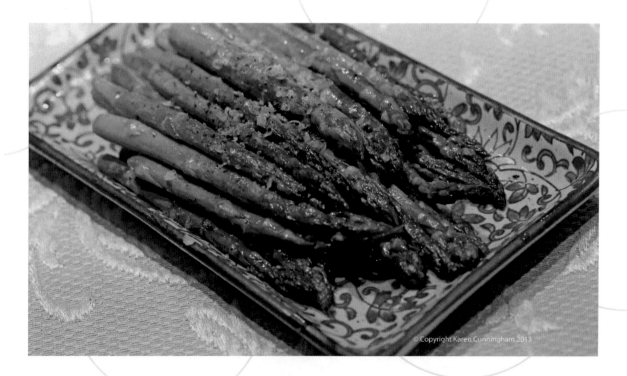

Roasted Beets ($)(Q)(E)

Serves: 2
Per serving: 100 Calories, 0.2g Fat, 22.9g Carbs, 2.2g Fiber, 2.5g Protein

Ingredients:

2 large beets
1 cup orange juice
1/4 tsp mineral salt
grated zest of 1 orange

Directions:

Heat oven to 350 and place your beets on a silpat or other cooking sheet on a cookie tray.

Bake until a cake tester goes through the beet without too much force. Let the beets cool in the oven.

Remove and peel and chop into sizes that are appealing to you

My favorite is roasted beets covered with orange juice and some grated orange rind.

You can add any nuts or seeds to the beets, but just do this before serving unless you want pink walnuts or pine nuts

Simple delicious beets are great marinated in orange juice for 3-4 days in the fridge.

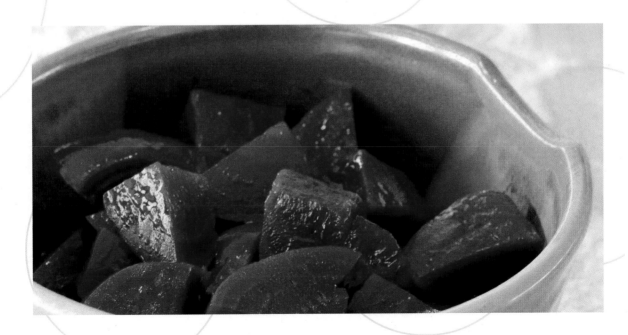

Cabbage with Roasted Root Vegetables ($)(E)

Serves: 6
Per serving: 214 Calories, 6g Fat, 33g Carbs, 7g Fiber, 6.7g Protein

Ingredients:

Use medium sized vegetables

2 carrots – peeled and chopped
2 Turnips– peeled and chopped
2 Rutabagas– peeled and chopped
2 Parsnips– peeled and chopped
2 sweet potatoes– peeled and chopped
2 Onions– peeled and chopped
2 Tbsp EVOO
1 tsp poultry seasoning
1 sprig Rosemary
6 cups vegetable broth
1 red bell pepper – chopped
1 tsp of your favorite herbs
pinch saffron

Directions:

Roasted root vegetables are such a hearty treat - simply chop as many root vegetables as you like into 1 inch pieces.

Place in a roasting pan and rub with EVOO, salt and pepper and sprinkle with poultry seasoning.

Add a sprig of rosemary and roast in the oven at 350 degrees until done.

Then make your most favorite vegetable broth, then throw in a little spice (if you like things on the hot side).

Add a pinch of Saffron, and 1 tsp poultry seasoning (usually a mix of parsley, sage, rosemary and thyme).

Chop up half a large cabbage and put into the broth along with chopped red peppers and carrot - simmer for ten minutes and ladle into bowls and serve with the roasted root vegetables over the top.

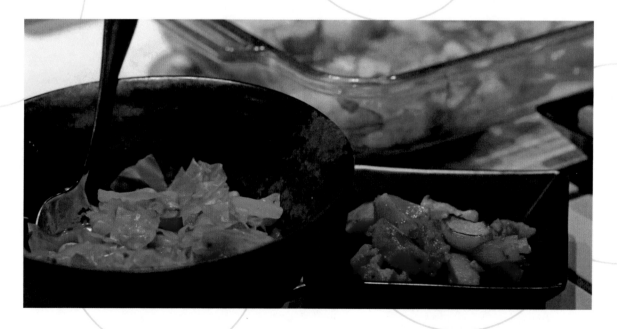

Zucchini, Tomato, Bell Pepper Gratin (Q)($)(E)

Serves: 6
Per serving: 113 Calories, 3.3g Fat, 19.6g Carbs, 6.1g Fiber, 5.7g Protein

Ingredients:

1 large sweet yellow onion
EVOO
Salt & Pepper
1 small branch of thyme
1 bunch basil
6-8 medium slicing tomatoes
1 red bell pepper
10 small green or yellow zucchini

Directions:

Peel and slice onions. Cut pepper into strips
Slice zucchini diagonally. Slice tomatoes as if for a
sandwich.

Rinse basil, shake dry and then remove leaves,
discarding the stems. Remove leaves from the thyme.

Sauté the onions until translucent in the EVOO on low
heat.

Turn heat to medium and add pepper, sauté until soft

Heat oven to 350.

Place all of the onions and peppers in a 9x12 glass
baking dish, spread evenly over bottom of pan.

Then spread all of the basil over that layer.

Then make layers alternatively of zucchini and
tomatoes, finishing with tomatoes – each layer should
be very lightly salted and peppered.

When you are finished layering, press the vegetables
down to firm the dish up a little.

Bake until cooked to your satisfaction.

If the tomatoes seem a little dry in the baking process,
remove from the oven and tilt the pan, scooping some
of the juices and spreading over the top layer.

This will also help infuse these great and very simple
flavors.

Finish with a sprinkle of pepper and apple cider
vinegar

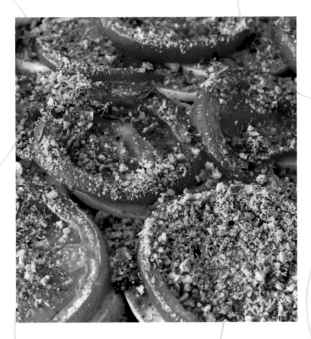

Coconut Broccoli (Q)($)(E)

Serves: 4
Per serving: 177 Calories, 12.1g Fat, 13.8g Carbs, 4.7g Fiber, 7.7g Protein

Ingredients:

6 cups broccoli – sliced lengthwise
½ cup unsweetened coconut milk
1 Tbsp Miso paste
1 tsp freshly grated ginger
1 clove garlic
½ cup vegetable stock
4 Tbsp raw or lightly toasted pumpkin seeds

Directions:

Heat the liquids in a medium fry pan.

Add the ginger, miso and garlic and mix well.

Bring to a slow boil and add the broccoli.

Cook for a few minutes turning often.

Remove from heat when the broccoli is bright green and just a little soft.

Place on a serving platter and spoon over the sauce and pumpkin seeds.

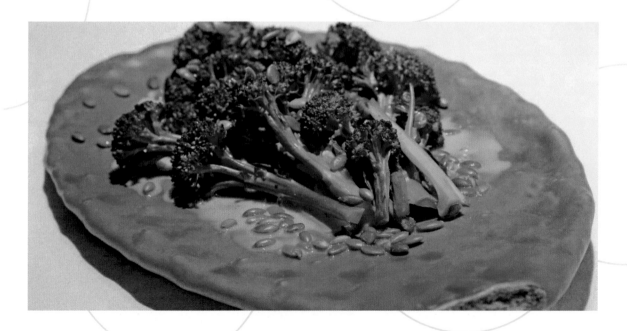

Grilled Eggplant and Vegetables (E)($)

Serves: 4
Per serving: 393 Calories, 13.2g Fat, 58.9g Carbs, 5.8g Fiber, 12.5g Protein

Ingredients:

1 small eggplant (about 1 pound) - cut into 1/4-inch rounds
2 small zucchini - cut lengthwise into 1/4-inch slices
1 red bell pepper - quartered
1 clove garlic - minced
3 Tbsp EVOO
3/4 tsp mineral salt
1/4 tsp fresh-ground black pepper
1/4 tsp grated lemon zest
4 tsp lemon juice
3 Tbsp fresh parsley - chopped
3/4 tsp ground cumin
3/4 pound brown rice pasta cooked according to directions on packet – set aside
pine nut parmesan cheese - for serving

Directions:

Light the grill or heat the broiler. In a large shallow bowl, toss the eggplant, zucchini, bell pepper, and garlic with 2 Tbsp of the oil, 1/4 tsp of the salt, and 1/8 tsp of the black pepper.

If using the broiler, arrange the vegetables in a single layer on one large or two smaller baking sheets, preferably nonstick. Grill or broil in batches, turning the vegetables once, until they are tender and lightly browned, 10 to 12 minutes. Cut the vegetables into 1 1/2-inch pieces.

In a small glass or stainless-steel bowl, whisk together the remaining 4 tablespoons olive oil, the lemon zest, lemon juice, parsley, cumin, and the remaining 1/2 tsp salt and 1/8 tsp pepper.
Toss pasta with 1 Tbsp of water, the oil-and-lemon-juice mixture, and the vegetables. Add more pasta water if the pasta seems dry. Top with some pine nut parmesan (see page for recipe).

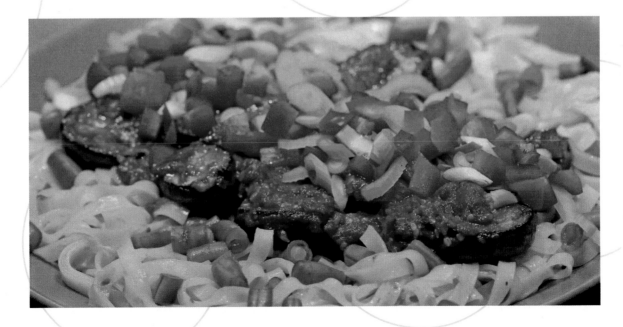

Broccoli with Garlic (Q)($)(E)

Serves: 4
Per serving: 47 Calories, 2.6g Fat, 5.2g Carbs, 1.8g Fiber, 2.0g Protein

Ingredients:

1 bunch broccoli - washed, trimmed and cut into pieces
3 cloves garlic - minced
Pinch of chili flakes
Zest of a lemon
1 Tbsp lemon juice
2 tsp EVOO
1/4 cup water or vegetable broth

Directions:

Heat 2 tsp EVOO in a skillet and add garlic and chili flakes.

Cook just until fragrant.

Add broccoli.

Stir for about 30 seconds.

Pour in water or broth and cover.

Cook about 3 minutes until broccoli is tender, but still bright green.

Top with lemon juice and zest. Season with mineral salt and pepper.

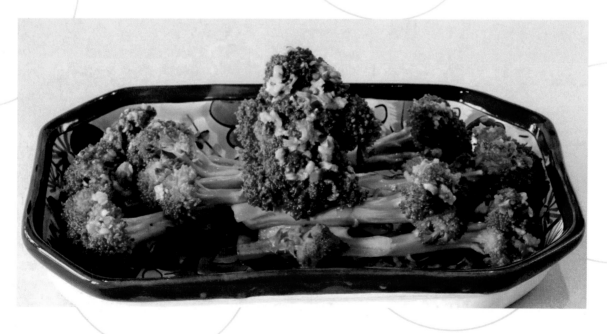

Crispy Butternut Squash (Q)($)(E)

Serves: 4-6
Per serving: 145 Calories, 12g Fat, 10g Carbs, 2g Fiber, 1g Protein

Ingredients:

1 medium Butternut Squash
4-6 cloves of garlic - chopped
3 ½ Tbsp EVOO
2 Tbsp roughly chopped sage
1Tbsp lemon juice
Mineral Salt and pepper

Directions:

Heat oven to 350 degrees.

Slice butternut squash into ½ inch thick slices.

Rub with EVOO .

Place on lined baking sheet.

Scatter sage, garlic and salt and pepper over each slice.

Bake 30 minutes or until soft and slightly browned.

Finish with the lemon juice and some additional sage if you like.

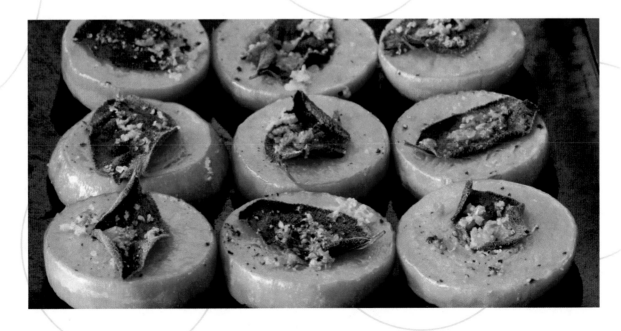

Broiled Cauliflower Fennel and Pumpkin Seeds (Q)($)(E)

Serves: 4
Per serving: 114 Calories, 9g Fat, 7g Carbs, 3.4g Fiber, 2.7g Protein

Ingredients:

½ head cauliflower – broken into florets
1 large fennel bulb – sliced horizontally
2 lemons - sliced and deseeded
2 Tbsp Grapeseed oil
cracked black pepper
2 Tbsp dry roasted pumpkin seeds
2 Tbsp lemon juice

Directions:

Turn broiler to medium-high.

Lay the vegetables on a covered cookie sheet and brush with the oil.

Crack as much pepper as you like over the tray and broil for about 10 minutes or until the cauliflower just starts to brown, as in the picture.

Remove from broiler and drizzle with the pumpkin seeds and lemon juice and serve.

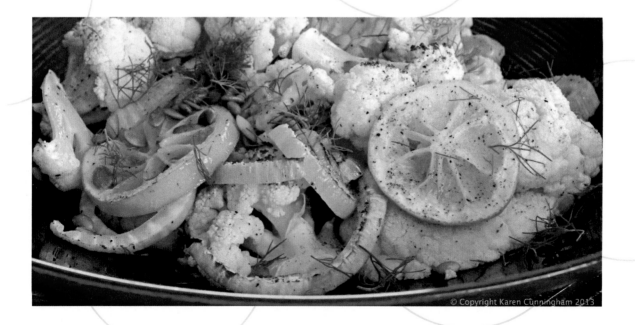

© Copyright Karen Cunningham 2013

Broiled Cauliflower with Orange and Olive (Q)($)(E)

Serves: 4
Per serving: 178 Calories, 10.6g Fat, 20.5g Carbs, 6.9g Fiber, 4g Protein

Ingredients:

1 medium sized cauliflower – cut into 2 inch vertical slices
2 Tbsp grapeseed oil – for brushing
mineral salt and black pepper
2 oranges – peeled, sliced and deseeded
1 cup kalamata or, if you are cleansing, salt cured olives

Directions:

Arrange the cauliflower slices on a lined cookie sheet.

Brush with the oil and sprinkle with salt and pepper.

Broil on medium heat for about ten minutes until the cauliflower starts to brown and crunch a little.

Remove from oven and serve with the orange slices and olives.

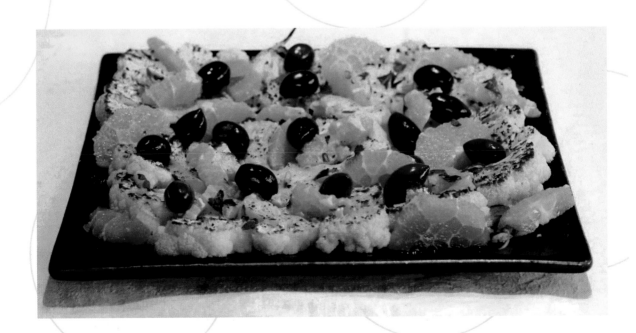

Garlic Grilled Artichoke (Q)($)(E)

Serves: 4

Per artichoke: 132 Calories, 7.2g Fat, 15g Carbs, 7.1g Fiber, 4.6g Protein

Ingredients:

4 medium sized artichokes – halved lengthwise
2 Tbsp grapeseed oil
4 tsp minced garlic
grated mineral salt
½ cup lemon juice

Directions:

Trim the ends of the artichokes, cut one third off the top of each artichoke, cut in half lengthwise, scrape the furry center bits out

Drizzle with a mix of garlic, mineral salt, and organic grape seed oil.

Turn on the grill and roast them cut side down.

When they look done (like in the picture) turn cut side up and roast a little longer on a plate and drizzle with lemon juice.

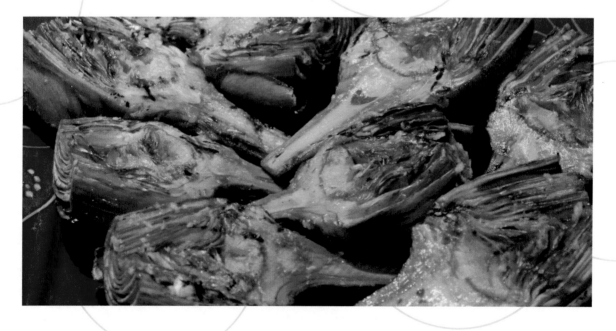

Garlicky Green Beans (Q)(E)($)

Serves: 6
Per serving: 46 Calories, 2.5g Fat, 5.9g Carbs, 2.6g Fiber, 1.5g Protein

Ingredients:

1 lb green beans – ends removed
2 Tbsp water
3 cloves garlic – crushed
1 tbsp lemon juice
1 Tbsp EVOO
1 tsp Nut 'N Seed Breading (see page 370) for the topping per person

Directions:

In a sauté pan, heat the EVOO to medium heat.

Add the garlic and sauté for a couple of minutes.

Add the green beans lemon juice and water and sauté just until the beans turn bright green – stirring all the time. This will just be a couple of minutes.

Remove and serve immediately topped with Nut N' Seed breading.

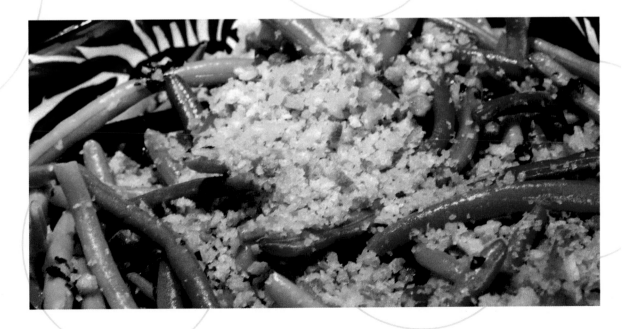

Orange Broccoli (Q)($)(E)

Serves: 4
Per serving: 56 Calories, 10.6g Carbs, 2.9g Fiber, 3.9g Protein

Ingredients:

5 cups broccoli
1/2 cup vegetable stock
½ cup orange juice
grated zest of 1 orange
¼ tsp mineral salt
ground coriander - optional

Directions:

Sauté the broccoli and the orange juice and vegetable stock for about 4-5 minutes.

Platter and sprinkle on the orange zest and then grind some coriander over the top.

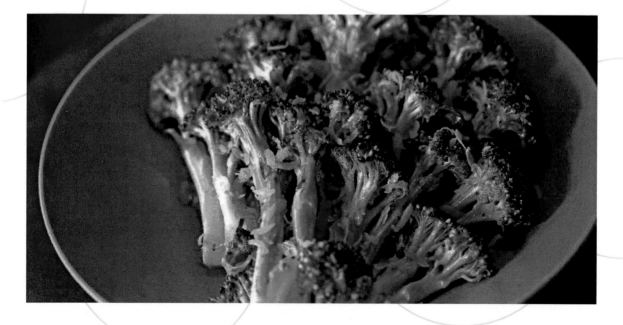

Peruvian Potatoes (Q)($)(E)

Serves: 5
Per serving: 231 Calories, 8.6 g Fat, 36g Carbs, 5.5g Fiber, 4g Protein

Ingredients:

2 1/2 pounds blue Peruvian potatoes*
3 cloves garlic - minced
2 Tbsp fresh cilantro -chopped
3 Tbsp EVOO
1/2 tsp salt
1/8 tsp ground black pepper
2 tsp fresh leaf thyme or 1/2 tsp dried leaf thyme

*use purple potatoes if not available

Directions:

Scrub potatoes – do not peel. Cut potatoes into 1-inch pieces.

Toss with the garlic, cilantro, EVOO, salt, pepper, and thyme.

Arrange in one layer in a large baking pan or roasting pan.

Cook, turning occasionally, for 20 to 25 minutes, or until browned and tender.

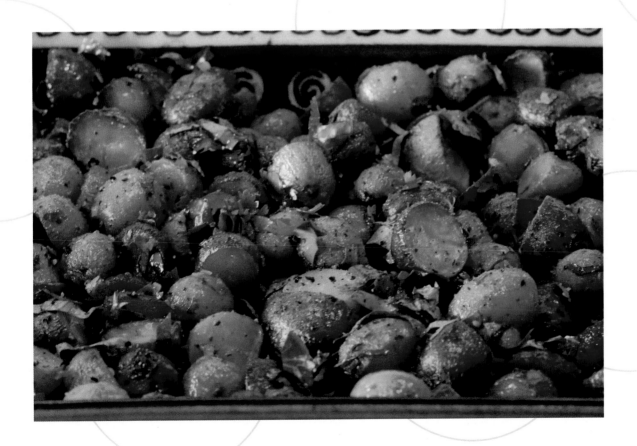

Edamame (Q)($)(E)

Serves: 2
Per serving: 80 Calories, 3g Fat, 6.5g Carbs, 2.5g Fiber, 6.5g Protein

Ingredients:

2 cups edamame in the shell

Directions:

Steam and serve with asian inspired marinade (see page 210) as a dipping sauce.

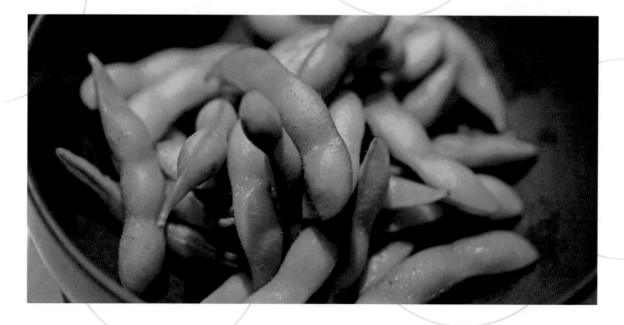

Parsnip Rice (Q)($)(E)

Serves: 3-4
Per serving: 184 Calories, 13g Fat, 16.4g Carbs, 4.5g Fiber, 2.8 Protein

Ingredients:

2 cups peeled fresh parsnips – roughly chopped into pieces of about the same size
3 Tbsp macadamia nuts
3 Tbsp pine nuts
1 Tbsp EVOO
3 tsp date syrup (dates blended with water)
3 tsp lemon juice
1 Tbsp white miso

Directions:

Pulse the parsnips in the food processor until the mix resembles rice grain.

Add the remaining ingredients and gently pulse until everything is combined.

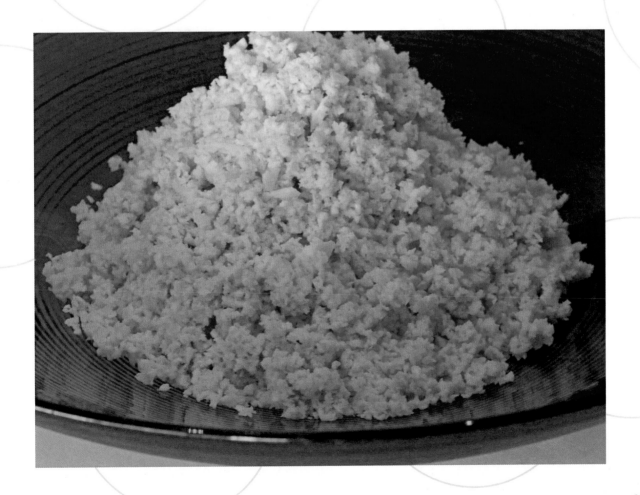

Cauliflower Artichoke Pepper Medley (Q)(E)($)

Serves: 4

Per serving: 73 Calories, 3.8g Fat, 7.8g Carbs, 3.2 Fiber, 2.3g Protein

Ingredients:

2 cups cauliflower florettes
8 oz jar of baby artichokes
1 yellow or orange bell pepper – sliced
1 Tbsp EVOO
½ tsp fresh ground black pepper
¼ cup sliced parsley
¼ cup vegetable stock

Directions:

In a sauté pan on medium heat sauté everything together for about 5 minutes.

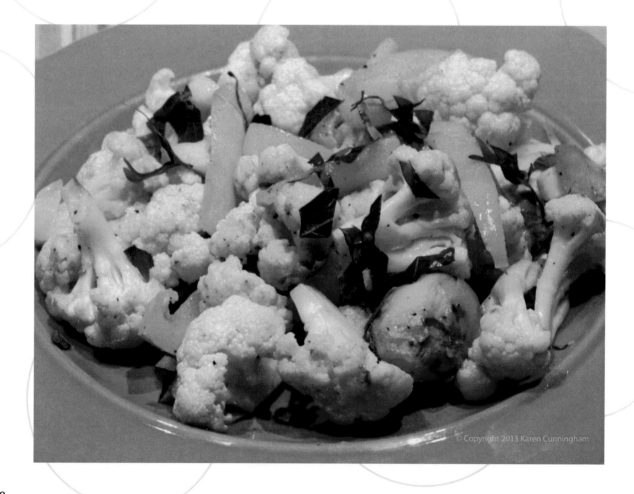

Crème Peas (E)($)

Serves: 4
Per serving: 141 Calories, 5.7g Fat, 16.4g Carbs, 5g Fiber, 6.5g Protein

Ingredients:

1 1/2 Tbsp grapeseed Oil
2 Tbsp white onions - diced
2 Tbsp GF flour
3/4 cup non-dairy milk or 3/4 cup vegetable broth
1 Tbsp nutritional yeast
2 cups frozen peas
mineral salt and pepper to taste

Directions:

Melt the oil on low heat in a pan. Add the onions and cook for about a minute.

Add the flour and stir until absorbed. Add the nutritional yeast.

Slowly stir in the milk or broth.

Turn up the heat and bring the broth to a boil.

Turn the heat down and once the broth has thickened add the peas.

Heat through.

NOTE:
Not suitable for freezing.

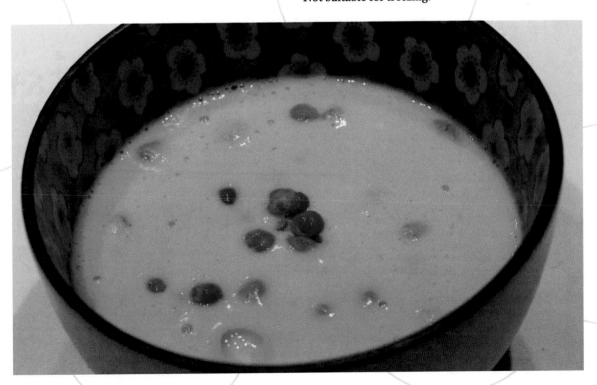

Sautéed Brussel Sprouts (Q)($)(E)
Serves: 6-8
Per serving: 98 Calories, 5g Fat, 12g Carbs, 4.7g Fiber, 4.1g Protein

Ingredients:

1 1/2 lb. fresh brussels sprouts
2 cloves garlic - peeled & sliced
1/4 cup white balsamic vinegar (apple cider vinegar if cleansing)
mineral Salt & pepper to taste
2 Tbsp EVOO
1 medium yellow onion - peeled & sliced
Nut 'N Seed breading for the topping (see page 370)

Directions:

Trim off the stems and remove any limp leaves from the sprouts.

Blanch the sprouts in boiling water to cover for 5 minutes.

Drain and rinse under cold water to stop the cooking.

Heat a large frying pan and add the olive oil, garlic and onion. Sauté until the onion just becomes tender.

Add the blanched, drained brussels sprouts. Sauté a few minutes until they are cooked to your liking.

Add the vinegar and toss. Add EVOO, salt and pepper and toss again.

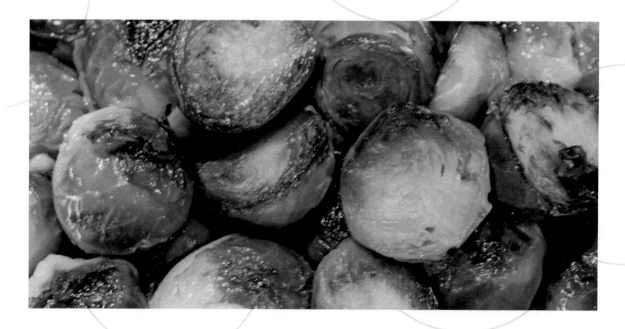

Roasted Asparagus and Fennel (Q)($)(E)
Per serving: 236 Calories, 18.8g Fat, 11.9g Carbs, 6.3g Fiber, 10.8g Protein

Ingredients:

1 lb asparagus – trimmed
1 medium fennel bulb – sliced vertically (keep a few fronds)
2 Tbsp lemon juice
1 cup walnuts – lightly toasted
mineral salt and pepper

Directions:

On a griddle preheated to medium-hot place asparagus and fennel .

Drizzle 1 Tbsp of the lemon juice over the top and grill for about 5 minutes turning occasionally.

Add a few of the fennel fronds in the last minute.

Transfer to a serving plate and sprinkle with the remaining lemon juice and then the walnuts.

Serve as a side or main alone or with horseradish cranberry sauce.

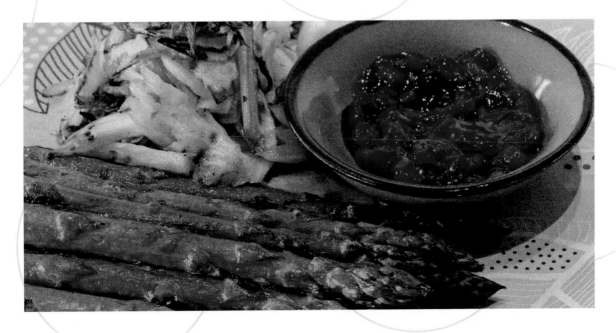

Marinated Mushrooms (E)($)

Serves: 4

Per serving: 77 Calories, 5.1g Fat, 6.7g Carbs, 3.2g Fiber, 3.3g Protein

Ingredients:

4 cups button mushrooms – sliced
8 cups baby spinach leaves
1 avocado – peeled and diced
1 large carrot - grated
4 green onions – thinly sliced
2 tsp sesame seeds – lightly toasted
Marinade - use asian inspired marinade (see page 210)

Directions:

Add slice mushrooms to marinade and coat mushrooms well in the sauce – leave at room temperature for about 2 hours – drain mushrooms, keeping the marinade for use over the salad.

Arrange salad on a platter and pour on marinade .

Arrange mushrooms over the top and sprinkle with the sesame seeds.

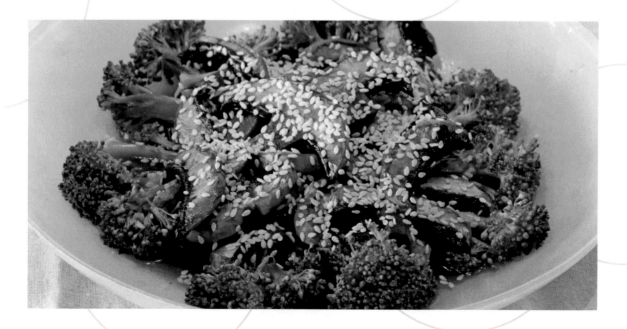

Beets with Pine Nuts (Q)($)(E)

Serves: 2
Per serving: 292 Calories, 21.2g Fat, 22.1g Carbs, 4.9g Fiber, 4.4g Protein

Ingredients:

2 cups roasted beets
zest of one orange
½ cup Orange Juice
½ cup lemon juice
2 Tbsp EVOO
mineral salt and pepper to taste
3 Tbsp lightly toasted pine nuts

Directions:

Chop the beets into 1inch pieces

Marinate them in the juice for about an hour

Serve with the zest and pine nuts

NOTE:
Sprinkle the pine nuts at the last minute or they will become pink

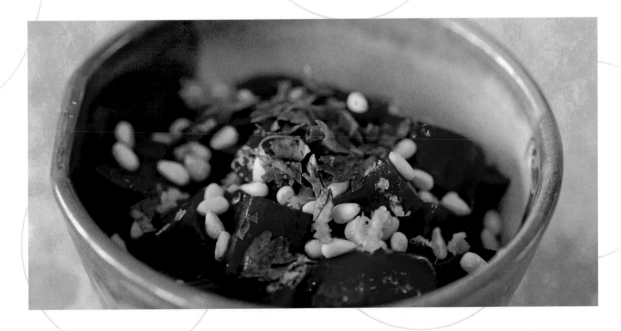

Roasted Peppers (Q)($)(E)

Per pepper: 37 Calories, 0.4g Fat, 7.2g Carbs, 2.5g Fiber, 1.2g Protein

Ingredients:

1 red bell pepper (or pepper of your choosing)
1 brown paper bag

Directions:

Place your bell pepper directly over the flame of a gas burner or on an outside BBQ on high.

Watch the pepper carefully as it will blacken – that is desired. Once one side blackens, using a pair of tongs, turn the pepper to blacken all sides.

Remove from the flame and place the pepper in a brown paper bag to sweat for about 15 minutes.

Gently remove the pepper from the bag and over a glass bowl, break the pepper open and collect the juice that will have formed inside

Take your pepper to the sink and remove all seeds and skin under running water. If the pepper is blackened well, the skin will just slip off.

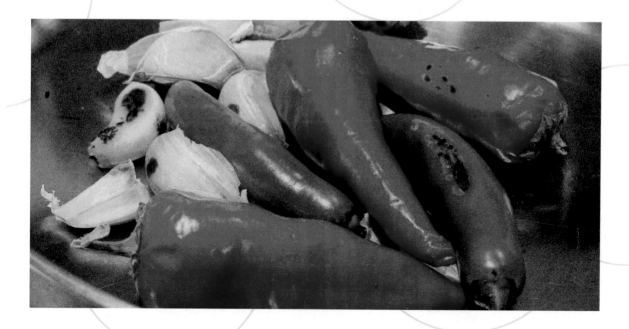

Spinach with Tahini (Q)($)(E)(R)

Serves: 2
Per serving: 206 Calories, 14.5g Fat, 14g Carbs, 7.2g Fiber, 10.7g Protein

Ingredients:

1 medium garlic clove - chopped
3 Tbsp well-stirred tahini (Middle Eastern sesame paste)
1 1/2 to 2 Tbsp fresh lemon juice (to taste)
1/4 tsp salt
3/4 cup water
15 oz loosely packed baby spinach
2 tsp sesame seeds (optional) -toasted

Directions:

Blend together garlic, tahini, lemon juice, salt, and 1/4 cup water in a blender until smooth.

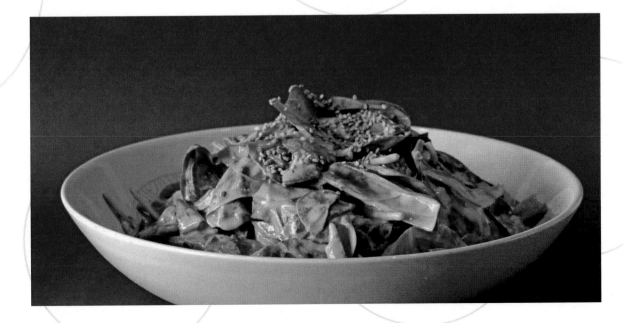

Sweet and Spicy Green Beans (Q)($)(E)

Serves: 2
Per serving: 120 Calories, 5.1g Fat, 18.6g Carbs, 6.3g Fiber, 3.8g Protein

Ingredients:

3/4 pound fresh green beans - trimmed
2 Tbsp Bragg's Liquid Aminos
1 clove garlic - minced
1 tsp garlic - minced
1 tsp red pepper flakes
2 tsp maple syrup
2 tsp grapeseed oil

Directions:

Arrange a steamer basket in a pot over boiling water, and steam the green beans 3 to 4 minutes.

In a bowl, mix the Bragg's, garlic, chili and brown rice syrup.

Heat the grapeseed oil in a skillet over medium heat. Add the green beans, and saute for 3 minutes.

Pour in the Bragg's sauce mixture. Continue cooking and stirring 30 seconds, Serve immediately.

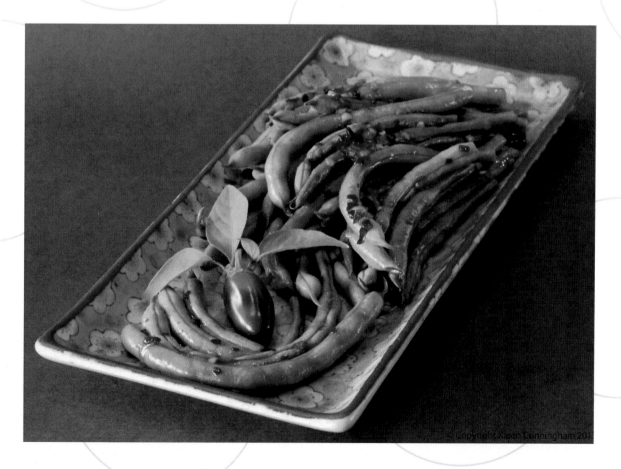

Braised Fennel with Tomatoes, Shallots and Onions (Q)($)(E)

Serves: 6
Per serving: 155 Calories, 9.7g Fat, 15g Carbs, 5.5g Fiber, 4g Protein

Ingredients:

3 fennel bulbs - cut into quarters
3 tomatoes - peeled and cut into quarters
3 Tbsp finely chopped shallots
1 tsp dill
1 tsp coriander seeds
1 Tbsp olive oil
1/2 cup pitted Kalamata (or your favorite) olives halved lengthwise
1 cup vegetable stock
Salt and Pepper to taste
1/2 cup roasted pine nuts
2 Tbsp celery leaves - finely chopped

Directions:

In a sauté pan, heat the oil over med heat.

Add the shallots and cook stirring until soft ~ about 1 minute.

Add the tomatoes, fennel, halved olives and vegetable broth. Reduce heat to low and cook for about 8 minutes.

Remove from the heat and stir in the dill and coriander seeds. Serve warm as an appetizer with pine nuts sprinkled on top.

Sprinkle celery leaves on top.

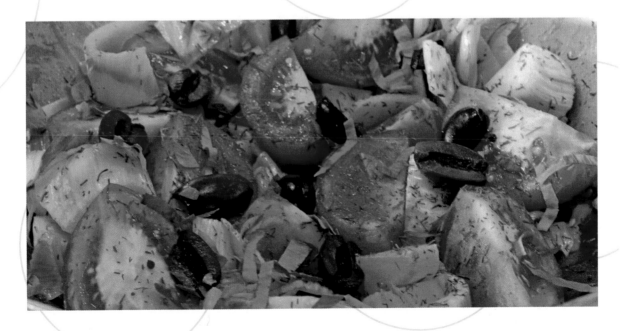

Braised Zucchini with Mint, Lemon and Pine Nuts (Q)($)(E)

Per serving: 96 Calories, 3 g Protein, 9g Carbs, 2 g Fiber; 7 g fat; 1 g Sat Fat

Ingredients:

2 pounds zucchini
2 Tbsp EVOO
1 cup onion - finely diced
2 cloves garlic - thinly sliced
Zest of 1/2 lemon
Salt
1 Tbsp chopped mint - divided
2 Tbsp lemon juice
2 Tbsp toasted pine nuts

Directions:

Cut the ends from each zucchini, slice the zucchini in quarters lengthwise and then cut the quarters in half crosswise. You'll have large pieces of zucchini about 2 to 3 inches long.

In a heavy-bottomed skillet, warm the olive oil and the onion over medium/low heat until the onion softens and becomes fragrant, 3 to 4 minutes.

Add the zucchini, the garlic, lemon zest, 1 tsp salt, 1 tsp mint and 2 Tbsp of water and stir well to combine. Reduce heat to low and cover.

Cook, stirring occasionally, until the zucchini is extremely tender and almost translucent, about 25 minutes. There should be some liquid still in the bottom of the pan.

Remove the lid, add the lemon juice and increase heat to high.

When the liquid begins to bubble, remove from heat and set aside uncovered.

When the zucchini is at warm room temperature, stir in the remaining 2 tsp mint and the pine nuts, then taste and add more salt and lemon juice if necessary.

Serve warm or at room temperature.

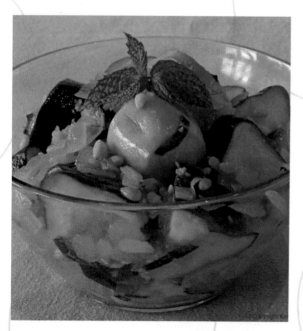

Broccoli with Toasted Tamari Sunflower Seeds (Q)($)(E)

Serves: 2
Per serving: 66 Calories, 1.9g Fat, 9.1g Carbs, 3.3g Fiber, 5.7g Protein

Ingredients:

8 oz broccoli
2 Tbsp toasted sunflower seeds
2 Tbsp tamari sauce
¼ cup water

Directions:

Mix the water and tamari together.

In a small saucepan place the broccoli and drizzle the water tamari mix over the top – bring to boil, turn heat down and simmer for two minutes.

Put broccoli into two serving bowls and sprinkle with the toasted seeds.

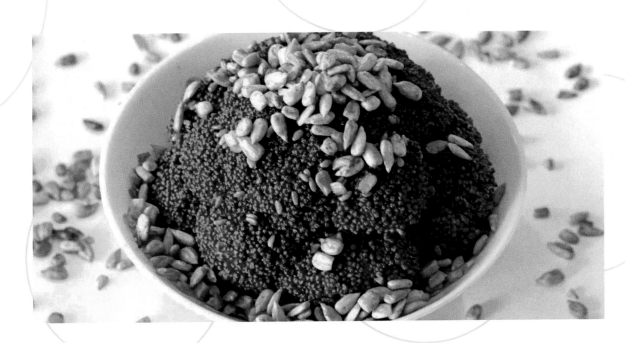

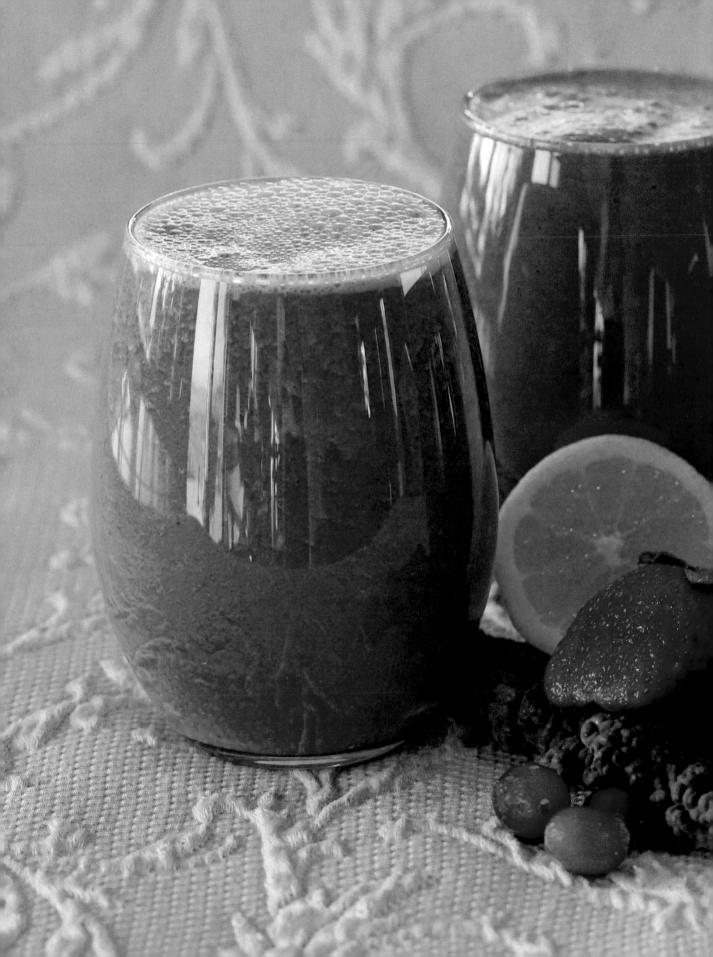

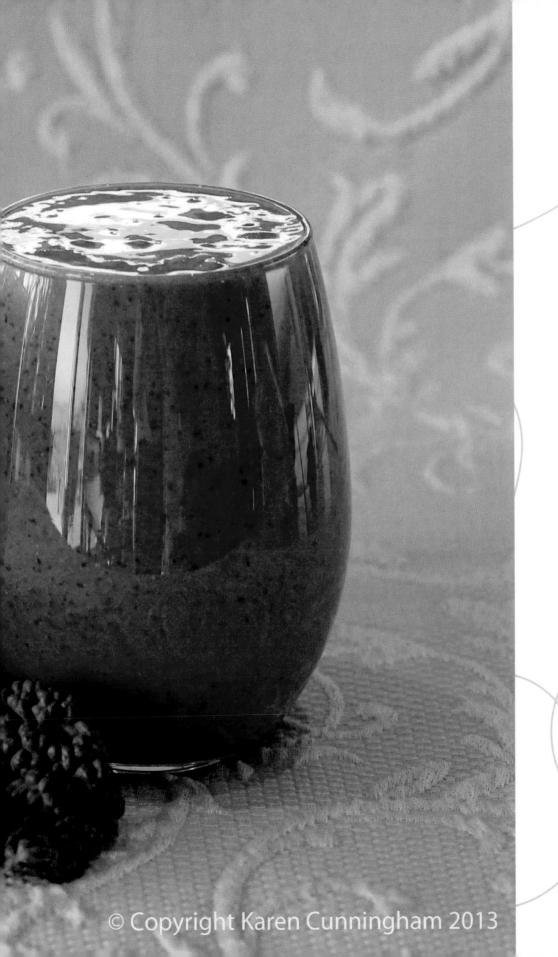

Drinks

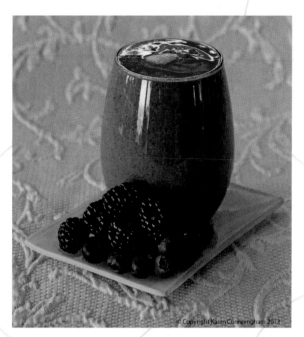

Purple Power Smoothie

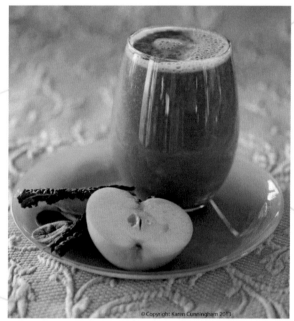

Green Meanie

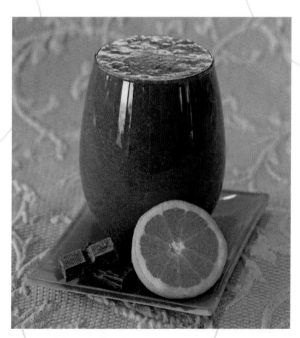

Chocolate Jaffa

Purple Power Smoothie (Q) (E)

Ingredients:

2 scoops chocolate pea, cranberry, rice protein powder
8 oz water
1 cup mixed purple berries – blackberries and blueberries
1 probiotic

Blend.

Per drink: 232 Calories, 5.2g Fat, 29g Carbs, 9.6g Fiber, 22g Protein

Green Meanie (Q)(E)
(concocted by Kwanua Robinson)

Ingredients:

2 scoops vanilla pea, cranberry, rice protein powder
1/2 scoop soluble fiber
4 stems organic kale – ribs removed
1/2 large green apple
8-10 oz water
add ice as desired

Blend.

Note:
This recipes works best if you have a high speed blender.

Per drink: 245 Calories, 4.7g Fat, 34g Carbs, 6g Fiber, 21g Protein

Chocolate Jaffa (Q)(E)

Ingredients:

2 scoops chocolate pea, cranberry, rice protein powder
8 oz water
1 medium sized orange – peeled
1 probiotic

Per drink: 232 Calories, 4.7g Fat, 30g Carbs, 5g Fiber, 21.2g Protein

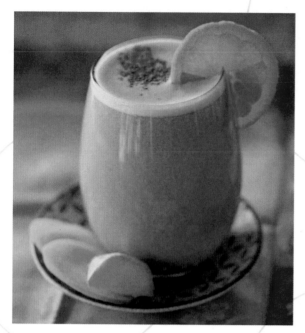

Spicy Apple Pie

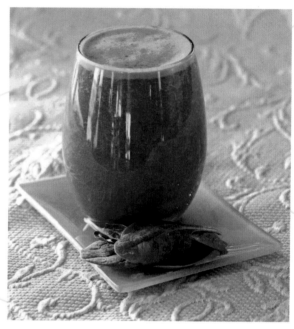

Popeye

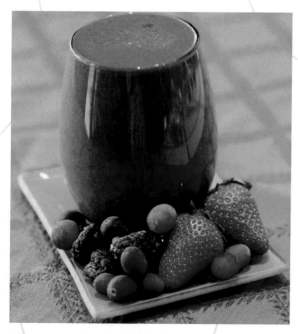

ChocoBerry Smoothie

Spicy Apple Pie (Q)(E)

Ingredients:

2 scoops vanilla pea, cranberry, rice protein powder
1 scoop soluble fiber
1 medium sized green apple chopped
sprinkle of nutmeg and cinnamon to taste
1/2 " piece fresh ginger
8 oz water or plant milk – almond, rice, hemp, coconut
plus your daily probiotic

Blend

Per drink: 289 Calories, 3.3g Fat, 44.9g Carbs, 15.1g Fiber, 25.5g Protein

Popeye (Q)(E)

Ingredients:

2 scoops vanilla or chocolate pea, cranberry, rice protein powder
1 scoop soluble fiber
8 oz water or plant milk – almond, rice, hemp
a large handful of baby spinach
plus your daily probiotic

Blend.

Per drink: 179 Calories, 3.1g Fat, 16.5g Carbs, 10.3g Fiber, 25.4g Protein

ChocoBerry Smoothie (Q)(E)

Ingredients:

2 scoops chocolate pea, cranberry, rice protein powder
1 scoop soluble fiber
1 cup mixed berries – strawberry, blackberry, blueberries
8 oz water or plant milk – almond, rice, hemp, coconut
plus your daily probiotic

Blend

Per drink: 246 Calories, 3.5g Fat, 33g Carbs, 15g Fiber, 25.5g Protein

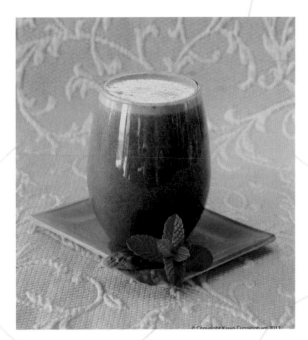

Chocomint Smoothie

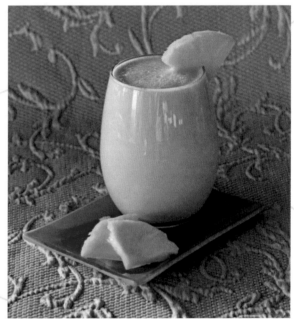

Proteina Colada

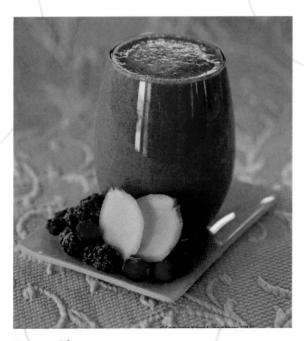

Berry Ginger

Chocomint Smoothie (Q)(E)

Ingredients:

2 scoops chocolate pea, cranberry, rice protein powder
1 scoop soluble fiber
1 small handful of fresh mint (spearmint) or chocolate mint
8 oz water or plant milk – almond, rice, hemp, coconut
plus your daily probiotic

Blend.

Per drink: 191 Calories, 3.1g Fat, 16.9g Carbs, 10.8g Fiber, 25.4g Protein

Proteina Colada (Q)(E)

Ingredients:

2 scoops vanilla pea, cranberry, rice protein powder
1 scoop soluble fiber
1 thick slice fresh pineapple
8 oz water or plant milk – almond, rice, hemp, coconut
plus your daily probiotic

Blend.

Per drink: 204 Calories, 3.g Fat, 23.4g Carbs, 10.8g Fiber, 25.3g Protein

Berry Ginger (Q)(E)

Ingredients:

2 scoops vanilla pea, cranberry, rice protein powder
1 scoop soluble fiber
1 cup mixed berries – strawberries
1" piece of fresh ginger
8 oz water or plant milk – almond, rice, hemp, coconut
plus your daily probiotic

Blend.

Per drink: 289 Calories, 3.9g Fat, 36.8g Carbs, 15.7g Fiber, 25.4g Protein

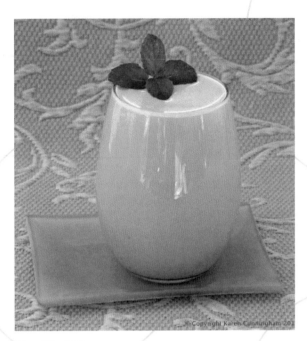

Vanilla Mint

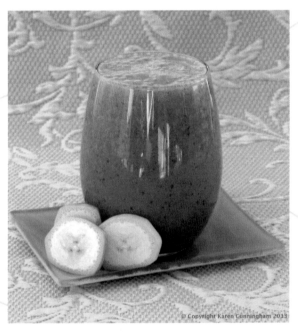

Strawberry banana Chocolate

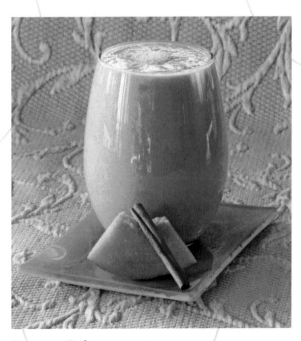

Papaya Spice

Vanilla Mint (Q)(E)

Ingredients:

2 scoops vanilla pea, cranberry, rice protein powder
1 scoop soluble fiber
a couple of sprigs of mint (spearmint)
1/2 " piece fresh ginger
8 oz water or plant milk – almond, rice, hemp, coconut
plus your daily probiotic

Blend.

Per drink: 196 Calories, 3.3g Fat, 20g Carbs, 10.8g Fiber, 25.4g Protein

Strawberry Banana Chocolate (Q)(E)

Ingredients:

2 scoops chocolate or vanilla cranberry, brown rice and pea protein
1/2 scoop soluble fiber
1/2 frozen banana
1/2 cup strawberries
8 oz water

Blend.

Per drink: 294 Calories, 3g Fat, 29g Carbs, 13.2g Fiber, 41g Protein

Papaya Spice (Q)(E)

Ingredients;

2 scoops vanilla pea, cranberry, rice protein powder
1 inch thick slice of fresh papaya
1/2 tsp ground cinnamon
1/4 tsp ground cardamom
1/4 tsp turmeric
1 citrus fizz stick
8oz water

Blend.

Per drink: 237 Calories, 3.2g Fat, 27.2g Carbs, 13.1g Fiber, 25.9g Protein

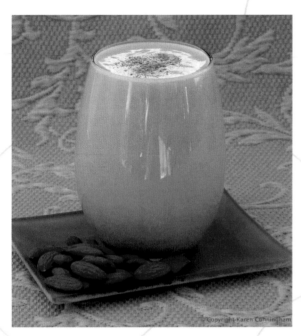

Almond Shake

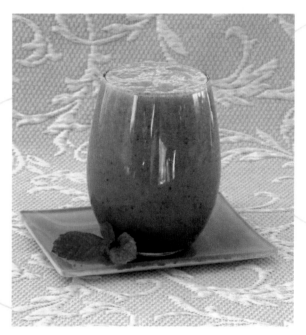

Berry Mint

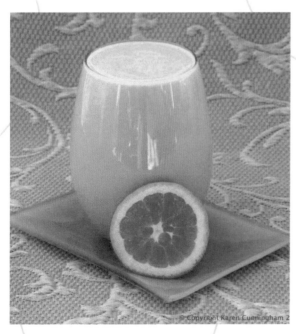

Orange Creamsicle

Almond Shake (Q)(E)

Ingredients:

1 scoops vanilla pea, cranberry, rice protein powder
1 scoops chocolate cranberry-rice-yellow pea protein
powder
1 Tbsp almond butter
pinch of ground cinnamon
1 scoop soluble fiber
8-10 oz water

Blend.

Per drink: 269 Calories, 9.6g Fat, 8.8g Carbs, 2.2g
Fiber, 36.3g Protein

Berry Mint (Q)(E)

Ingredients:

2 scoops vanilla pea, cranberry, rice protein powder
1 scoop soluble fiber
a couple of sprigs of mint (spearmint)
1 cup strawberries
plus your daily probiotic

Blend.

Per drink: 192 Calories, 1.5g Fat, 21g Carbs, 8.1g Fiber
22g Protein

Orange Creamsicle (Q)(E)

Ingredients:

2 scoops vanilla cranberry, brown rice and pea protein
oranges
6 oz water
1 whole orange

Blend.

Per smoothie: 290 Calories, 1.9g Fat, 47g Carbs, 9.8g
Fiber, 24.5g Protein

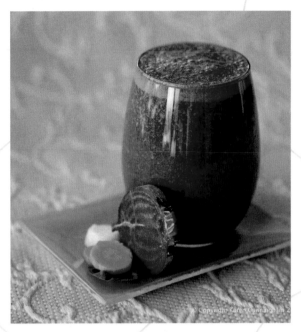

Beet It

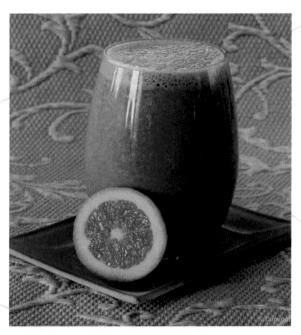

Spinach Orange Milkshake

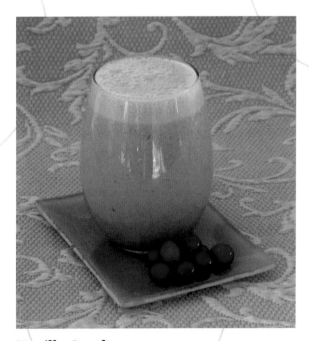

Vanilla Cranberry

Beet It (Q)(E)

Ingredients:

2 scoops vanilla pea, cranberry, rice protein powder
1 whole beet
1 carrot
slice of fresh ginger
1 probiotic
8 - 10oz water

Blend.

Per drink: 251 Calories, 2.7g Fat, 23.1g Carbs, 5.4g Fiber, 33.9g Protein

Spinach Orange Milkshake (Q)(E)

Ingredients:

1 handful spinach
1 whole orange peeled
1 cup almond milk

Blend.

*Serve over ice

Per drink: 133 Calories, 3.8g Fat, 24g Carbs, 6.1g Fiber, 3.6g Protein

Vanilla Cranberry (Q)(E)

Ingredients:

2 scoops vanilla pea, cranberry, rice protein powder
1 scoop soluble fiber
a couple of sprigs of mint (spearmint)
plus your daily probiotic
8 oz water
1/2 cup unsweetened cranberries

Blend.

Per drink: 157 Calories, 1.5g Fat, 13.5g Carbs, 6.5g Fiber, 21g Protein

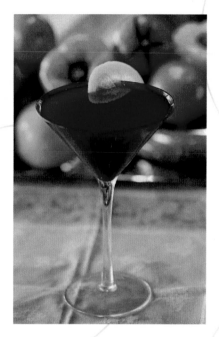

A Niner

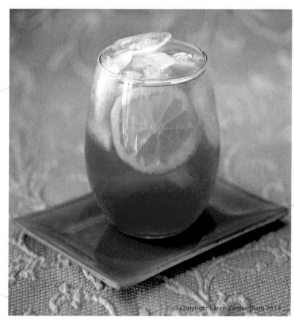

Lemon Detoxifying Tea

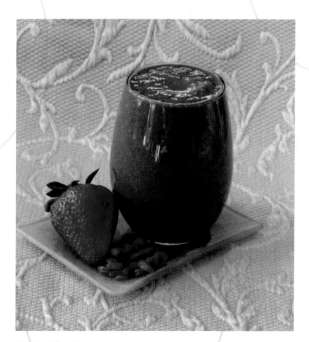

Goji Shake

Niner Cocktail (Q)(E)

Ingredients:

1 tomato,
1/4 red pepper
juice of one lemon,
6 oz water
a couple of drops of liquid Stevia or ½ tsp maple
syrup
1 tsp pomegranate powder
*The rest is up to your imagination.

Blend.

Per drink: 46 Calories, 0.7g Fat, 8.4g Carbs, 1.6g
Fiber, 1.3g Protein

Lemon Detoxifying Tea (Q)(E)

Choose your favorite detoxifying tea and make a pot.

Add slices of lemon and serve hot or cold.

You can also add a slice of ginger root.

*Nutrition information

Goji Shake (Q)(E)

Ingredients:

2 scoops vanilla pea, cranberry, rice protein powder
¼ cup dried goji Berries
1 cup strawberries
7oz water

Blend.

Per drink:194 Calories, 1.9g Fat, 21.8g Carbs, 4g Fiber,
23g Protein

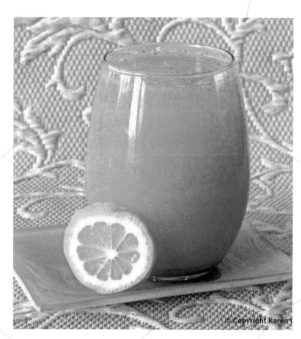

Golden Elixir

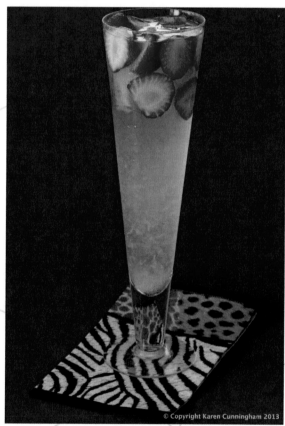

Strawberry Limeade Spritzer

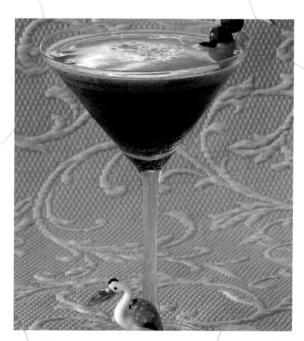

Blueberry Spritzer

Golden Elixir (Q)(E)

Ingredients:

1 cup hot water
1 Tbsp lemon juice
1/8 tsp turmeric
1/8 tsp ground ginger
1/8 tsp cayenne
1/2 tsp maple syrup

Per drink: 13 Calories, 2.7g Carbs, 0.1g Protein

Strawberry Limeade Spritzer (Q)(E)

Ingredients:

½ cup fresh squeezed lime juice
12 strawberries halved
2 tsp maple syrup
12 oz spritzer water

Gently combine in two separate glasses.
Add ice before the strawberries

Per serving (½ recipe): 57 Calories, 0.1g Fat, 15g Carbs, 1.2g Fiber, 0.8g Protein

Blueberry Spritzer (Q)(E)

Ingredients:

3 oz blueberry juice
3 oz favorite immunity tonic
spritzer water
fresh blueberries

Mix.

Per drink: 46 Calories, 0.1g Fat, 11.1g Carbs, 0.1g Protein

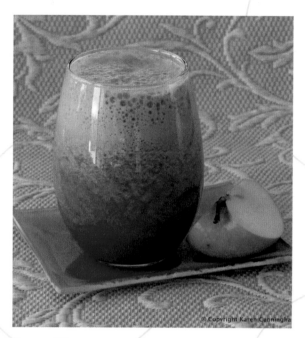

Super Hero

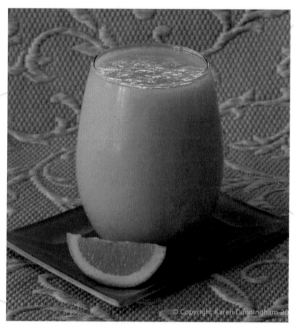

Calma Karma

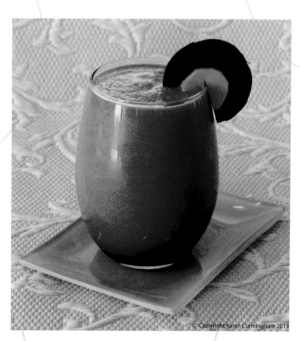

Immunity Kick Start

Super Hero (Q)(E)

Ingredients:

1 apple
1 1/2 spinach,
energy booster
8 oz water

Blend.

Per drink: 111 Calories, 0.1g Fat, 24g Carbs, 4.7g
Fiber, 0.4g Protein

Calma Karma (Q)(E)

Ingredients:

8 oz orange juice
daily probiotic

Mix.

Per drink: 117 Calories, 0g Fat, 27.6g Carbs, 1g Fiber,
1.6g Protein

Immunity Kick Start (Q)(E)

Ingredients:

1 cup grated raw beet
2 cups grated raw carrot
½ inch piece of fresh ginger
1 serve of your favorite immunity support drink

Blend.

Per drink: 171 Calories, 1g Fat, 39.3g Carbs, 9.8g
Fiber, 5.1g Protein

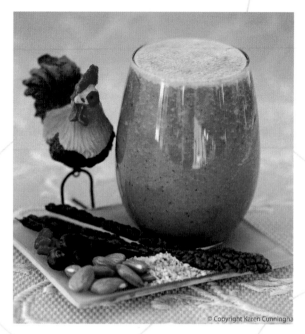

364 Days

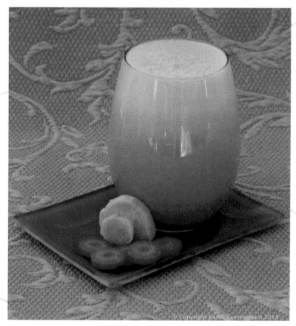

Carrot Ginger Smoothie

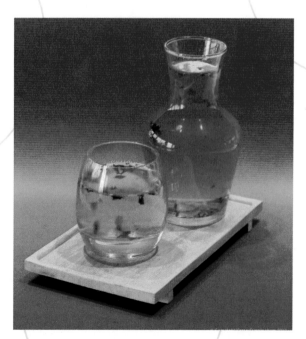

Mixed Mint Tea

364 Days (Q)(E)

Ingredients:

2 scoops vanilla pea, cranberry, rice protein powder
2 stalks kale
½ green apple
1 Tbsp hemp seeds
½ cup unsweetened blueberry juice
1 Tbsp goji berries
1 Tbsp blueberries
2 Tbsp almonds
8 oz water

Blend.

Per drink: 332 Calories, 10.9g Fat, 33.7g Carbs, 5.4g Fiber, 26.5g Protein

Carrot Ginger Smoothie (Q) (E)

Ingredients:

2 scoops pea, cranberry, rice protein powder - vanilla
1 scoop soluble fiber
1 carrot
1/2 " piece fresh ginger
8 oz water or plant milk – almond, rice, hemp, coconut
plus your daily probiotic

Blend.

Per drink*: 180 Calories, 5g Fat, 11.7g Carbs, 15g Fiber, 22g Protein

*using almond milk

Mixed Mint Tea (Q)(E)

Ingredients:

1 serving of your favorite detoxifying Tea
2 Tbsp mixed mints
8 oz hot water

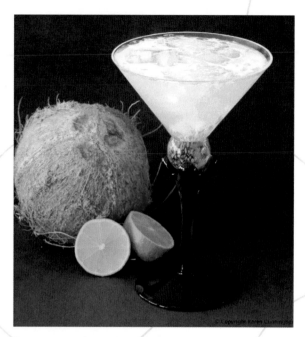

Coconut Lime Spatina

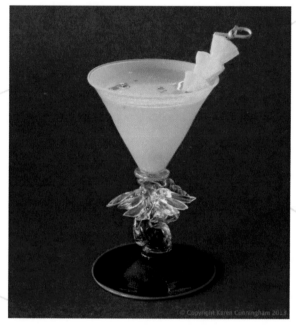

Nojito

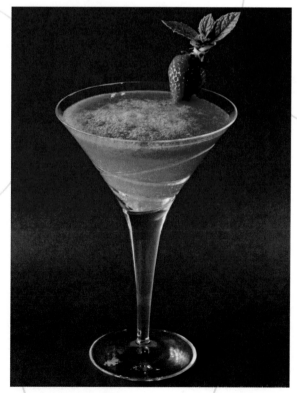

Strawberry Mint Julep

Coconut Lime Spatini (Q)(E)

Ingredients:

1 Tbsp Lime Juice
3 oz coconut water (preferably from a fresh coconut)
2 drops vanilla extract
1 tsp coconut flakes for garnish

Share over ice and serve in your favorite glass.

Per drink: 38 Calories, 0.7g Fat, 5.2g Carbs, 1.1g Fiber,
0.7g Protein

Nojito (Q)(E)

Ingredients:

4 oz unsweetened pineapple juice
4 oz coconut water (preferably from a fresh coconut
1 Tbsp lime juice
1 Tbsp chopped spearmint - bruised (=mash it a little
to release the flavors)

Shake over ice and serve with a pineapple skewer.

Per serving (1/2 drink): 42 Calories, 0.2g Fat, 10.4g
Carbs, 1.6g Fiber, 0.8g Protein

Strawberry Mint Julep (Q)(E)
- Contributed by Alex Caspero

Ingredients:

4 oz strawberries
1 tsp. lemon juice
2 tsp mint leaves - crushed
1 cup crushed ice
1/3 cup sparkling water

In a blender combine strawberries, lemon juice, and
mint leaves. Blend into smooth. Pour into a glass with
crushed ice and top with sparkling water. Garnish
with mint sprig and whole strawberry

Per drink: 41 Calories, 0.1g Fat, 8.9g Carbs, 1.8g Fiber,
0.9g Protein

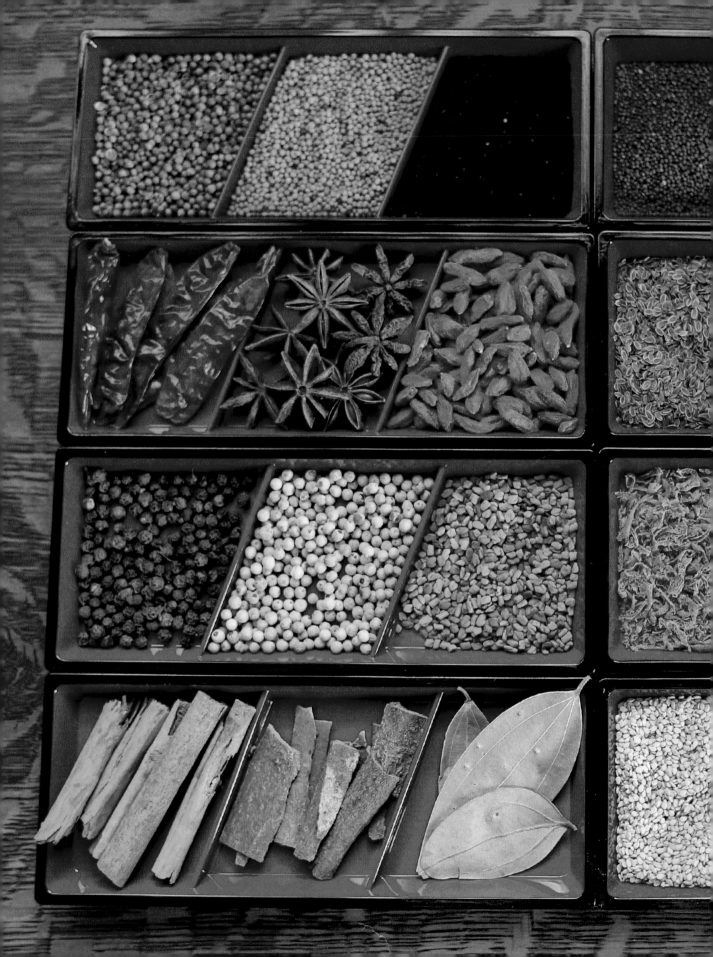

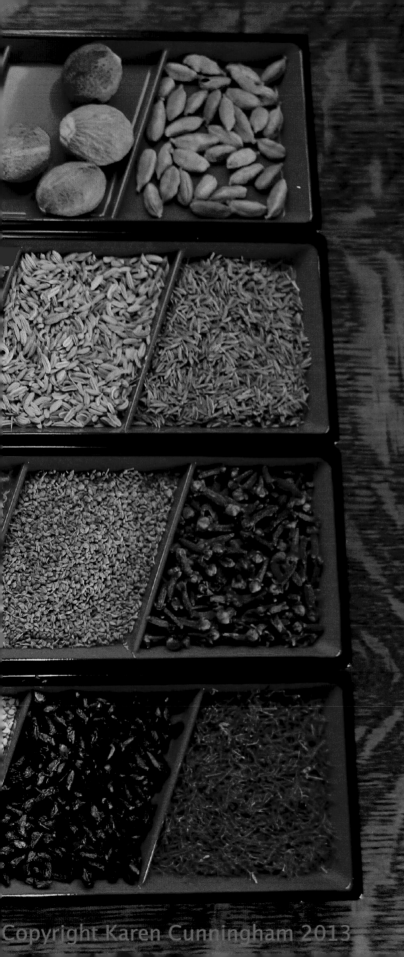

Herbs and Spices

Black Sesame Otsu (E)($)

Per serving (1/4 recipe): 305 Calories, 16.7g Fat, 28.5g Carbs, 4.8g Fiber, 11.8g Protein

Ingredients:

1 tsp pine nuts
1 tsp sunflower seeds
1/2 cup black sesame seeds
1 ground Stevia leaf
1 1/2 Tbsp Bragg's Liquid Aminos or tamari
Scant 1 Tbsp toasted sesame oil
2 Tbsp brown apple cider vinegar
1/8 tsp cayenne pepper
Fine-grain sea salt
1 cup white cabbage - shredded to resemble fettuccine
12 oz spaghetti style rice noodles or bean threads
12 oz extra-firm organic tofu
EVOO
1 bunch green onions, white and light green parts-thinly sliced

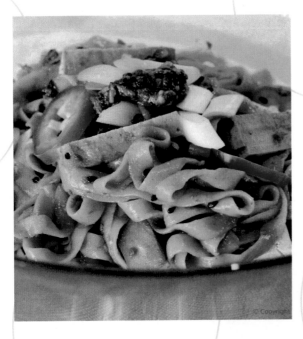

Directions:

Toast the pine nuts and sunflower seeds in a large skillet over medium heat until golden, shaking the pan regularly.

Add the sesame seeds to the pan and toast for a minute or so. It's hard to tell when they are toasted; look closely and use your nose.

Remove from the heat as soon as you smell a hint of toasted sesame; if you let them go much beyond that, you'll start smelling burned sesame.

Transfer to a food processor. Stir in the stevia, Bragg's, sesame oil, brown apple cider vinegar, and cayenne pepper. Taste and adjust if needed.

Bring a large pot of water to a boil. Salt generously, add the noodles, and cook according to the package instructions until tender.

Drain, reserving some of the noodle cooking water, and rinse under cold running water.

While the noodles are cooking, drain the tofu, pat it dry, and cut into matchstick shapes.

Season the tofu with a pinch of salt, toss with a small amount of oil, and cook in a large skillet over medium-high heat for a few minutes, tossing every couple minutes, until the pieces are browned on all sides.

Reserve a heaping Tbsp of the sesame paste, then thin the rest with 1/3 cup of the hot noodle water.

In a large mixing bowl, combine the soba, half of the green onions, and the black sesame paste. Toss until well combined.

Add the tofu and toss again gently. Serve topped with a tiny dollop of the reserved sesame paste and the remaining green onions.

Seedy Sprinkles (Q)(E)($)

Per serving (1 Tbsp): 48 Calories, 3.9g Fat, 2.4g Carbs, 1.4g Fiber, 2.5g Protein

Ingredients:

2 Tbsp dried onion bits
2 Tbsp dried garlic bits
2 Tbsp sesame seeds
2 Tbsp poppy seeds
2 Tbsp flax seeds
2 Tbsp hemp seeds
2 Tbsp chia seeds
1 Tsp mineral salt

Directions:

Mix ingredients together.

Store in your fridge in an airtight container.

Sprinkle on everything.

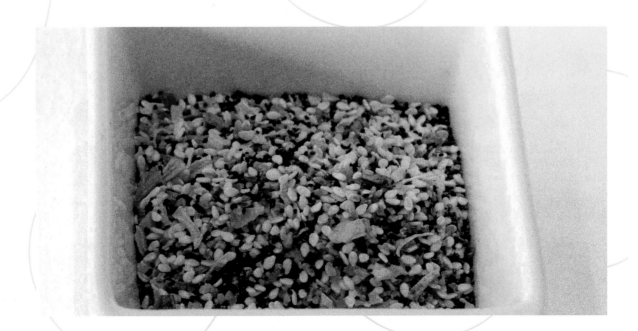

Celery Salt (Q)(E)($)
Entire recipe: 11 Calories, 0g Fat, 3g Carbs, 2.2g Fiber, 0.7g Protein

Ingredients:

½ cup of the finest Mineral salt you can find
1 bunch celery that still has its leaves attached*

*We tend to throw out the leaves but they have more nutrition than the stalk! Surprisingly, the leaves contain much more fiber than the stalk! 100 grams of celery stems contains 1.2 grams of fiber compared to 100 grams of celery leaves which contain 2.2 grams of fiber. The leaves also contain more vitamin A, C, magnesium & selenium. In addition to this recipe, enjoy the leaves in salads or as a garnish on soups.

Directions:

Take the leaves from the celery and place them either on dryer sheets for the dehydrator or on covered cookie sheets

Dry in the dehydrator at 100 degrees until leaves are dried – about 4 hours or at the lowest temperature in your oven – this will vary from 30 minutes to an hour.

Leaves should be completely crumbly. Mix with your salt and use for any savory dish

Berbere (Q)(E)($)
Per serving (about 1/8th recipe): 10 Calories, 2g Carbs, 0.5g Fiber, 0.4g Protein

Ingredients:

1/3 cup red chili pepper flakes
2 1/2 tsp garlic powder
1 tsp dried onion flakes
1 tsp ground ginger
1 tsp ground cloves
1 tsp salt 1/2 tsp ground cumin
1/2 tsp ground fenugreek
1/2 tsp ground cinnamon
1/2 tsp ground cardamom
1/2 tsp ground black pepper

Directions:

Combine all ingredients.

Mix thoroughly.

Store mixture in an airtight container.

Niter Kibbeh (Q)(E)($)
Per serving (~ 2 Tbsp): 98 Calories, 10.9g Fat, 0.3g Carbs, 0g Protein

Ingredients:

2 cups grapeseed oil
1/4 cup onion - chopped
2 cloves garlic - minced
2 tsp fresh ginger - peeled and grated
1/2 tsp turmeric
4 cardamom seeds, crushed
1 cinnamon stick
2 cloves, whole
1/8 tsp nutmeg
1/4 tsp ground fenugreek
1 Tbsp fresh basil or dried basil

Directions:

In a small saucepan, heat grapeseed oil on medium heat add the other ingredients and reduce the heat to a simmer.

Gently simmer, uncovered, on low heat for about 20 minutes

Remove from heat and pour the liquid through a cheesecloth into a heat-resistant container. Discard the spices and solids.

Covered tightly and store in the refrigerator.

Niter kibbeh will keep for up to 2 months.

Za'atar (Q)(E)($)
Per serving (3 Tbsp): 92 Calories, 7.1g Fat, 6.4g Carbs, 3.5g Fiber, 2.9g Protein

Ingredients:

3 parts toasted sesame seeds
2 parts dried thyme
1 part dried marjoram or oregano (oregano has a slightly stronger flavor)
1/2 - 1 part powdered sumac (available at middle eastern grocery stores)
salt, optional

Directions:

Crumble the thyme and marjoram as fine as possible.

Uses: Drizzle a good quality EVOO over the top, add some tomatoes or olives and you have a wonderful appetizer. Split socca bread then coat the rough side of the round with EVOO, then sprinkle with Za'atar (and salt if desired)before baking in the oven at about 450 degrees until crisp. Sprinkle over salads for a zesty lift. Fabulous sprinkled sparingly over tofu scramble. Use when baking any savory breads

Dukkah - Egyptian Spice Blend (Q)(E)($)
Per serving (1/16th recipe): 61 Calories, 5.2g Fat, 2.7g Carbs, 1.4g Fiber, 2g Protein

Ingredients:

½ cup almonds - lightly toasted
½ cup hazelnuts – lightly toasted
1/2 cup sesame seeds – lightly toasted
2 tsp ground coriander - lightly toasted
2 tsp ground cumin - lightly toasted
2 Tbsp freshly ground black pepper
1 tsp mineral salt

Directions:

Put all ingredients except for the sesame seeds into the food processor and process until nuts resemble breadcrumbs.

Place in a bowl and mix in the sesame seeds.

Store in the fridge in an airtight container.

Sprinkle over vegetables, pastas, on top of sandwiches and dips.

Gomasio (Q)(E)($)
Per Tbsp: 53 Calories, 4.5g Fat, 2.3g Carbs 1.2g Fiber, 1.7g Protein

Ingredients:

¼ cup Sesame seeds – lightly toasted
1 tsp dulse flakes
½ tsp mineral salt

Directions:

Mix together and enjoy over soups, salads, vegetables, rice etc.

Note: This is a powerful Anti Acid blend that alkalizes your blood.

Lemon Pepper (Q)(E)($)
Entire recipe: 49 Calories, 0.6g Fat, 13g Carbs, 5g Fiber, 2g Protein

Ingredients:

3 medium sized lemons
6 tsp whole black peppercorns

Directions:

Zest the lemons – yellow skin only
In a blender – crack the while peppercorns until they are crushed.
Add zest and blend until mixture looks even.
Lay mix on a large plate or dehydrator sheet and allow to dry.
Air dry 2- 4 days – then seal into a container.
Dehydrate on lowest temp for about 6 hours.
Sprinkle on anything that needs a little spicing up.

Togarashi (Q)(E)($)
Entire recipe: 124 Calories, 5.8g Fat, 16.5g Carbs, 5.8g Fiber, 5.9g Protein

Ingredients:

2 Tbsp black peppercorns
1 Tbsp dried tangerine peel
1 Tbsp ground red chili pepper
2 tsp flaked nori
2 tsp black sesame seeds
2 tsp crushed hemp seeds
2 tsp minced garlic

Directions:

Blend together and use on anything that needs spicing up.

Nut 'N Seed Breading (Q)(E)($)
Per 2 Tbsp: 85 Calories, 6.6g Fat, 2g Carbs, 3.8g Fiber, 3.6g Protein

Ingredients:

½ cut finely chopped pistachios
½ cup ground flax seeds
1 tsp mineral salt
1 tsp lemon zest – fine grate
1 Tbsp ground dried sage
1 Tbsp dried parsley
1 tsp ground dried thyme
1 Tbsp Grapeseed Oil

Directions:

Mix everything together and store in an airtight container in the refrigerator

Ras el Hanout (Q)(E)($)
Makes ~ 8 Tbsp
Per 1 tsp: 5 Calories, 0.2g Fat, 0.9g Carbs, 0.6g Fiber, 0.1g Protein

Ingredients:

1 tsp salt
1 tsp ground cumin
1 tsp ground ginger
1 tsp ground turmeric
3/4 tsp ground cinnamon
3/4 tsp freshly ground black pepper
1/2 tsp ground white pepper
1/2 tsp ground coriander seed
1/2 tsp ground cayenne pepper
1/2 tsp ground allspice
1/2 tsp ground nutmeg
1/4 tsp ground cloves

Directions:

Mix.

Garam Masala (Q)(E)($)
Per serving: 55 Calories, 2.3g Fat, 9.8g Carbs, 4.1g Fiber, 2g Protein

Ingredients:

1 Tbsp ground cumin
1 1/2 tsp ground coriander
1 1/2 tsp ground cardamom
1 1/2 tsp ground black pepper
1 tsp ground cinnamon
1/2 tsp ground cloves
1/2 tsp ground nutmeg

Directions:

Mix

*CHEF TIP: Storing Fresh Ginger

Ginger is such a wonderful healthful spice, so we use it liberally in many recipes.

When I buy fresh ginger, I bring it home and immediately peel and slice the whole piece into small pieces. It goes into a bag into the freezer for use at any time.

Ginger is also much easier to grate when frozen.

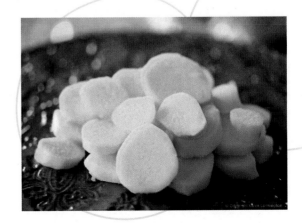

Super-Nu (Q)(E)($)

Entire recipe: 224 Calories, 15.3g Fat, 15.2g Carbs, 4.5g Fiber, 9.8g Protein

Ingredients:

One bunch of kale (about 10 leaves) - de ribbed (or a large handful of baby kale)
2 sheets of Nori (calcium/mineral packed seaweed) easiest to get as well
zest of 2 lemons
1/4 cup sunflower seeds - gently dry toasted in a skillet
2 Tbsp sesame seeds - gently dry toasted

Directions:

Lay the kale on cookie sheets or dehydrator sheets so it does not overlap.

On a second sheet lay the Nori sheets

On a third lined sheet the lemon zest

Either in a dehydrator at 145 degrees or in your oven at the lowest setting place the cookie/dehydrator sheets and toast/dry until the kale and Nori are crunchy/crumbly and the lemon zest is dried - this will vary from 30 minutes onwards so keep checking. Remove trays as they become ready and leave to cool.

Once all ingredients are dried and crumbly simply crumble into a bowl and mix well.

Store in an airtight container and keep a small bottle in your bag for instant nutrition on the run.

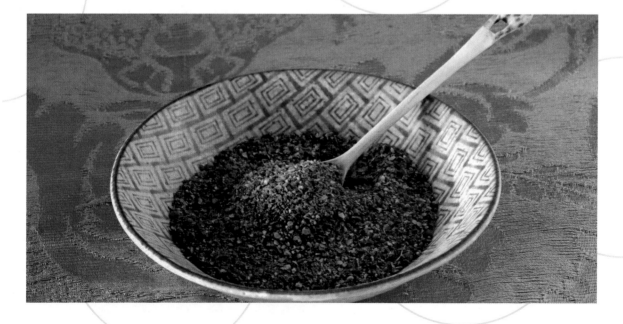

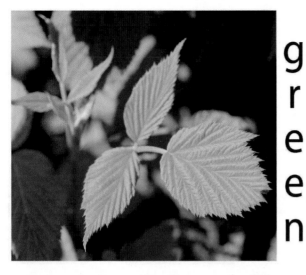

g
r
e
e
n

green

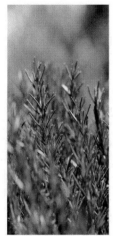

green

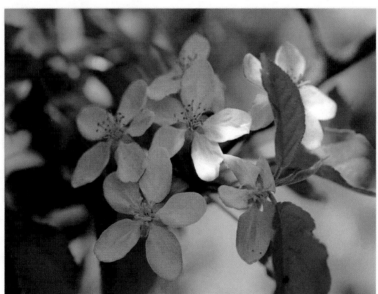

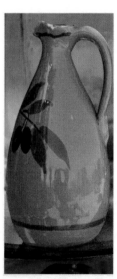

green

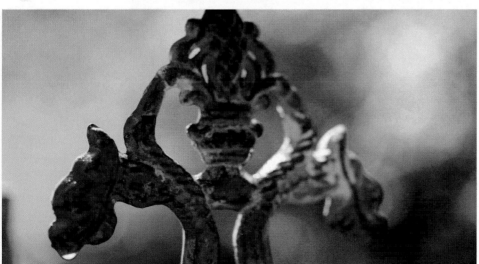

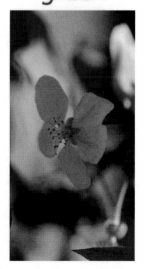

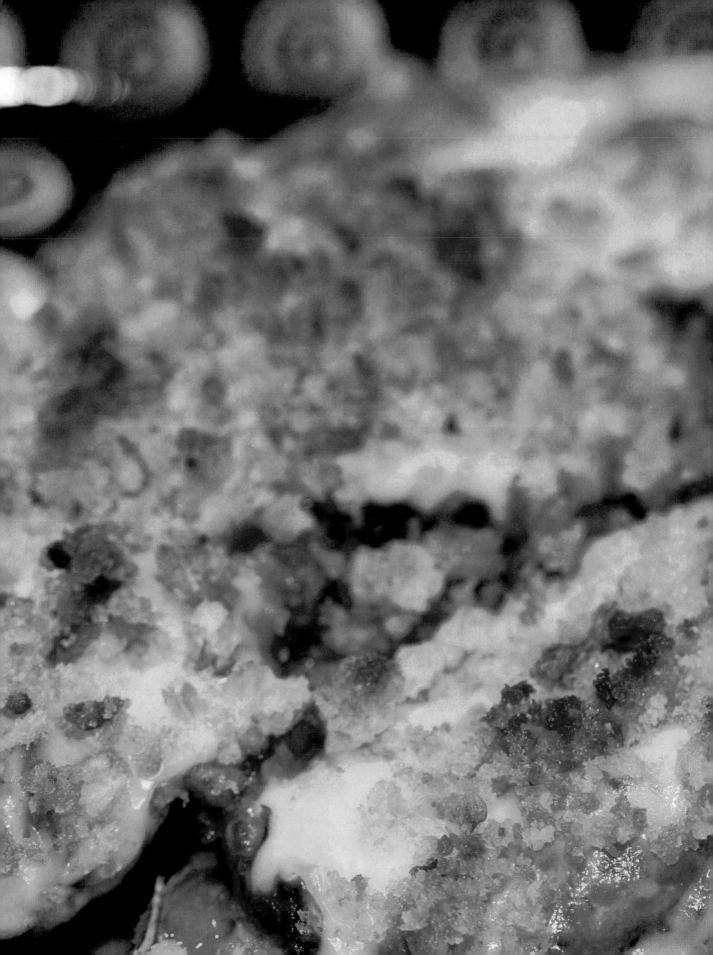

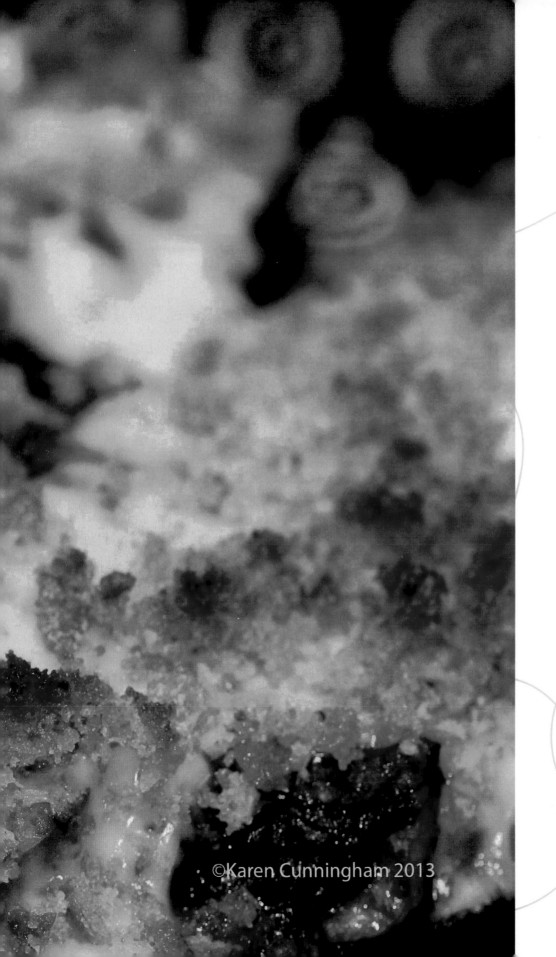

Day 365

Baked Eggplant Stuffed with Mushrooms (NCF)

Serves: 4- 6
Per serving (when serving 4): 516 Calories, 44g Fat, 28.6g Carbs, 8.7g Fiber, 8g Protein
Per serving (when serving 6): 344 Calories, 29.5g Fat, 19g Carbs, 5.8g Fiber, 5.3g Protein

Ingredients:

1 medium sized eggplant (aubergine)
1/2 cup EVOO
1 large red or brown onion – finely chopped
4 oz (113g) of your favorite Mushrooms (I love to mix them) - chopped
1/2 cup pesto
1 cup grated DaiyaCheese – Mozzarella or a mix
Garlic GF Breadcrumbs
2 Tbsp EVOO
2 cloves garlic
Salt and Pepper
Parsley or Basil as a garnish.

Directions:

Preheat oven to 400F

Slice one big eggplant into two halves lengthwise, scoop out the center flesh with a tsp, leaving about a 1/2 inch thick eggplant all round.

Keep the extra flesh aside, sprinkled with a little salt.

Place the two pieces in a bowl and spread a little EVOO inside both halves of the eggplant, sprinkle with a little salt, then place face down on a cookie sheet in the oven and cook for about 10 minutes at 400F.

Put the onions into a medium sized fry pan and cook until golden brown, add the flesh that you scooped out of the eggplant, plus with the mushrooms.

Cook for about 5-7 minutes until the mushrooms give up their water and look soft.

Add a little salt, pepper and pesto. Mix well. Taste and adjust seasonings to suit you.

Breadcrumbs:

Remove the slices of eggplant from the oven, and fill with the sauteed vegetables.

Put the Garlic Breadcrumbs and Daiya cheese on top

Put back into the oven face up this time and leave for another 10-15 minutes, or until the cheese is melted and has a golden color.

*Keep and eye on the dish as the oven is hot and you do not want to burn the breadcrumbs or the cheese

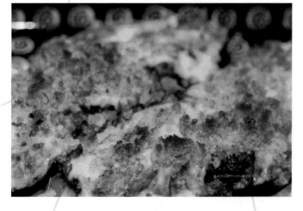

Curry Baked Fries (NCF)(Q)($)(E)

Serves: 4
Per serving: 161 Calories, 3.8g Fat, 29.6g Carbs, 4.8g Fiber, 3.2g Protein

Ingredients:

2 Large potatoes (preferably purple) – higher nutrition – scrubbed and cut into large wedges
1 Tbsp EVOO
1 tsp mineral salt
2 tsp mild curry powder

Directions:

Lightly coat the potato wedges with EVOO and salt and then coat with the curry powder.

Bake in the oven at 350 degrees until crunchy and cooked through – 30 minutes or so.

Enjoy with Cashew sour crème (see page 238) or coconut yoghurt with a dash of cayenne pepper.

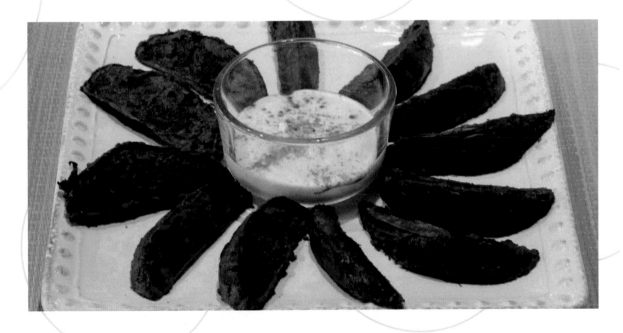

Not Mac and Cheese (NCF)(E)
Serves: 4
Per serving: 415 Calories, 25.3g Fat, 38.5g Carbs, 5.3g Fiber, 14.2g Protein

Ingredients:

1 ½ cup raw cashews - soaked then drained
2 Tbsp Miso paste
3 Tbsp lemon juice
2 cups water
¼ cup nutritional yeast
1/2 tsp. chili powder
1/2 clove garlic
pinch of turmeric
pinch of cayenne pepper
1/2 tsp mustard (dijon or yellow)
8 oz pasta noodles (rice or quinoa) cooked to
directions – keep slightly firm
*A high speed blender makes this recipe very easy. If
you do not have a high-powered blender use your food
processor, it will just take a little more time and you
will have to scrape down the edges of the processor.

Directions:

Blend all the ingredients in the blender, and blend
until smooth and creamy.

Once the pasta is done, combine the ingredients
gently and heat in a 300 degree oven for about 30
minutes.

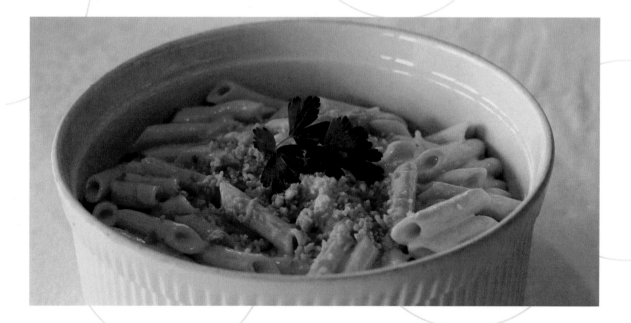

Oven Roasted Root Vegetable Chips (NCF)(E)($)

Serves:
Per serving (1/2 cup): 84 Calories, 3.7g Fat, 12g Carbs, 2.6g Fiber, 1.3g Protein

Ingredients:

1 medium sweet potato
1 medium russet potato
1 parsnip
1 turnip
1 carrot
1 beet
2 Tbsp EVOO
1 tsp M\mineral salt
1 tsp cumin
½ tsp paprika
1 tsp turmeric

Directions:

Heat oven to 400 degrees.

Peel sweet potato and slice very thin – a mandolin would make this easy.

Slice other vegetables very thinly.

Toss slices in a bowl with the spices (used gloved hands to coat – no gloves=orange stained hands).

Layer on a cookie sheet and bake 20 – 25 minutes. Flip half way through the cooking and make sure they are crisp when done

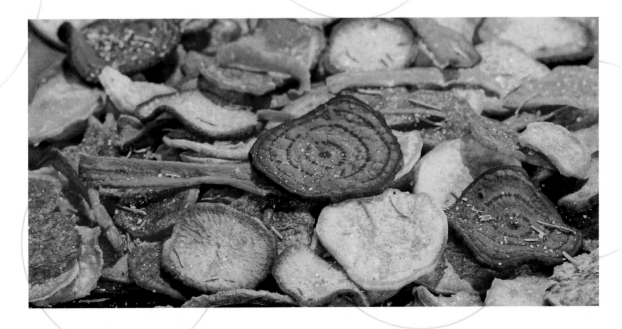

Fire Roasted Corn (NCF)(E)(Q) ($)

Serves: 6

Per serving: 68 Calories, 2.4g Fat, 11.6g Carbs, 0.8g Fiber, 1.7g Protein

Ingredients:

2 cobs corn
1 tsp chopped Jalapeno pepper
1 Tbsp chopped parsley
½ tsp mineral salt
1 tsp sweet paprika
1 Tbsp EVOO

Directions:

Roast the corn in the husk on the BBQ until husks are blackened and when you pull them away from the corn, the corn looks like it has been boiled. It does not matter if the corn is undercooked.

Once the corn is done, remove from the heat and wait until it is cool enough to handle.

With a sharp blade, remove the corn kernels from the husk and place in a bowl with all the other ingredients – you can eat at room temperature or re-heat in a small pan.

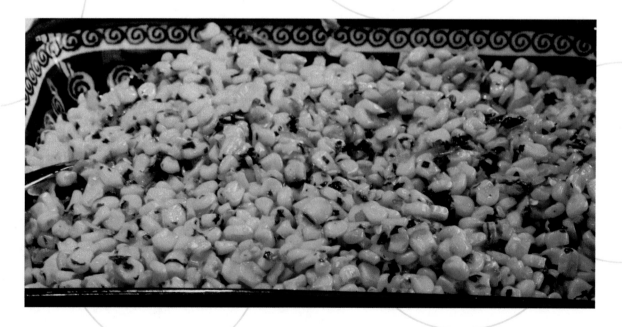

Artichoke Mushroom Pizza (NCF)

Serves: 6
Per serving: 169 Calories 11g Fat, 13.8g Carbs, 6.2 8.1g Protein

Ingredients:

1 cauliflower pizza crust (see page 301)
½ cup sweet tomato sauce (see page 192)
½ cup cashew cheese (see page 243)
½ cup baby spinach leaves
½ cup chopped mushrooms of your choice
½ cup halved baby artichokes (I use jarred artichokes in water)

Directions:

Top cauliflower pizza crust with ingredients and bake for 15 minutes.

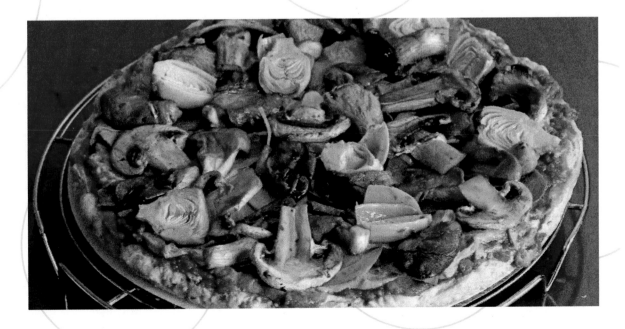

Not Pizza (NCF)

Serves: 6

Per serving: 153 Calories, 9.9g Fat, 12.2g Carbs, 5.2g Fiber, 7.1g Protein

Ingredients:

1 cauliflower pizza crust (see page 301)
½ cup sweet tomato sauce (see page 192)
2 Tbsp basil pesto
1/2 cup baby spinach
½ cup unsweetened pineapple chunks – fresh is best
1 chopped tomato

Directions:

Top cauliflower pizza crust with ingredients and bake for 15 minutes.

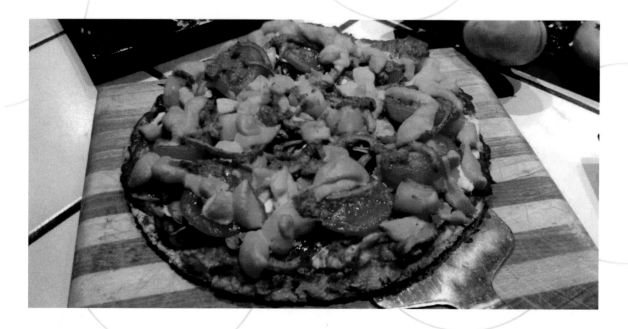

Walnut Mushroom Pizza (NCF)

Serves: 4 as a main, 8 as a starter
Per serving (as a main): 379 Calories, 31.8g Fat, 19.1g Carbs, 4.1g Fiber, 10.2g Protein
Per serving (as a starter): 190 Calories, 15.9g Fat, 9.6g Carbs, 2.1g Fiber, 5.1g Protein

Ingredients:

TOPPING
2/3 cup cashew cheese (see page 243)
½ cup chopped walnuts
a handful basil leaves
freshly ground pepper

MUSHROOM MIX
2 large Portobello mushrooms - peeled and sliced into ¾ inch strips
1 cup of another mushroom – your choice (I used trumpet mushrooms for the pizza in the photo) – sliced
2 cloves garlic – crushed
1 Tbsp grape seed oil
¼ tsp mineral salt

Directions:

Preheat oven to 450 degrees.

Start with a finished socca crust (See page 297).

On a medium to hot griddle drizzle the grape seed oil and sauté the mushrooms until just browned Sprinkle with the garlic and salt and then remove from the heat to a plate

Layer the mushrooms over the Socca crust and then drizzle with the cashew cheese and the walnuts Cook for about ten minutes

Remove the pizza from the oven, drizzle with a few drops of Evoo, sprinkle with pepper and torn basil, and serve.

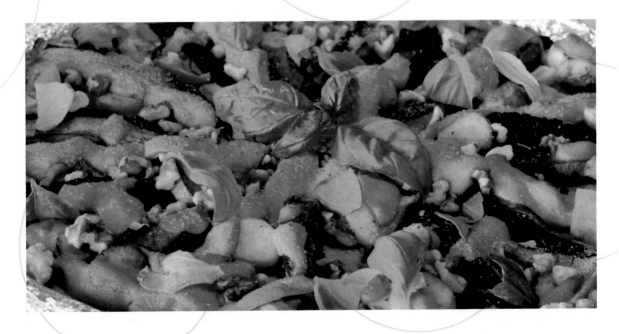

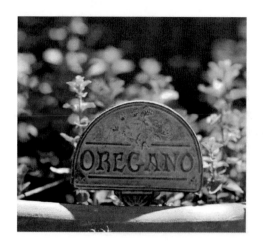

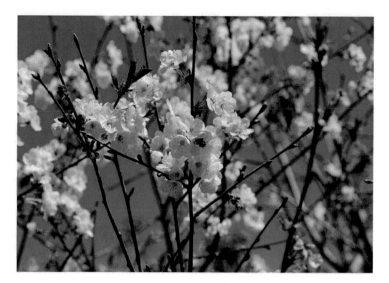

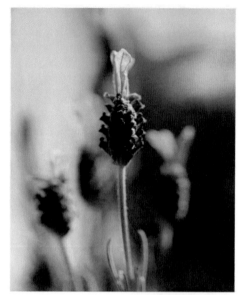

serenity

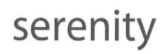

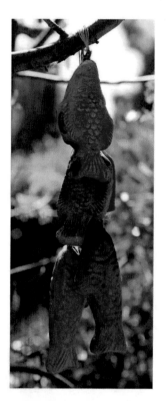

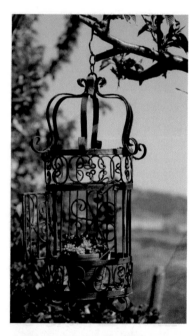

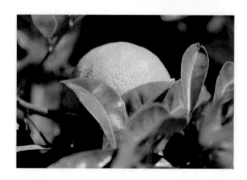

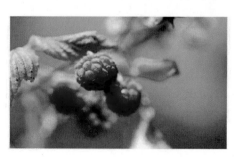

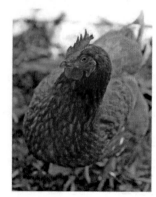

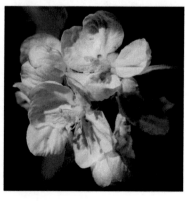

Additional Information

GMO: A Dietitian's Perspective

Let's get some terminology down first. GMO stands for Genetically Modified Organisms, an organism that has been changed using genetic engineering. GMO's are used in research, agriculture, and gene therapy. While some research methods may use GMOs for positive outcomes, the ones found in our food supply are not.
The problem:

1. Safety: There are very few authentic studies done on the safety of GMOs. For one, the FDA does not require testing when a gene is transferred to a plant that is a common allergen. The fact that my specialty is in food sensitivities, I find this to be alarming. If you are allergic to soy, you may not know that the corn you're eating has been implanted with soy genes. I have clients who tell me that when they eat food in other countries, their allergies/sensitivities disappear or lessen. When they eat the exact same item in the USA, they have a reaction. So is an apple really an apple? If it's genetically modified, probably not. GMOs are not required to pre-market safety testing (like other food additives are). In the United States, most soybeans, cotton, and corn are genetically modified.

2. Labeling: Unfortunately, as of now, companies don't have to state that their product contains GMO's. Most soybeans are genetically modified. Unless it says 'Organic Soybeans' or Non-GMO soybeans used, I would bet that it is a genetically modified organism.

3. To me, the most important: the environment. Besides the monopoly that GMO seeds have on the small farmer (check out Food, Inc. for more on that). GMOs also have an damaging effect on cross-pollination. The inability for plants to cross-pollinate creates super weeds, which then creates the need for more toxic pesticides to be used to kill them. It also severely limits biodiversity, we need weeds!

For these reasons, we highly encourage non-GMO produce. Organic produce will be GMO free. For products such as corn and soy, always choose organic to ensure that you are not having GMO corn and soy.
For more information check out these publications:

Farmageddon: Food and the Culture of Biotechnology (Brewster Kneen: New Society Publishers, 1999)
Genes in the Field: On Farm Conservation and Crop Diversity (Stephen Brush: Lewis Publishers, 1999)
Seeds of Deception: Exposing Industry and Government Lies about the Safety of the Genetically Engineered Foods You're Eating (Jeffrey Smith: Chelsea Green, 2003)

Complete vs. Incomplete Proteins:

"Where do you get your protein?" is one of the most common questions that plant-based eaters hear. There is a lot of confusion about the need to eat meat, especially for protein needs. Most of this comes from the difference between complete vs. incomplete proteins. Rest assured, there is no need to get protein from animal sources. We will explain the difference between plant and animal proteins in the next section.

All proteins are made from 20 different amino acids. Some amino acids, called non-essential, are made from the body. Others, called essential amino acids cannot be produced by the body and must be consumed in food.

There are nine essential amino acids (histidine, isoleucine, leucine, lysine, methionine, valine, phenylalanine, threonine, and tryptophan for our bio-chem fans). Plant foods do contain at least some of every essential amino acids, but have a lower percentage of at least one. This is what makes them "incomplete". You could get enough essential amino acids by just eating one food, like black beans, but you would have to eat cups of black beans a day. While we love our beans, that's not exactly practical or enjoyable.

Instead, we emphasize a variety of plant foods to ensure that you are getting all of your protein needs. This is where the idea of protein combining comes into play. When we first starting analyzing vegetarian diets, it was thought that each meal and snack must combine the right pairings of foods to make a complete protein. For example, beans and rice, pasta and peas or peanut butter and whole wheat bread. While that thinking wasn't necessarily wrong, it's proven to be unnecessary. Our bodies are able to store essential amino acids and combine when necessary. Which gives us just another reason to eat a wide variety of foods.

Anytime we talk protein, we must talk about the importance of legumes. I personally think that legumes are one of the most nutritious foods we can consume. Rich in fiber, protein, iron, magnesium, calcium, and other important minerals, they include foods like beans, peas, lentils, soybeans, and peanuts.

The big reason to include these foods in your diet is that they are one of the few plant sources of the essential amino acid Lysine. Diets that are mostly vegetables, fruits, and grains can be too low in lysine. I recommend at least 2-3 servings of legumes a day, mostly for this reason. Black beans in your morning vegetable scramble, a bowl of lentil soup for lunch, and almond butter and apple for snack will provide enough lysine for a 140# adult.

If you don't like beans, try to find other lysine-rich foods to enjoy on a daily basis. quinoa, cashews, walnuts, pistachios, peanuts, oatmeal and some vegetables are alternative options.

Vegan Nutrition: A Starter Guide

What is a vegan diet?
A vegan diet is one that is completely devoid of animals or animal products. While this may sound restrictive, many vegans feel like they eat a more varied diet than omnivores. Fruits, vegetables, beans, grains, and nuts are all vegan! Favorite foods like pizza, tacos, burritos, pasta, lasagna, BBQ, sandwiches, ice cream, and mac and cheese can all easily be prepared vegan! If you enjoy ethnic food, you're in luck! Lots of ethnic foods are naturally vegan, enjoy Indian, Ethiopian, Chinese, Thai, Mexican & more! With a vegan diet, you are only limited by your imagination! If it can be made vegan, I guarantee someone, somewhere has tried it!

What is a healthful vegan diet?
That being said, just like a omnivore diet, if you eat primarily junk it doesn't matter if you are vegan or not! A balanced vegan diet is made up of these four food groups: 1) legumes, nuts, and seeds; 2) grains; 3) vegetables; and 4) fruits. Because individual nutrient needs and energy requirements vary due to age, activity level, and one's state of health, this guide should only be considered a broad blueprint for a balanced vegan diet. Consult a dietitian familiar with vegan nutrition for a personalized set of recommendations.

LEGUMES, NUTS, AND SEEDS (4+ servings per day)
The legume-nut-seed group includes beans, split peas, lentils, nuts, seeds, and soy products. These nutrient-dense foods are packed with protein, fiber, minerals, B vitamins, protective antioxidants, and essential fatty acids. Consider ½ cup cooked beans, 4 ounces of tofu or tempeh, 1 cup almond, coconut or hemp milk, 1 ounce of nuts or seeds, or 2 tablespoons of nut or seed butter as a serving.

GRAINS (4-6+ servings per day)
Whole grains provide B vitamins, fiber, minerals, protein, and antioxidants. Whole, intact grains are recommended over refined as they retain the nutrients and the fiber. Think of a wheat kernel as three parts, the fibrous outer layer, the bran, starchy middle, endosperm, and the nutrient-packed core, the germ. Whole grains keep all of these parts, refined grains remove the bran and the germ. We love intact whole grains--such as brown rice, oats, wheat berries, millet, and quinoa and prefer them nutritionally to whole grain flours and puffed or flaked whole grains. Serving size examples include one slice of bread, ½ cup cooked grain, or 1 ounce of ready-to-eat cereal. Vary your intake based on your individual energy needs.

VEGETABLES (4+ servings per day)
Eat a Rainbow! There is no limit to the amount of vegetables you intake! Those who are looking to lose weight or reduce calories should consider increasing non-starchy vegetables while decreasing grains. Eating a wide variety of colorful vegetables every day will ensure that you're getting an assortment of protective nutrients in your diet. Leafy greens like kale & collards are packed with calcium! Eat at least 1-2 servings a day. Steam and have as a side for breakfast, shred and at to a salad, stuff in a sandwich, or stir-fry with dinner. Dark leafy greens are one of the best foods you can eat! A vegetable serving is ½ cup cooked, 1 cup raw, or ½ cup vegetable juice.

FRUITS (2+ servings per day)
Most fruits, especially citrus fruits and berries, are a great source of vitamin C; all fruits provide antioxidants and fiber. While juicing has become very popular, it's not always the best choice as it leaves out the fiber. Both soluble and insoluble are important here. Insoluble is found mostly in the skin, think apples, pears, and seeds of berries. It helps to increase transit time in the gut and add bulk!

Soluble fiber has been shown to reduce cholesterol levels and aid in fullness. A serving size is one medium piece, 1 cup sliced fruit, ¼ cup dried, or ½ cup of juice.

A few words about fats
Concentrated fats, such as oils and oil-based spreads, do not fall under a food group. They are not required for optimal health, as essential fats are found naturally in whole foods like avocados, olives, nuts, and seeds. Like any category, we prefer a whole-food version of fats but that's not to say that oils are unhealthy! Check out our Which Oil is Best article to determine which oil to use when. Choose oils and spreads that are minimally processed and limit your intake.

How healthy is a vegan diet?
Dare we say the healthiest? According to the American Dietetic Association's 2009 Position Paper on Vegetarian Diets, vegan diets "are healthful, nutritionally adequate, and may provide health benefits in the prevention and treatment of certain diseases." A healthy vegan diet helps reduce your risk of heart disease, cancer, obesity, and diabetes(5).

The scoop on some important nutrients
Everyone, regardless whether you are vegan or not need to be mindful of consuming all the nutrients needed order to be healthy. Three nutrients that everyone needs to pay attention to are vitamin B12, vitamin D, and omega-3 fatty acids.

Vitamin B12 is necessary for proper red blood cell formation, neurological function, and DNA synthesis. It is manufactured by certain types of bacteria found in nature. Because plants vary widely in their levels of this bacteria (and most of us favor our food scrubbed squeaky clean), we cannot rely on plant foods to meet our B12 needs. This is an important distinction as many vegans falsely believe that you don't need to supplement with Vitamin B12. We can ensure our dietary needs are met by consuming supplements and/or fortified foods. Our suggestion is to supplement with a vegan source of 2000 micrograms once a week or 10-100 micrograms a day. It's best to get a blood test if you think you might be deficient. It doesn't take long for sources to deplete in our bodies, especially if you were vegetarian or limiting animal products before becoming vegan. In this case, you may already be low. A MD can check for B12 and homocysteine levels. B12 is a tricky vitamin because it is absorbed in the large intestine. If you have any gut issues along the way, the amount you are taking might not be the amount you are absorbing. For this reason, a homocysteine test is advised as levels will be high if B12 intake is low, even if B12 shows up falsely high. Low B12 levels can be dangerous, they often mimic as dementia or Alzheimer's, especially in aging persons. Some vegan food is fortified with B12, but I still recommend that my clients take a supplement.

Vitamin D, the "sunshine vitamin", is also a hormone, not a true vitamin; our skin manufactures it from the ultraviolet rays of the sun. It plays an important role in bone health and supports normal neuromuscular and immune function. Be cautious of vitamin D levels if you always wear sunscreen, limit outdoor exposure, and/or live in a northern part of the country. I recommend all my clients test Vitamin D stores in the winter. Schedule a 25(OH)D (25-hydroxyvitamin D) blood test, and your healthcare provider can offer supplement guidelines based on the results.
Vitamin D blood levels are an international public health concern. Getting enough of it is not as easy as we may think. The body's ability to produce vitamin D from sun exposure varies based on skin pigmentation, sunscreen, clothing, time of year, latitude, air pollution, and other factors, and the vitamin is found naturally in only a handful of foods. This is why all people--not just vegans--need to be mindful about vitamin D. The latest research suggest that getting even 100% of the current Recommended Dietary Allowance (RDA) for vitamin D may be insufficient for many people. To

ensure adequate vitamin D intake, take 1000-4000 International Units (IU) per day, depending upon your age and other individual needs.

Most non-dairy milks are fortified with vitamin D, so be sure to check your favorite brands. Adequate vitamin D status is linked to a lowered risk of osteoporosis, certain cancers, and other chronic diseases. Supplemental vitamin D comes in two forms: vegan D2 (ergocalciferol), usually synthetic or manufactured from yeast, and non-vegan D3 (cholecalciferol), manufactured from lanolin (from sheep's wool)(12).

Omega-3 fatty acids. A proper balance of essential fats is important for optimal brain function, heart health, and infant/child development. Alpha-linolenic acid (ALA) is an omega-3 fatty acid that partly converts to DHA and EPA in the body. It is present in several plant foods, including flax products, hemp products, canola oil, walnuts, and leafy green vegetables. Aim to consume 2 to 4 grams of ALA per day:

food/serving size	ALA (grams)
Flaxseed oil, 1 Tbsp.	8.0
Flaxseed, whole, 2 Tbsp.	5.2
Flaxseed, ground, 2 Tbsp.	3.8
Hempseed oil, 1 Tbsp.	2.7
Walnuts, 1 oz (1/4 cup)	2.6
Canola oil, 1 Tbsp.	1.6
Tofu, firm, ½ cup	0.7
Greens (mixed), 2 cups	0.2

If you aren't sure whether your intake is adequate, you may wish to take up to 300 milligrams of algae-based DHA or DHA-EPA blend per day.
What about calcium?
Calcium is naturally widespread in the plant kingdom, and so our calcium needs can be met with whole plant foods or fortified calcium foods. Adults need about 1000 milligrams per day, though the amount depends on one's stage in the lifecycle, periods of growth require more calcium. We recommend choosing several calcium-rich foods in each food group each day. Some of the richest plant sources of calcium are: leafy green vegetables, figs, almonds and other nuts, sesame and other seeds, beans, calcium-set tofu, fortified nondairy yogurt, fortified soy products, fortified breakfast cereals, and fortified fruit juice.

Food/serving size(16)	Calcium (mg)
Calcium-set tofu, ½ cup	140-420
Fortified soy milk, 1 cup	200-370
Collard greens, 1 cup cooked	270-360
Fortified orange juice	300-350
Soy yogurt, 1 cup	150-350
Amaranth, 1 cup (cooked)	275
Broccoli rabe/Rapini, ½ bunch (cooked)	260
Sesame seeds (unhulled), 2 Tbsp.	175
Blackstrap molasses, 1 Tbsp.	80-170
Navy beans, 1 cup (cooked)	160
Bok choy, 1 cup (cooked)	160
Figs, 5 large (raw)	110

Almonds, 1 oz   70
Note: Calcium content varies depending on variety, brand, and origin.

What about iron?

Iron is a mineral used by the body to carry oxygen from our lungs to the rest of the body, among other functions. Iron deficiency can present as fatigue, cognitive impairment, and other health problems. Iron deficiency is the most common nutrient deficiency in the U.S. vegans and non-vegans need to be mindful about their iron intake.

The Recommended Dietary Allowance (RDA) for iron is as follows (by age and sex)[17]:

Group	Age	Iron (mg/day)
Infants	0-6 months	0.27*
	7-12 months	11
Children	1-3 years	7
	4-8 years	10
Males	9-13 years	8
	14-18 years	11
	19 and up	8
Females	9-13 years	8
	14-18 years	15
	19-50 years	18
	51-70 years	8
	>70 years	8
Pregnant Women	14-50 years	27
Lactating Women	14-18 years	10
	19-50 years	9

*This value is an Adequate Intake (AI) value. AI is used when there is not enough information known to set a Recommended Dietary Allowance (RDA).

Iron sourcesIron can be found in many plant foods, particularly beans, including:

Food, standard amount[16][17][18]	Iron (mg)
Soybeans, mature, cooked, 1/2 cup	4.4
Pumpkin and squash seed kernels, roasted, 1 oz	4.2
White beans, canned, 1/2 cup	3.9
Blackstrap molasses, 1 tbsp	3.5
Lentils, cooked, 1/2 cup	3.3
Spinach, cooked from fresh, 1/2 cup	3.2
Amaranth, cooked 1/2 cup	2.6
Kidney beans, cooked, 1/2 cup	2.6
Chickpeas, cooked, 1/2 cup	2.4
Soybeans, green, cooked, 1/2 cup	2.2
Navy beans, cooked, 1/2 cup	2.2
Refried beans, 1/2 cup	2.1
Black beans, cooked, 1/2 cup	1.8
Pinto beans, cooked, 1/2 cup	1.8

Notes on iron

While the form of iron found in plants (non-heme) is absorbed differently than the majority of iron in meat (heme), vegans' intakes can be as high or higher than meat eaters. That said, while a separate

Recommended Daily Allowance has not been set for vegans, it is stated that, to compensate for absorption differences, vegans may need to double the RDA for iron while still being careful to avoid over consuming it. The benefit of only absorbing non-heme iron is that your body will rarely absorb too much iron. Iron deficiency is just as dangerous as iron toxicity.

Iron absorption is inhibited when you consume calcium supplements or foods high in oxalates, coffee, and black and green tea at the same time as a foods containing iron. Spinach is very high in oxalates so why it is a good source of iron, it will not be absorbed well. To increase non-heme iron absorption at meals, consume with foods high in vitamin C, such as citrus fruits, bell peppers, and green leafy vegetables.(18) It is widely observed that cooking non-heme foods in a cast iron skillet can improve iron content as well.

What about protein?

Protein contributes to healthy muscles and bones, tissue repair, a healthy immune system, and more. Since 10-20% of calories in most plant foods (legumes, vegetables, and grains especially) are from protein, and humans need only about 10-15% of their calories from protein, requirements are easily met with a diet consisting of a variety of whole plant foods. More is not better when it comes to protein. Many people falsely believe that we need abundant amounts of protein to grow and develop muscle. That notion has also been at the corner store for many popular low-carb diets. Not true, any nutrient in excess will be stored into energy, mostly adipose tissue. Excess protein can also be hard on the body as protein takes more energy to digest than carbohydrates.

It was once believed that vegetarians needed to consume "complementary" proteins to be complete. After years of research, we know this is not accurate. The body stores amino acids, the building blocks of protein, so that complete proteins can be manufactured from the diet over the course of the day. Isn't the body amazing?

The RDA for protein is age and gender dependent. Pregnancy, activity level, and health status also affect your needs. However, to get a general sense of what your daily protein intake is in grams, take your weight in pounds and multiply it by .36 (a 150 pound adult would want to consume about 55 grams of protein per day). For comparison sakes, the average American consumes 80-100 grams of protein a day!

The following sample meal plan easily reaches that goal, at 77 grams of protein:

Breakfast:
1.5 cups oatmeal (9g) + cinnamon combined with
1 oz walnuts (4g)
1 small banana (1g)

Lunch
1.5 cups of three bean chili (16g)
½ organic spelt english muffin (2.5g)
2 cups southwestern vegetable salad (4g)
Dinner:
2 cups stir fried sweet potato, onion, bok choy, and broccoli (5g)
4 oz sesame orange baked tofu (7g)
2 cups brown rice (9g)

Snack

2 tbsp peanut/almond butter (8g) on whole grain crackers (3g) and fruit (1g
2 oz trail mix (8g)

Don't I need some cholesterol?
Though vegan diets are 100% cholesterol free, this is 100% fine. There is no Daily Recommended Intake for cholesterol because it is not an essential nutrient. The body (specifically the liver) manufactures all the cholesterol a person needs to be healthy

What about food allergies?
There are numerous healthy grain alternatives for vegans with a wheat allergy or gluten intolerance. In fact, many grains are nutritionally superior to wheat, including quinoa and millet. Products that were once only available in wheat varieties (such as bread and crackers) are now available wheat- and gluten-free. A soy allergy is also workable; soybeans are just one food. Soy-based meat analogs can be replaced with nut- or wheat-based varieties (such as seitan). Nut allergies are usually isolated; few people are allergic to all nuts and seeds. Testing can determine which nuts and seeds are safe. Substitutions usually work well in recipes and in foods such as granola, trail mix, and nut/seed "butters."

I tried a vegan diet and felt unhealthy. What did I do wrong?
Sometimes when we make positive changes to our diet—such as eliminating animal products or replacing processed junk food with whole plant foods—we may encounter some temporary bodily complaints, such as cravings, fatigue, or digestive discomfort. These are not uncommon during a major dietary transition, especially if fiber intake increases dramatically in a short period of time. If symptoms continue more than 2-3 days, you may want to see a doctor to rule out coincidental health conditions.

Sometimes a well-intentioned change to eating vegan can backfire when the diet is not properly balanced. One common mistake when transitioning to a vegan diet is eating too few calories, especially if you start out with a high raw-diet. Healthful vegan diets tend to be big on volume–your plate should be overflowing with fresh food, especially when you include lots of raw vegetables. If you continue eating the same volume of food as before, you might not get enough calories, leaving you tired, hungry, and irritable. Another common mistake is simply replacing meat with meat analogs, dairy products with soy alternatives, and regular sweets with vegan sweets; going heavy on these and light on the vegetables, fruits, and whole grains is not a healthy approach. To learn how to best reap the benefits of a healthful vegan diet, sign up for a vegan nutrition or cooking class, or pick up a reliable book on vegan nutrition such as Becoming Vegan, by Brenda Davis and Vesanto Melina.

Too much of a good thing?
Many vegans enjoy some soy products to mimic the flavors and textures of meat and dairy products. Is it possible to consume too much soy? Yes, it is. It's possible to eat too much of many kinds of foods. Eating too many processed soy products, in particular, means that other foods are being displaced, which throws off a healthful balance of foods. A reasonable daily limit of *processed* soy products is 2 servings per week, but the healthiest soy products are the least processed and/or those that are fermented: edamame, miso, tempeh, tofu, and fortified soymilk made from whole organic soybeans.

VEGAN PROTEIN INFORMATION
by Dr. Kelly Martin, B.S., Pharm.D.

Cranberry protein is unique in that it is the only 100% plant protein that contains 25% complete protein including all essential amino acids. Cranberry protein is extracted using cold-pressing technology preserving natural balances and naturally occurring fatty acids, which increases the absorption of the other nutrients.

- Powerful detoxifier and diuretic (flushes out the kidneys)
- Treats bladder, kidney and urinary problems
- Boosts immune system, protecting against influenza and the common cold
- Increases "good" cholesterol (HDL), and reduces "bad" cholesterol (LDL)
- Improves circulation and reduces risk of heart disease
- Helps to relieve stress & depression
- Treats skin conditions such as: acne, dermatitis, psoriasis, burns & wounds
- Also considered one of the best remedies for REDUCING CELLULITE!

A high fiber, low calorie, nutrient dense vegetarian SUPERFOOD, **Peas are also a remarkable source of plant-based proteins and amino acids!** Protein from peas satisfies all FAO essential amino acid requirements. The amino acids found in peas include **Lysine, Arginine, Glutamine, Leucine, Isoleucine & Valine** (Branched Chain Amino Acids - BCAAs)

- Aid muscle tissue maintenance
- Comparable to egg and milk proteins
- BCAAs are higher in pea protein than any other vegetable protein
- Helps restore nitrogen balance after intense physiological stress
- Increases muscle mass while reducing body fat during intense exercise
- Improves vasodilatation and promotes a healthy heart
- Assists in maintaining lean body mass
- Facilitates calcium absorption (promoting healthy bone development in children)
- Boosts the immune system: producing antibodies, hormones, enzymes, collagen, and tissue-repair
- Low in sulfur proteins (sulfur proteins speed up the aging process)
- Increases metabolism and satiety (helping you to feel "full")
- Recent studies show that consuming pea protein results in fewer calories consumed at the next meal.
- Natural tonic for preventing and treating high blood pressure
- Promotes healthy kidney function

Rice Protein Health benefits of Rice Protein Rice Protein effect on cholesterol and triglyceride metabolism

Standard cooked rice has a protein content of only 5%-7%. To make concentrated rice protein, whole brown rice is ground into flour, and then mixed with water. Natural enzymes are then added sequentially to break down and separate out the carbohydrates and fibers from the protein portion of the slurry. Since the process is enzyme based, temperature must be kept low to preserve the enzyme activity levels. Low temperature and chemical free processing prevents the denaturing of amino acids, as is seen in soy and dairy processing. The end product is 80-90% pure, hypoallergenic, easily digested protein. After four hours, the body digests over 86% of all ingested rice protein, compared with about 57% for soy. In the end, rice protein has a biological value of between 70-80, a net protein utilization of about 76, and a total absorption ration of some 98%.

Note: rice protein is high in the amino acids cysteine and methionine, but tends to be low in lysine, which negatively impacts its bioavailability. If you can raise its lysine levels, you can dramatically increase its bioavailability.

Pea Protein

When it comes to perception, more people have a problem with the "idea" of pea protein than with rice protein. But in fact, pea protein has a very mild, pleasantly sweet taste. It's one of the better tasting proteins. Pea protein is the concentrated natural protein fraction of yellow peas. The process used for concentrating pea protein is water based, making the end product very "natural."

The Beneficial Combination of Rice and Pea Proteins

As mentioned above, rice protein is high in cysteine and methionine, but tends to be low in lysine. Yellow pea protein, on the other hand, tends to be low in the sulfur containing amino acids, cysteine and methionine -- but high in lysine. The bottom line is that when used in combination, rice protein and yellow pea protein offer a Protein Efficiency Ratio that begins to rival dairy and egg -- but without their potential to promote allergic reactions. In addition, the texture of pea protein helps smooth out the "chalkiness" of rice protein. Like rice protein, it is hypoallergenic and easily digested.

On a different note, the rice/pea combo also has a nice branch chain amino acid profile -- only slightly less than whey. **Whey Rice/Pea Leucine (percent of total)** 8 7 **Isoleucine (percent of total)** 6 4 **Valine (percent of total)** 5 4

Common Misconceptions: Eating Healthy is Expensive:

Going plant-based won't automatically save you money, but it might! Right now, the most expensive items in your grocery cart are probably meat, dairy, and processed foods. Removing those three items alone can make a significant cut in your grocery bill. With any diet, plan within your budget. The best way to cut back on food-associated expenses is to limit eating out and convenience items. While we include some exotic ingredients in our recipes, most of the ingredients you can find at your neighborhood store or might already have in your pantry. After you purchase the basics, stocking your fridge each week will include a few trips to the market primarily for fresh items like fruits & vegetables.

We encourage you to locate a few markets to comparison shop. Living in Northern California, it's budget friendly to join a CSA (community supported agriculture) and head to the farmer's market a few times a week for produce. I can usually get local, organic produce much cheaper at the market than I can at the store! However, I know that's not the case for everyone. Do some research on options in your area. www.localharvest.org is a great resource to identify local markets at CSAs in your area. Another tip? Head down to your local ethnic market. While curry pastes, coconut milk, and spices can be 'gourmet' in regular grocery stores, most ethnic markets will carry these items for less. I head down to my asian market to stock up on exotic spices, tempeh, fresh made tofu, rice noodles and miso.

Buying in season will help cut down on produce costs. While blueberries are delicious, buying them fresh outside of July or August can be an expensive delicacy. Look to frozen fruits and vegetables as well. Most frozen produce is frozen at the peak of ripeness, ensuring a concentrated amount of vitamins and antioxidants. This is a great budget-friendly option if you are going to cook your vegetables anyway. It also cuts down on prep time, perfect for last-minute dinners or lunches. I use organic, frozen berries in my smoothies. It's an inexpensive way for me to enjoy the nutrients of berries all year long. Other budget friendly vegan food? Grains and legumes! Vegetarian sources of protein tend to be pretty inexpensive, most bags of dried beans sell for $1 a pound!

Convenience foods, by nature, tend to be more expensive. While these products are great in a pinch, relying on them all the time can really add up. Decide which item are easier to make yourself. Salad dressings, hummus, nut butters, don't take much time to create and are healthier and less expensive than packaged versions. A pressure cooker is a great tool for dried legumes. I make a big batch of dried beans for the week in mine and freeze portion-sized bags of what I don't need. When I need beans, I just take them right from the freezer and into whatever dish I am making.

Lastly, try out your green thumb! Herbs are key in flavorful, low fat dishes plus they contain lots of nutrients! Since a little goes a long way, you don't need much to make a dish really pop. Most markets, grocery stores, and hardware stores will sell potted herb gardens in the spring and summer. Water often and enjoy! Even those will tiny, city apartments can enjoy a windowsill herb garden.

Fats & A Heart-Healthy Lifestyle:

Remember back in the '80's and early '90s when everything was 'fat-free?" Bagels were touted as an uber-healthy breakfast, along with Snackwells cookies, fat-free salad dressings, and pasta. Fast forward three decades and we now know that not only is fat good for you, but essential in a healthy diet.

For food manufacturers, it comes down to one of two choices for flavor: fat or sugar. For baked goods, if I am going to cut down on the fat, I need to up the sugar to keep the flavor. For sugar-free foods, you increase the fat. It's a lose-lose for processed foods and for our health. If a food naturally contains fat, consuming a fat-free version likely means you are consuming a product that is higher in sugar and not any healthier.

You shouldn't fear healthy fats. Eating a plant-based diet means that your diet is naturally cholesterol free and low in saturated fats. When all types of fat in the diet are replaced with carbohydrates, both LDL (not good) and HDL (good) cholesterol drop. But, replacing saturated fats with healthy plant fats lowers LDL (not good) cholesterol and doesn't affect HDL (good) cholesterol. In fact, replacing monounsaturated fats with saturated fats in the diet can improve glucose control with people with diabetes.

For these reasons, we recommend a diet that is cholesterol-free, low in saturated fat, but not too low in plant-based fats. Think nuts, avocados, and plant oils. This way of eating is the traditional "Mediterranean Diet".

Carbohydrates & a Heart-Healthy Lifestyle:

All carbohydrates, whether from a zucchini or a cookie are digested, absorbed into the bloodstream as glucose (blood sugar). After eating, as glucose levels rise, the hormone insulin is also released into the blood. Insulin allows cells to uptake glucose from the blood, to use as energy.

Some carbohydrates are digested and converted to glucose more quickly than others, mostly due to the fiber, protein, and fat in the meal as all of these factors slow glucose release. The glycemic index (GI) measures how quickly carbohydrates are broken down and absorbed. Carbohydrates are found in all plant foods, fruits, vegetables, grains, beans, and legumes. They should be the cornerstone of our diet, making up 55-65% of our total caloric intake. While some of our recipes are high in carbohydrates, they are also high in fiber and come only from whole grain sources, fruits, vegetables, beans are legumes. In other words- the healthiest foods on the planet!

Which oils are best?

Some oils are very healthful, others not so much — and for different reasons. How do you know what's really important when choosing a cooking oil?

First things first:

1.   All saturated fats are not created equal. While coconut oil is 90% saturated fat, it also provides cardiovascular benefits. Lard, also high in saturated fat, does not provide any benefits and increases heart disease risk.

2.   Oils high in Omega-6 fatty acids should be limited. These include corn, soybean, and cottonseed. High intake of omega-6 fatty acids, which are highly concentrated in the above oils have been linked to cellular inflammation, a driving force behind degenerative disease. That's not to say we don't need Omega-6 fatty acids, they are an essential part of our diet. Get them the natural way- through nuts and seeds!

3.   Partially hydrogenated oils (trans-fats) should be avoided at all cost. Reading the label is the best way to determine whether or not the produce contains trans-fats, no matter what the front of packing says. If you see the words "partially-hydrogenated"... kindly put it back on the shelf!

4.   Monounsaturated fats are heart-healthy as they increase HDL cholesterol. Oils with high monounsaturated fats amounts are considered to be great choices. Oleic acid is a monounsaturated fat.

5.   While oils are a healthy way to get fat in your diet, whole food choices are better. Raw avocados contain more nutrition than avocado oil, walnuts contain more nutrients than walnut oil, and so on.

Best Choices:
Unrefined Safflower, Hazelnut, Flax, Hemp, Olive (buy in tin cans or dark glass bottles. EVOO fraud is very common. If it's very inexpensive for a large amount, it's probably not EVOO), Virgin, Unrefined Coconut Oil, Macadamia, Avocado, Almond, Pecan, Peanut, Hazelnut

Second Best Choices: Sunflower (tends to be refined and bleached, high oleic is better than linoleic), Rice oil, Walnut, Sesame, Grapeseed

Kindly Avoid: Soybean (usually refined and GMO unless organic), Non-organic Canola (Rapeseed), Cottonseed, Hydrogenated Coconut, Corn, Palm, Palm Kernel

Cheat Sheet to which oils to use:

Best for cold foods, like salads. Have a low smoke-point:
 Flaxseed oil, unrefined safflower, hazelnut oil, walnut, pumpkin seed oil
Best for baking, low-heat cooking (less than 320 F):
 Hemp, Unrefined Coconut, Olive, unrefined peanut and semi-refined safflower
Best for stir-fry, 320 F +
 Coconut oil, Macadamia, semi-refined walnut oil, high-quality (low acidity) EVOO, sesame oil, grape seed oil, virgin EVOO, hazelnut oil, peanut oil, unrefined avocado oil, almond oil
 For the real gourmet, I would like to give a plug to Rick at Sapore Messo. Sapore Messo Foods brings to you exceptional Extra Virgin Olive Oils from all over the world and a wide variety of Aged Balsamic Vinegars, including both red and white vinegars imported from Modena, Italy.
Premium, first cold press premium oils focusing on freshness and purity, retaining all the benefits of the Omega-3 fatty acids and polyphenols you expect from pure Extra Virgin Olive Oils. We offer Arbequina from California, Hjiblanca from Spain, a GreekKoroneiki, citrus and savory blends from Tunisia, Chile, Spain and Italy and much more
www.saporemesso.com

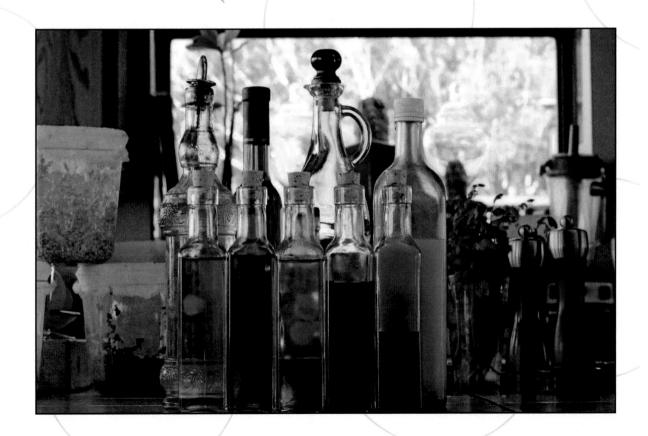

The Dirty Dozen and the Clean Fifteen:

No doubt you have heard of the two lists of produce affectionately called "the dirty dozen" and "the clean 15." These titles represent produce that is either the most contaminated with pesticides, the former, and those that have little pesticide residue, the latter. These two lists were put together by the Environmental Working Group to help consumers determine which foods to buy organic and which to purchase conventionally. The foods are listed from most pesticides (celery) or cleanest (onions) downward.

The Dirty Dozen:	The Clean Fifteen:
Celery	Onions
Peaches	Avocados
Strawberries	Sweet corn
Apples	Pineapples
Domestic blueberries	Mango
Nectarines	Sweet peas
Sweet bell peppers	Asparagus
Spinach or Kale	Kiwi fruit
Cherries	Cabbage
Potatoes	Eggplant
Imported grapes	Watermelon
Lettuce	Grapefruit
	Sweet potatoes
	Sweet onions

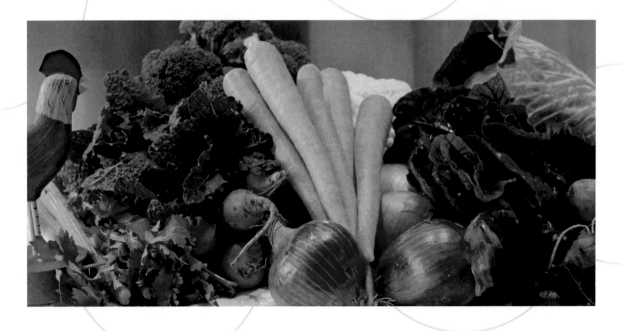

Comparing the two lists, you can see that the ones on the dirty dozen list are mostly fruit, items which are very porous and open to absorbing more pesticides. Most of the items on the clean fifteen have tough skin that can be tough to penetrate, like avocados, pineapples, and grapefruit.

While we would prefer that you purchase everything organic, we also understand that might not be a possibility for everyone. Yes, organically grown produce are typically more expensive than conventionally grown produce. This is not always the case, but more so than not. I tell my clients to try and buy organically those foods on the dirty dozen your family eats the most of. For example, potatoes contain less contaminates than peaches. However, if a family typically eats potatoes 2-3 times a week and peaches 4-5 times a year, buying potatoes organically as much as you can afford would be better than buying peaches organically since you don't consume peaches as often.

Frozen produce can also be labeled organic and is often less costly than it's fresh counterparts. When using fruit that doesn't need to be fresh, as in a smoothie or cooked dish, try purchasing the organic frozen item, just thaw and use as you normally would. It should be noted that labeling items "Certified Organic" is a long and expensive process, something that a lot of small farms cannot afford to do even if their produce is grown organically. Head to your local farmers market and talk with farmers, even if their produce isn't labeled as such, it may very well be organic. And, since you are paying the farmer directly, farmers market produce is often less expensive than what you will find at the grocery store.

In addition to preservative use, organic produce is also GMO-free. We highly recommend that you do not consume GMO foods; please note that corn, sugar beets, and soy are almost always GMO unless they are labeled organic.

Herbs and Spices

Hear the word "antioxidants" and you probably think of deeply colored produce like blackberries, blueberries, kale, or even chocolate. If might surprise you that spices and herbs contain just as many, if not more, antioxidants. In fact, one teaspoon of ground cinnamon has the equivalent level of antioxidants as a half cup of blueberries and one cup of pomegranate juice. Herbs, including basil and parsley, are from plants and plant parts. Spices often come from the seeds, berries, bark, or roots of plants.

We use spices and herbs in every dish of this book, in addition to their antioxidant amounts they add tons of flavor without fat, salt, or sugar. Flavorful, healthy cooking relies on the creative combinations of both herbs and spices.

Antioxidant power: Antioxidants -- found in foods like fruits and vegetables --protect cells against the effects of free radicals. Free radicals are molecules produced when your body is exposed to toxins or by environmental exposures like tobacco smoke and pollution. Antioxidants can protect you against heart disease, cancer and other diseases. They include beta-carotene, lutein, lycopene, selenium and vitamins A, C, and E.

Anti-inflammatory properties: Inflammation has been identified as a precursor to many chronic diseases, such as heart disease, allergies, and Alzheimer's to name a few. Antioxidants in cinnamon have been linked to lower inflammation, as well as reductions in blood glucose concentrations in people with diabetes.

Weight loss: There is some research that shows spices can promote satiety, aid in weight management and enhance the overall quality of a diet. The capsaicin in peppers are believed to have metabolic boosting properties. In addition, if the food you eat is flavorful and satisfying, like the recipes in this book, there is a good chance you will eat less and therefore consume fewer calories.

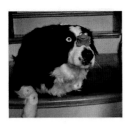
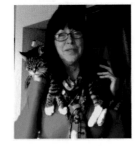
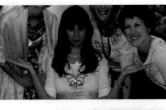
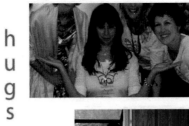

h
u
g
s

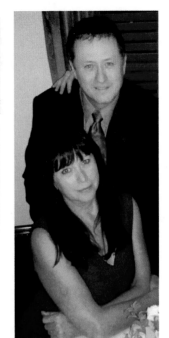

m
e
a
n

m
o
r
e

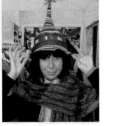
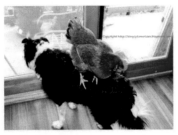
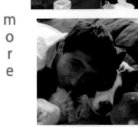

food?

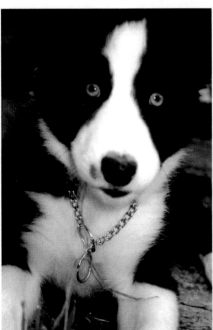
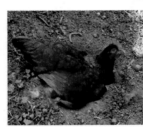
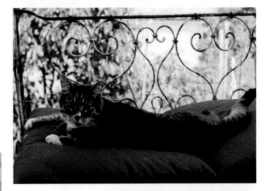

k
i
n
d
n
e
s
s

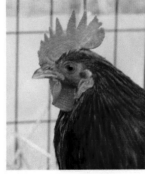
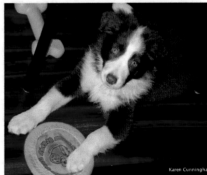

my best friend
is a chicken

l
o
v
e
m
e
t
o
o

love me

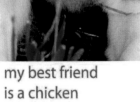
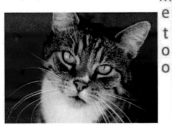
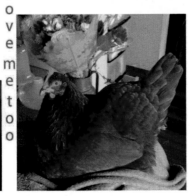
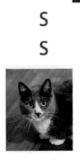
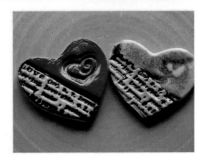

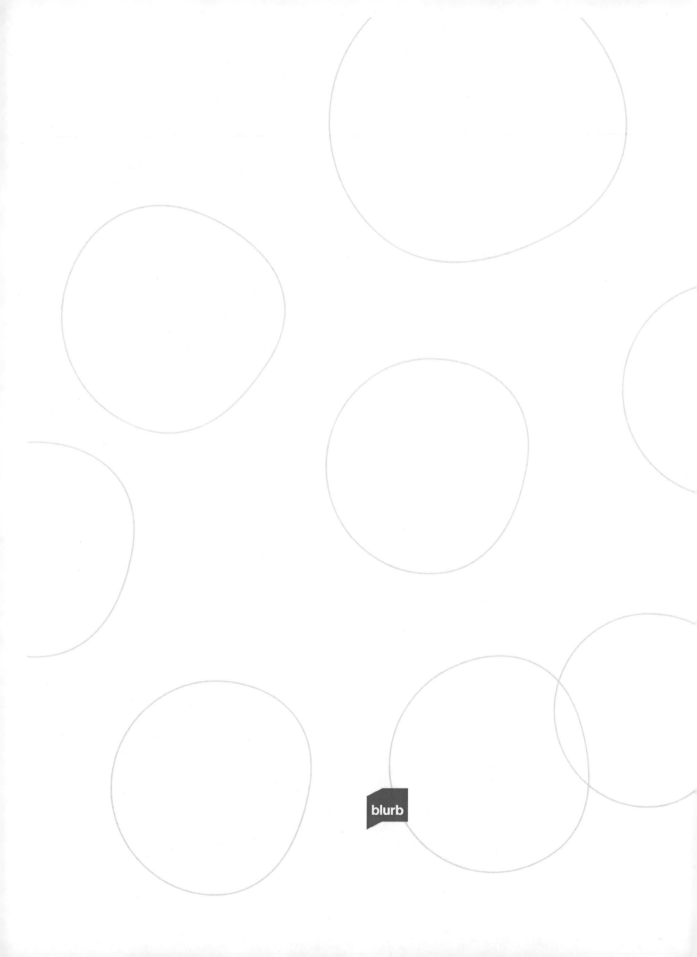

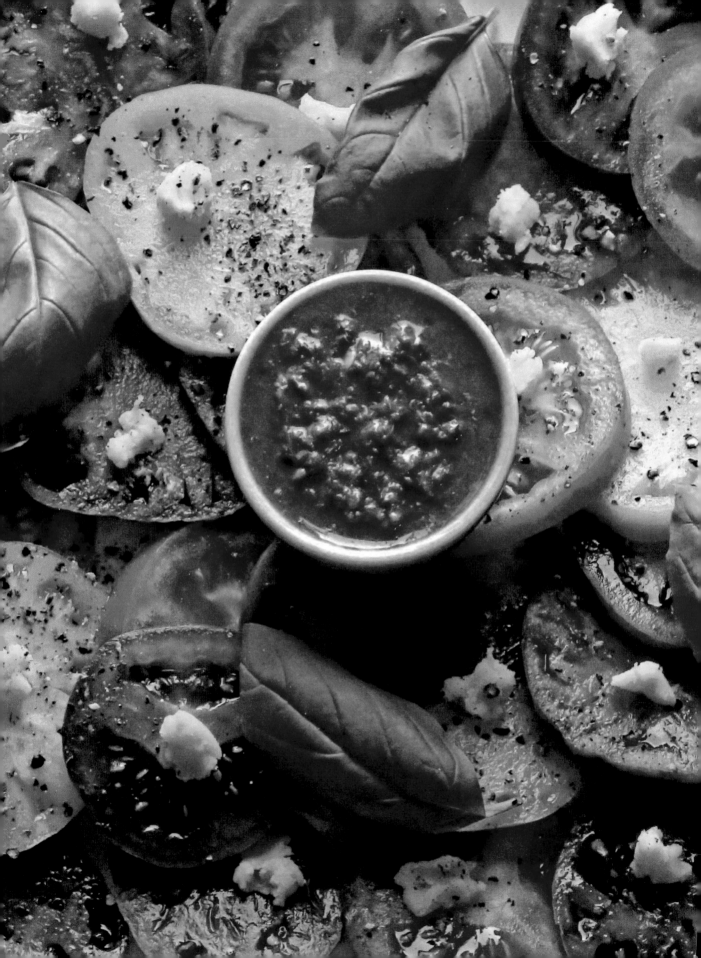

Made in the USA
Las Vegas, NV
05 April 2024

88238630R10255